WALKING ALBUQUERQUE

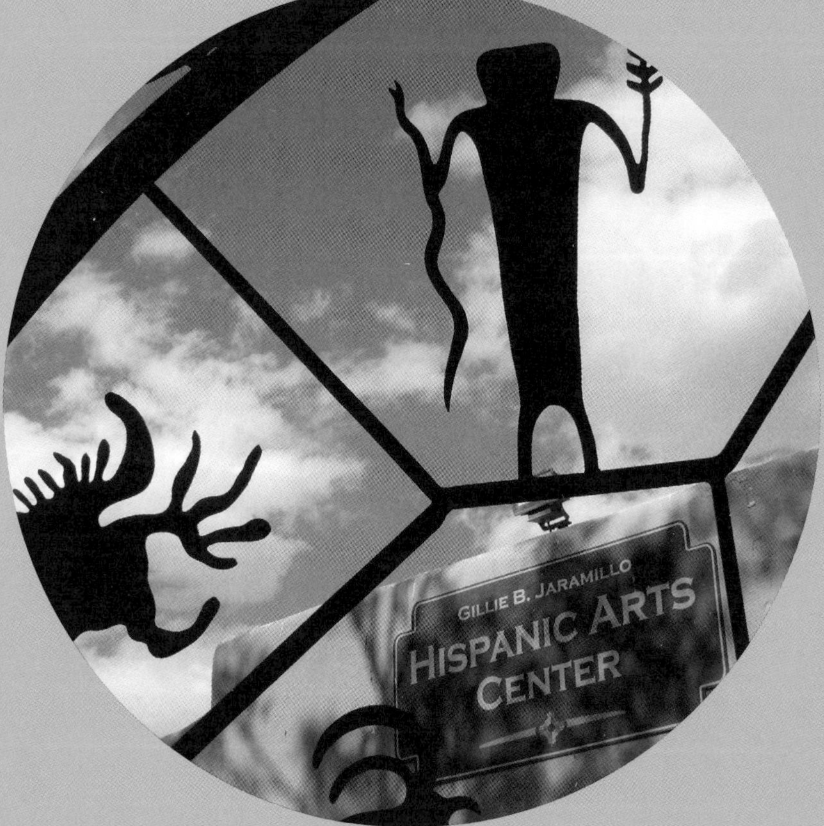
GILLIE B. JARAMILLO
HISPANIC ARTS
CENTER

WALKING ALBUQUERQUE

30 tours of the Duke City's historic neighborhoods, ditch trails, urban nature, and public art

Stephen Ausherman

WILDERNESS PRESS *. . . on the trail since 1967*

Walking Albuquerque: 30 Tours of the Duke City's historic neighborhoods, ditch trails, urban nature, and public art

Editors: Holly Cross and Kate Johnson
Cover and interior photos: Copyright © by Stephen Ausherman
Cartographer: Scott McGrew
Cover and book design: Larry B. Van Dyke and Lisa Pletka
Indexer: Sylvia Coates

ISBN: 978-0-89997-767-6; eISBN: 978-0-89997-768-3

Manufactured in the United States of America

Published by: **WILDERNESS PRESS**
An imprint of Keen Communications, LLC
PO Box 43673
Birmingham, AL 35243
800-443-7227; fax 205-326-1012
info@wildernesspress.com

Visit **wildernesspress.com** for a complete listing of our books, and for ordering information.

Distributed by Publishers Group West

Cover photos: *Front, clockwise from bottom center:* rattlesnake sculpture on University Blvd. median, Mesa del Sol; Barr Canal, Mountain View; Chevy 3100 at Tappan House, El Rancho Plaza; Lobo sculpture, UNM South Campus; Explora! Science Center and Children's Museum, Museum and Courthouse; San Ignacio Catholic Church, Martineztown–Santa Barbara; Anderson-Abruzzo Albuquerque International Balloon Museum, Balloon Fiesta. Back, clockwise from top: El Santuario de San Lorenzo, Bernalillo; Routes Rentals & Tours, Old Town; goats grazing at Los Chavez, Los Duranes.

Frontispiece: Detail from *Petro Circle* by Doug Weigel (see Walk 27)

acknowledgments

My sincere thanks to those who shared their knowledge and contributed to the diverse local perspectives expressed throughout this guidebook: Joe Abbin, Lance Anderson, Rick Brittain, Rudolfo Carrillo, Martin Garcia, Claudia Infante, Camilla Jaquette, Jennifer Owen-White, David Ryan, Susan Schwartz, Michael Scialdone, Mike Smith, Scott Smith, Bob Tilley, Mark Weaver, Steven J. Westman, and Michael Wolff.

And as always, special thanks to Betsy.

author's note

The art of walking involves a particular sense of relating to the cityscape and connecting to its natural and cultural environment on levels that cannot be reached by any other mode of transport. Walking is storytelling in motion, a narrative unfolding not in chronological order, but rather as a spacial sequence of layered events. Consider this book as a kind of bridge between specific places at the present moment and those who occupied it at various times. The purpose is not so much to guide you on specific routes but to take you off predictable paths. Like Zen labyrinths, these routes are designed to lead you into a new awareness of the urban landscape and the lives of those who pass through it. Follow the directions with that in mind. More important, follow your instinct. Feel free to drift off course in any direction that interests you. Likewise, steer clear of areas your gut tells you to avoid. Ideally, you'll find these walks as starting points for much greater urban expeditions in a marvelous, mystifying town known as Albuquerque.

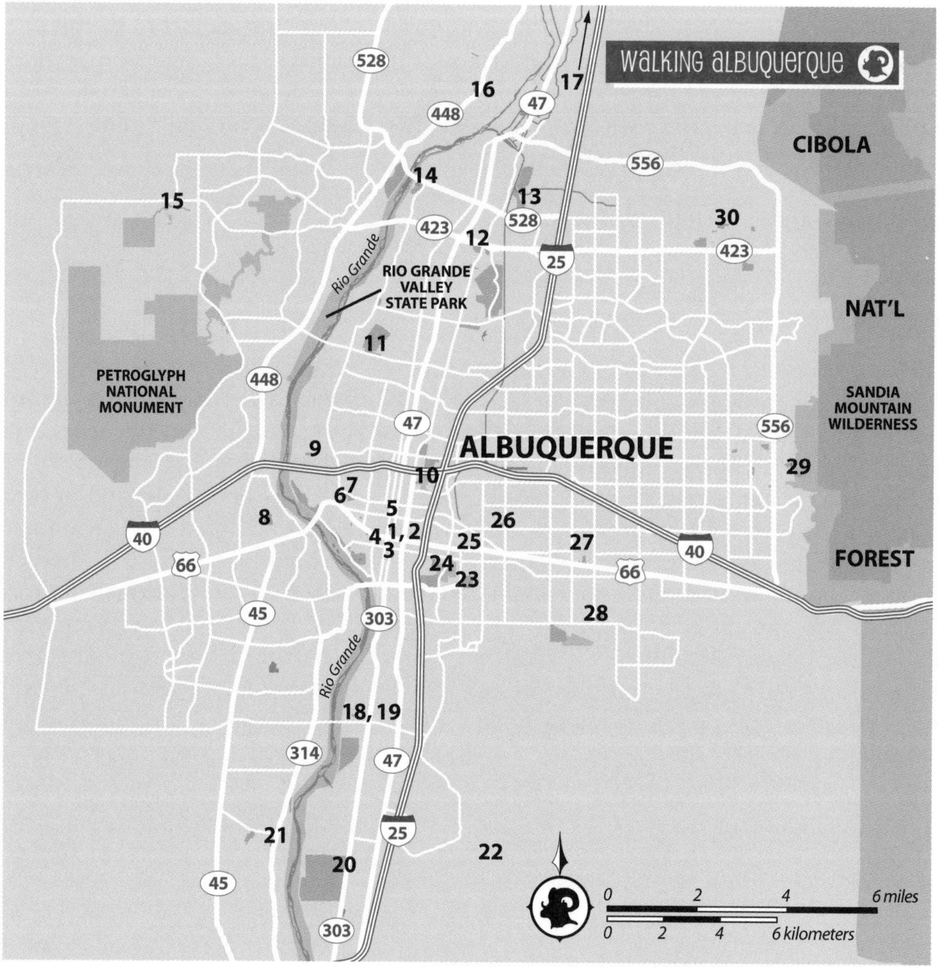

NUMBERS ON THIS LOCATOR MAP CORRESPOND TO WALK NUMBERS.

Table of Contents

INTRODUCTION

"Even for Albuquerque, this is pretty Albuquerque."
—Kirk Douglas, *Ace in the Hole*

People have walked in this area for the past 12,000 years. The earliest established walking routes date back at least a thousand years. For nearly two centuries following its founding, the Villa de Alburquerque was, by lack of choice, a pedestrian town.

The City of Albuquerque mushroomed in response to the AT&SF Railroad, Route 66, and Kirtland Air Force Base. With so much of its early industry catering to planes, trains, and automobiles, Albuquerque didn't exactly develop as a perambulator's paradise. However, that doesn't mean the art of walking has met its demise here. Far from it. A surge in renovations and redevelopment projects is currently ushering the city into a walking (and bicycling) renaissance.

Yet there's never been a shortage of places to explore on foot, and each step brings you that much closer to the best aspects of the city's richly diverse culture. Cuisine features prominently into many routes where restaurants tempt you with aromas both exotic and native. Art is often quickly accessible not just in nearby galleries and museums but also outdoors. With hundreds of public artworks—sculptures, murals, mosaics—the city is essentially a museum without ceilings. And with nearly 3,000 square feet of parkland per person, Burqueños (Albuquerqueans) have more open space than any other city dwellers in America. And plenty of sunny days to enjoy it. On average, Albuquerque basks in 310 days of sunshine per year.

A walk just about anywhere in this multifaceted town reveals layers of its history, which exceeds 300 years. These 30 walks delve into the city's past and ponder its future, all the while encouraging you to go out now and experience its quirky nuances at a leisurely pace.

One of the greatest challenges in writing this book was predicting what readers might find absent from or added to any given route. For updates and other useful bits of information, visit **restlesstribes.com/walq.**

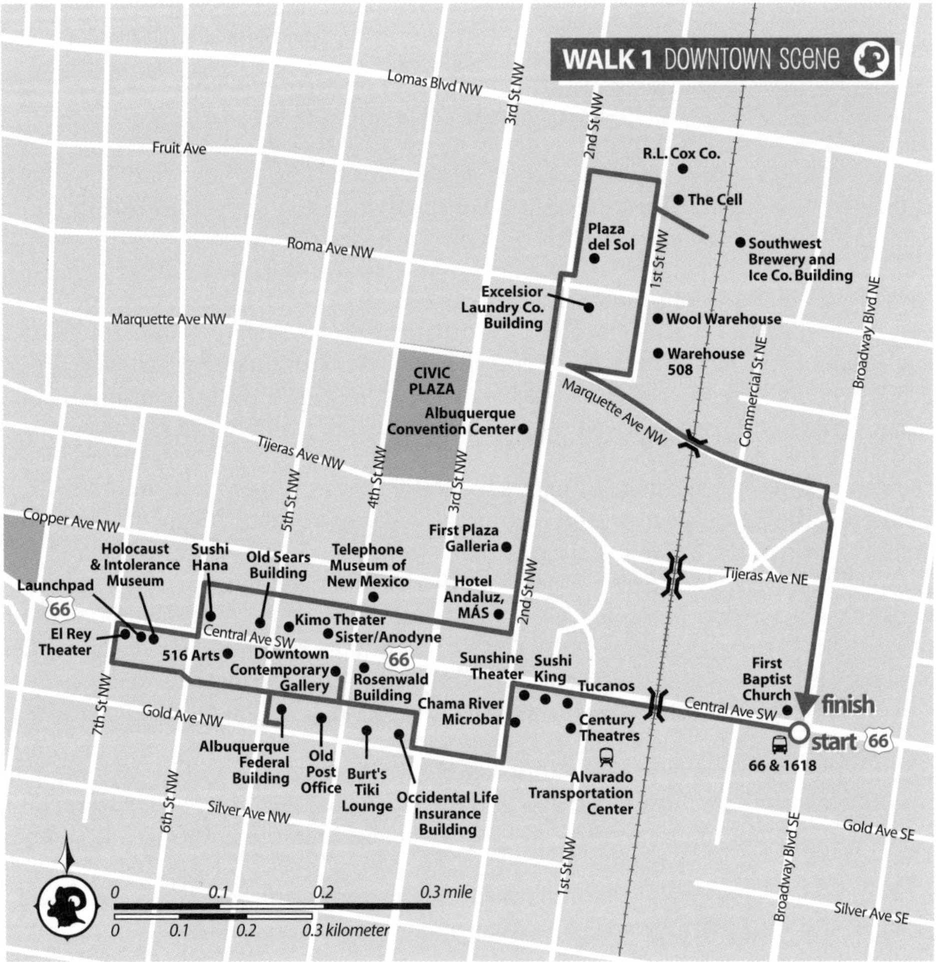

WALK 1 DOWNTOWN SCENE
Lomas Blvd NW
Fruit Ave
Roma Ave NW
Marquette Ave NW
Tijeras Ave NW
Copper Ave NW
Central Ave SW
Gold Ave NW
Silver Ave NW
Tijeras Ave NE
Gold Ave SE
Silver Ave SE
7th St NW
6th St NW
5th St NW
4th St NW
3rd St NW
2nd St NW
1st St NW
Commercial St NE
Broadway Blvd NE
Broadway Blvd SE
R.L. Cox Co.
The Cell
Southwest Brewery and Ice Co. Building
Plaza del Sol
Excelsior Laundry Co. Building
Wool Warehouse
Warehouse 508
CIVIC PLAZA
Albuquerque Convention Center
First Plaza Galleria
Hotel Andaluz, MÁS
Telephone Museum of New Mexico
Old Sears Building
Sushi Hana
Holocaust & Intolerance Museum
Launchpad
El Rey Theater
Kimo Theater
Sister/Anodyne
516 Arts
Downtown Contemporary Gallery
Rosenwald Building
Sunshine Theater
Sushi King
Tucanos
Chama River Microbar
Century Theatres
Alvarado Transportation Center
First Baptist Church
finish
start
66 & 1618
Albuquerque Federal Building
Old Post Office
Burt's Tiki Lounge
Occidental Life Insurance Building
66
0 0.1 0.2 0.3 mile
0 0.1 0.2 0.3 kilometer

1 THE DOWNTOWN SCENE: (AND WHAT'S BEHIND IT)

BOUNDARIES: **Broadway Blvd., Gold Ave., 7th St., Lomas Blvd.**
DISTANCE: **2 miles**
DIFFICULTY: **Easy**
PARKING: **Numerous lots and free street parking north of Central Ave., west of Broadway Blvd.**
PUBLIC TRANSIT: **Buses 66 and 1618 on Central Ave. at Broadway Blvd. Numerous routes serve the area. Railrunner station is on 1st St. south of Central Ave.**

Albuquerque is geographically divided into four quadrants that are officially part of any street address: NE (northeast), NW (northwest), SE (southeast), and SW (southwest). Central Ave. delineates north and south, the BNSF Railway tracks divide east and west. This walk hits all four quadrants, following a route as creative as the area it explores. Inspiration for this walk comes largely from expert wanderer David Ryan, author of the book and blog *The Gentle Art of Wandering*, who said, "When I walk in cities I hope to find a combination of interesting streets, alleys, paths, stairs, and whatever else is available along the way to make the walk special." With that in mind I sketched out a route using the alleys, an underpass, and the viaduct; then David and I set out to walk it. As expected we wandered off course, dropped in on businesses where we had no business, talked to strangers, gazed upon murals, waved at security cameras, debated the purpose of seemingly pointless structures, reminisced about what used to be here, took guesses on what might be there in the near future, and generally spent an entire afternoon in awe of everything around us. In these mere 2 miles (an abbreviated version of our meander that day) are enough sites and stories to fill volumes. What follows then are the briefest possible descriptions of 30 or so random things that captured our attention.

- **Start at the southwest corner of Central Ave. and Broadway Blvd. First Baptist Church looms on the northwest corner with 87,000 square feet of building space on 7 acres of land. It sustained severe fire damage in 2010 and was on the market for $7.5 million in 2014 and was acquired by Innovate ABQ, an idea incubator that links local high-tech institutions with start-up companies to create innovative businesses.**

- **Walk west on Central. These first two blocks to the underpass are the only part of the walk in Albuquerque's southeast quadrant. Much like Four Corners Monument, where Arizona, Colorado, New Mexico, and Utah meet, the center line of Central beneath the** railroad tracks is where you could straddle Albuquerque's four quadrants at once, but that's not advised. Also in this underpass are a series of panels featuring historical photos and interpretive information. The translucent panels seem to light up as you approach or leave, depending on the angle of the sun. In 2014, the city announced plans to elevate the underpass, so you may find yourself crossing over the tracks instead.

- Once you cross the tracks, the site on your right (a parking lot in 2014) is slated to become downtown's premier entertainment hub. On your left, the first building you pass in the southwest quadrant is the Alvarado Transportation Center, a feature in Walk 3. For now continue past the neon signs for Century Theatres and Tucanos Brazilian Grill. The smoky aroma on this corner is difficult to resist for those who crave unlimited servings of charred and skewered meats. For those who prefer delicate fare, Sushi King is right next door. The next door down is Sunshine Theater, the hottest downtown spot to catch concert tours. Memorable shows in past years include CocoRosie and Insane Clown Posse. The six-story Sunshine Building, a reinforced concrete construction with a yellow brick façade, was designed by Henry C. Trost to house Albuquerque's first movie palace, which opened in 1924. It's one of a dozen or so buildings on this route that are listed on the National Register of Historic Places.

- Turn left on 2nd St. Blink and you'll miss the Chama River Microbar tucked in the southwest corner of the Sunshine Building. The mural across the street is *Mother Road,* a tribute to Route 66 (Central Ave.) by Working Classroom. Poke your head in the alley ahead for Ernest Doty's raven composition in aerosol and house paint, *We Exist Somewhere Between Limbo and Purgatory.* Past that is my personal favorite, *Totem of the Ancient Ones*, a triptych mural by Thomas Christopher Haag.

- Turn right on Gold Ave. The first building on your left housed the National Institute of Flamenco for 15 years before it burned down at the end of 2013. Sidewalk cafés, art venues, and other hip ventures come and go on this quiet block. Vacancies are common and soon filled with pleasant surprises. Ahead at the northwest corner of 3rd St. stands the distinctive Occidental Life Insurance Building. Henry C. Trost designed this 1917 masterpiece to resemble Doge's Palace in Venice. A fire in 1933 destroyed its mahogany and Circassian walnut interior, but its glazed white terra-cotta tile façade of Venetian Gothic arches remains largely intact.

- Cross 3rd St. and turn right; then take a left into the alley on the north side of the Occidental Building. The most colorful mural on this block belongs to Burt's Tiki Lounge, a Polynesian-themed faux dive that was inexplicably placed on *Esquire* magazine's list of best bars in America. At the end of the block and fronting Central Ave. is the Rosenwald Building. Another creation of Henry C. Trost, this former department store opened in 1910 to carry the wares of Aron and Edward Rosenwald, German merchants who arrived in Albuquerque in 1878. The reinforced concrete structure is considered New Mexico's first fireproof building, despite the fire that gutted it in 1921.

- Before ducking down the alley in the 400 block, take a few steps south to see the plaque embedded in the sidewalk. It marks the geographic center of Albuquerque in 1912. (Over the century that followed, the geographic center shifted 1.5 miles north and about a quarter mile east. The 2012 plaque is on the north side of Coronado Park, between 3rd and 4th Streets.)

- Now take a quick detour north to the Downtown Contemporary Gallery in the historic Yrisarri Block. This building was completed in 1909 and has housed the gallery and numerous artist studios since 1996.

Other buildings you'll sneak behind on the 400 block include the Old Post Office and the Albuquerque Federal Building, both fronting Gold Ave. The post office was built in the Spanish Colonial Revival style in 1908. Since 2000, it has housed Amy Biehl High School, a charter school named for a high-spirited social activist from Santa Fe who, in 1993 at the age of 26, was murdered near Cape Town, South Africa. The six-story, 63,000-square-foot building by its side displays a marvelous assortment of Southwestern motifs throughout the exterior detailing. Take a detour to its front entry to check out the assortment of randomly placed terra-cotta petroglyphs inlaid around the archway, keeping in mind that swastikas were a distinctly Navajo motif when the building was completed in 1930.

The eight-story, block-long former federal office on the south side of the alley ahead was probably built in the 1970s and has spent most of the current century echoing the sentiments of that era. In 1978 Susan Dewitt wrote in *Historic Albuquerque Today*, "Off Central, pedestrians are often faced by blank-walled buildings, menacing and uninviting." No doubt she had this structure in mind. Apparently immune to arson, the

Modern monstrosity sold in an online federal auction in 2007 for $1.51 million and as of 2014 remains vacant.

On your right the wall art really starts to pop. Whether it's vandalism or public art often depends on who funded it. For example, stencils indicate which works are sponsored by 516 Arts. This unassuming art gallery fronting Central is a powerhouse for generating citywide events. It also hosts exhibitions by renowned international contemporary artists and occasionally displays masterpieces by the author of this book. Continue straight through the 600 block ahead, enjoying yet another hidden showcase of wall art.

- Turn right on 7th St. at the end of the last alley and go a half block north.

- Turn right on Central. Standing here on the southeast corner and named for its former owner Luigi—not his cousin, the legendary opera composer Giacomo—the Puccini Building housed both Puccini's Golden West Saloon and the El Rey Theater, built in 1929 and 1941 respectively. The latter is noted for hosting such music legends as Ella Fitzgerald and Arlo Guthrie. In 2008, shortly after major restorations to the historic structure, a fire gutted the Golden West, but the El Rey survived and received another round of restorations in 2012. The neighboring club, Launchpad, also survived and remains the best bet in town for cheap drinks and cutting-edge music acts. Underground music legends hosted here include Melt-Banana and Agent Orange. The next door down is the Holocaust & Intolerance Museum, a sobering reminder of human atrocities committed throughout the world.

- Turn left on 6th St., crossing Central and entering Albuquerque's northwest quadrant. Sushi Hana is on the northeast corner, in case you skipped Sushi King. Go half a block north.

- Turn right into the alley in the 500 block. The last building on the right is commonly referred to as the Old Sears Building. Expanded in 1955 following an interior fire and renovated in 1990, the 56,000-square-foot office building was on the market in 2014 for a mere $2.75 million. Its Streamline Moderne style stands in stark contrast to its Pueblo Deco neighbor to the east. The KiMo Theater, the pièce de résistance of downtown architecture, was commissioned by Oreste and Maria Bachechi, parents of Carlo Bachechi, whose family farm is featured in Walk 14. A boiler explosion in 1951 demolished the original lobby and killed 6-year-old Bobby Darnall, who allegedly haunts the theater to this day. A fire in 1963 destroyed the original stage. The KiMo dodged the wrecking ball in 1977 and has since undergone extensive restorations.

Also on the 400 block, Sister is a relatively new hipster bar with patio seating, pub games, and live music. The significantly older yet equally hip Anodyne pool hall is directly above it. Both have a fantastic beer selection. At the end of the block, across 4th St., the brick building ahead on the left was built in 1906 and has housed the Telephone Museum of New Mexico since 1997. Hundreds of phones are on display, along with switchboards, teletype machines, and a 2,000-pound, 7-foot bronze medallion. Hours are Monday, Wednesday, and Friday, 10 a.m.–2 p.m.

- Continue down the alleyway another two blocks.
- Turn left on 2nd St. Hotel Andaluz, the ten-story tower on the nearest corner, was built in 1939 as the first Hilton in New Mexico. At the time it was the tallest and the only air-conditioned structure in the state. Tapas and other exotic fare are available at MÁS, the elegant restaurant on the ground floor, and at Ibiza, the casual patio bar above it.
- Continue north past the First Plaza Galleria and the Convention Center. The southeast corner of 2nd St. and Roma Ave. has been the site of various laundry operations for more than a century. The present building was designed by Louis Hesselden in the early 1940s. Often mistaken for a vintage cinema or bus station, the Moderne-style structure is commonly referred to as the Excelsior Laundry

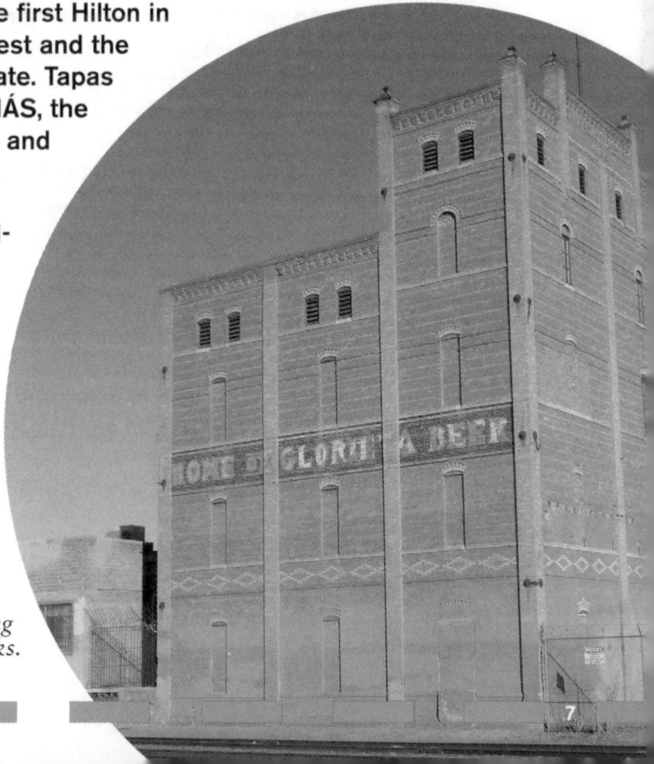

Southwest Brewery and Ice Co. Building overlooks the railroad tracks.

Company Building, also known as the American Linen Supply Building and the Ameri-Pride Building. Murals on its exterior walls illustrate its history.

- Turn right into the second parking lot entrance north of Plaza del Sol (the building shaped like a Mayan pyramid), and then walk east to 1st St. The arrow ahead indicating a "drive in fur & hide" is a bit misleading. It's simply an old drive-in sign partially painted over and relocated to R.L. Cox Co., which boasts an impressive inventory of animal-based materials. Their neighbor to the south is a black box known as The Cell, where the FUSION Theatre Company has been producing and performing great American plays since 2001.

- Turn right on 1st St. and detour into the parking lot for a closer look at the Southwest Brewery and Ice Co. Building. The trackside operation began in an adobe structure that was destroyed by fire in 1887. The brick-tower complex replaced it in 1902. When the state enacted prohibition in 1917, the brewing permanently ceased, but ice production continued until 1997. Real estate mogul Joe Maloof snapped up the vacant building allegedly because his mom thought it was one of the prettiest buildings she had ever seen. An adjacent warehouse burned down months later, slightly damaging the tower.

  Warehouses near the south end of 1st St. are the city's last remnants of an era when sheep surrounded the city and wool was a major industry. Youth Development Inc. occupies the Wool Warehouse, offering such services as after-school tutoring, gang intervention, and public housing assistance. Warehouse 508 is the town's biggest arts and entertainment center for youth. Serving as both a practice and performance space, it's likely the place to find the great local artists, actors, poets, DJs, dancers, and musicians of tomorrow. Walk-ins are welcome to tour the 26,000-square-foot facility. The mural on its south-facing wall is *Quantum Bridge,* described by artist Aaron Noble as "a semi-abstract time travel epic with aesthetic roots in comics, graffiti, and hip-hop."

- Turn right at the end of 1st St. and follow the sidewalk west toward 2nd St.

- Take a sharp left onto the viaduct and stay on the sidewalk until you cross back over the tracks, this time entering the northeast quadrant. Admittedly the view is better walking west, so look back every so often to admire the skyline. The eastbound view provides a dramatic illustration of the vast amounts of space we dedicate to parking lots. Try to enjoy the mountain vistas as well. The Sandias peak about 12 miles east. The tracks below appear to be on a collision course with the Jemez Mountains rising about 40 miles north.

- Turn right on Broadway and use the crosswalks to safely navigate your way back to where you started. For reference, First Baptist Church is the big brick building one block south.

Expert wanderer David Ryan recaps the walk accordingly: "I didn't know what to expect at the start of the walk, but as we kept going we ran into something interesting at almost every turn. The unique designs on the old Federal Building were a total surprise. It's worth a visit on its own. When I lived in Albuquerque in 1969, the Old Sears Building is where preinduction physicals were held by the military. Sears was long gone from downtown and located in Coronado Mall. Coronado and Winrock malls ended major retail downtown. Another unexpected highlight was when we took the elevator to the top of a parking deck at 3rd and Copper and had uninterrupted views of the Sandias to the east, the Manzanos to the south, and downtown all around us. This is a walk I would be happy to do over and over again."

POINTS OF INTEREST

Century Theatres cinemark.com/theatre-447, 100 Central Ave. SW, 505-243-9555

Tucanos Brazilian Grill tucanos.com, 110 Central Ave. SW, 505-246-9900

Sushi King sushikingnm.com, 118 Central Ave. SW, 505-842-5099

Sunshine Theater sunshinetheaterlive.com, 120 Central Ave. SW, 505-764-0249

Chama River Microbar chamariverbrewery.com, 106 2nd St. SW, 505-842-8329

Burt's Tiki Lounge 313 Gold Ave. SW, 505-247-2878

Downtown Contemporary Gallery downtowncontemporary.com, 105 4th St. SW, 505-363-3870

516 Arts 516arts.org, 516 Central Ave. SW, 505-242-1445

El Rey Theater elreytheater.com, 622 Central Ave. SW, 505-242-2353

Launchpad launchpadrocks.com, 618 Central Ave. SW, 505-764-8887

Holocaust & Intolerance Museum of New Mexico nmholocaustmuseum.org, 616 Central Ave. SW, 505-247-0606

Sushi Hana sushihananm.com, 521 Central Ave. NW, 505-842-8700

KiMo Theater kimotickets.com, 421 Central Ave. NW, 505-768-3522

Sister Bar sisterthebar.com, 407 Central Ave. NW, 505-242-4900

Anodyne theanodyne.com, 409 Central Ave. NW, 505-244-1820

Telephone Museum of New Mexico telecomhistory.org, 110 4th St. NW, 505-842-2937

Hotel Andaluz hotelandaluz.com, 125 2nd St. NW, 505-242-9090

MÁS hotelandaluz.com, 125 2nd St. NW, 505-923-9080

The Cell fusionabq.org, 700 1st St. NW, 505-766-9412

Warehouse 508 warehouse508.org, 508 1st St. NW, 505-296-2738

route summary

1. Start at the southwest corner of Central Ave. and Broadway Blvd. and walk west on Central Ave.
2. Turn left on 2nd St.
3. Turn right on Gold Ave.
4. Turn right on 3rd St. and go half a block north.
5. Turn left into the alley.
6. Turn right on 7th St.
7. Turn right on Central Ave.
8. Turn left on 6th St. and go half a block north.
9. Turn right into the alley.
10. Turn left on 2nd St.
11. Turn right into the second parking lot entrance north of Roma Ave.
12. Turn right on 1st St.
13. Turn right at the end of 1st St.
14. Take a sharp left onto the viaduct.
15. Turn right on Broadway Blvd.

CONNECTING THE WALKS

Walk 2 begins on the southeast corner of Central and Broadway. Walk 3 begins on 3rd St. one block south of Gold. To connect with Walk 4, continue one block west from the alley south of Central. For Walk 5, turn left on 4th St. from the alley north of Central and go two blocks north.

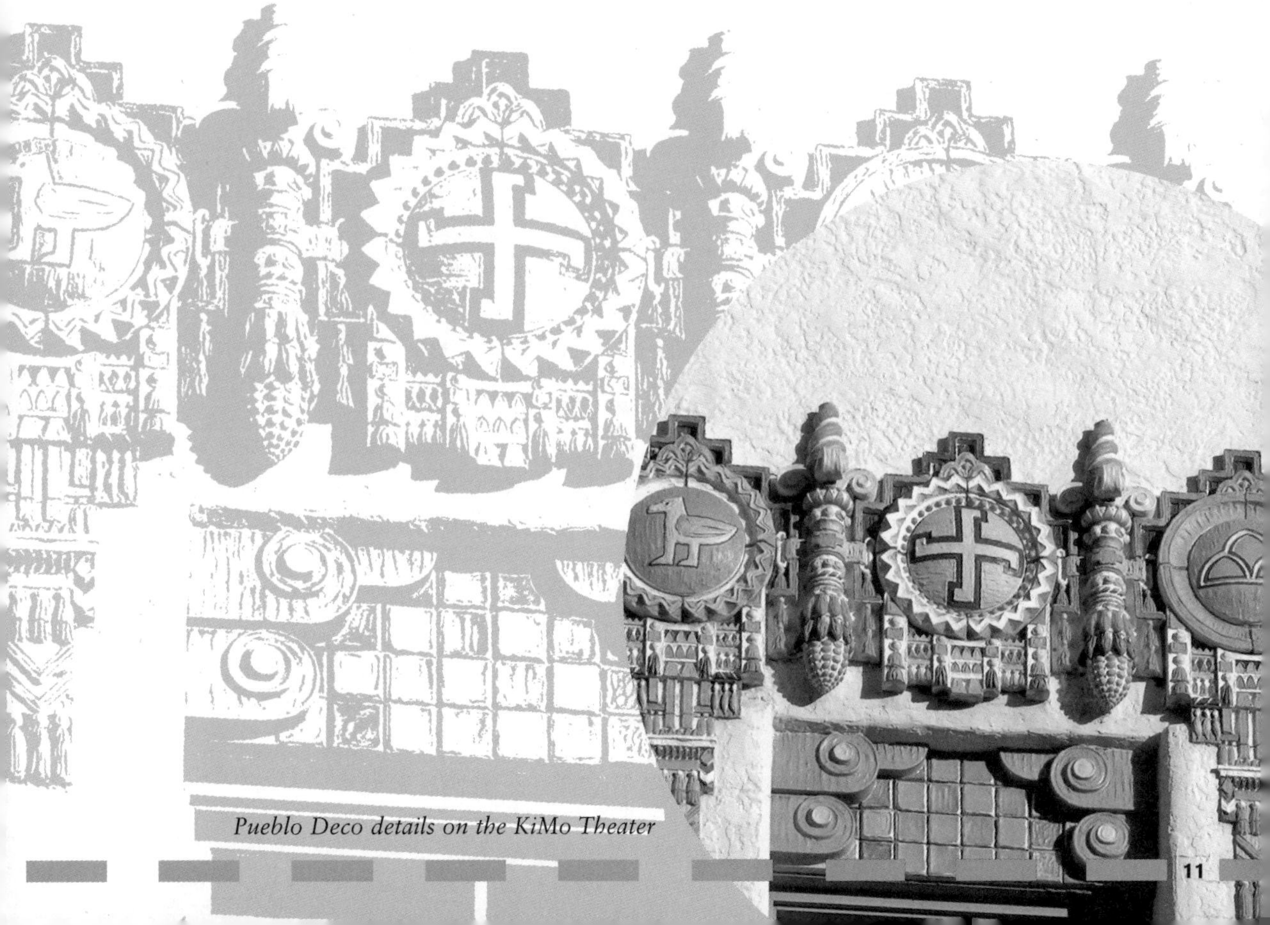

Pueblo Deco details on the KiMo Theater

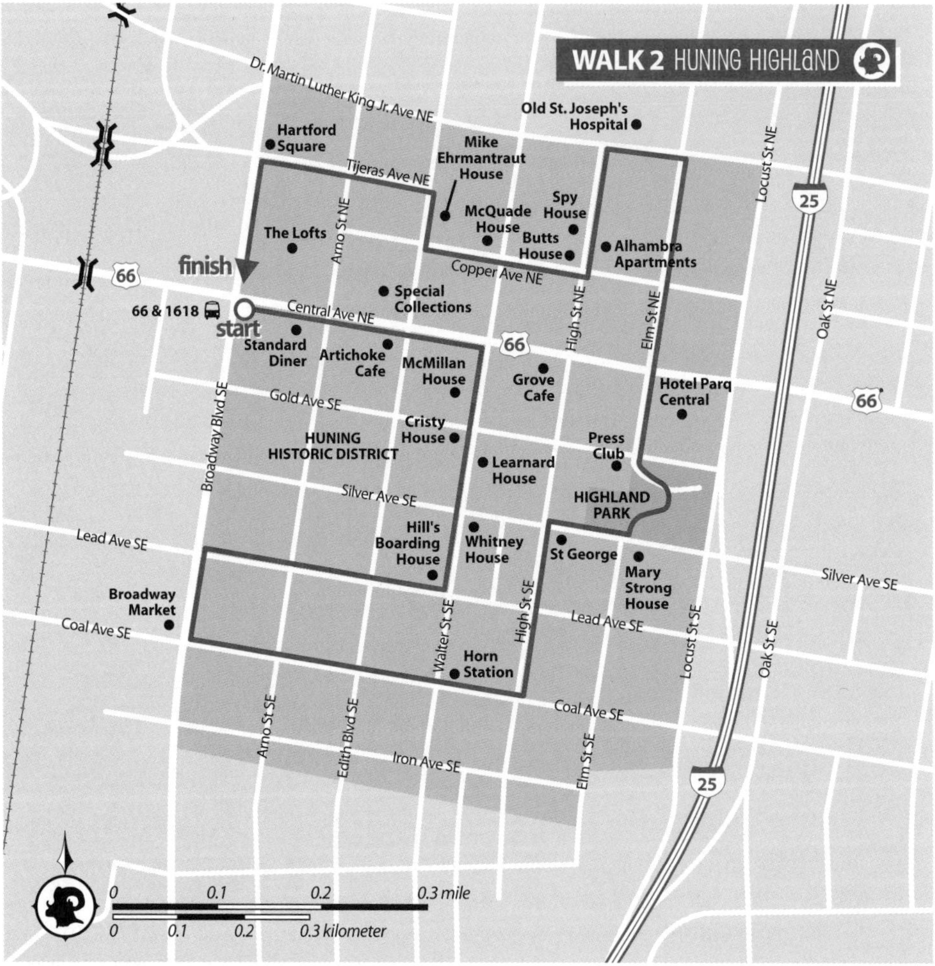
WALK 2 HUNING HIGHLAND
Dr. Martin Luther King Jr. Ave NE
Old St. Joseph's Hospital
Hartford Square
Mike Ehrmantraut House
Tijeras Ave NE
Spy House
McQuade House
Butts House
Alhambra Apartments
The Lofts
Arno St NE
Locust St NE
Copper Ave NE
finish
start
66 & 1618
Special Collections
Central Ave NE
High St NE
Elm St NE
Oak St NE
Standard Diner
Artichoke Cafe
McMillan House
Grove Cafe
Hotel Parq Central
Gold Ave SE
Broadway Blvd SE
Cristy House
HUNING HISTORIC DISTRICT
Press Club
Learnard House
HIGHLAND PARK
Silver Ave SE
Lead Ave SE
Hill's Boarding House
Whitney House
St George
Mary Strong House
Broadway Market
Coal Ave SE
Walter St SE
High St SE
Locust St SE
Oak St SE
Horn Station
Arno St SE
Edith Blvd SE
Iron Ave SE
Elm St SE
0 0.1 0.2 0.3 mile
0 0.1 0.2 0.3 kilometer

2 HUNING HIGHLAND: LEGACY OF THE RAILROAD AND ROUTE 66

BOUNDARIES: **Broadway Blvd., Coal Ave., Elm St., Dr. Martin Luther King Jr. Ave.**
DISTANCE: **2 miles**
DIFFICULTY: **Easy**
PARKING: **Free parking on Broadway Blvd., Coal Ave., Elm St., Dr. Martin Luther King Jr. Ave.**
PUBLIC TRANSIT: **Buses 66 and 1618 on Central Ave. at Broadway Blvd. Numerous routes serve the area. Railrunner station is on 1st St. south of Central Ave.**

In 1880 German immigrant/merchant/entrepreneur Franz Huning platted the lots east of the newly arrived railroad. By 1888, he'd already sold 63 percent of the 536 lots. Huning's Highland Addition, Albuquerque's first Anglo neighborhood, reflects Anglo-American values and Victorian tastes in home design. Architectural examples include Queen Anne, Italianate, and Colonial Revival—all styles that could be ordered prefabricated in factories and delivered via the railroad. A growing fascination for and dependence on automobiles contributed to the neighborhood's decline. The 1937 realignment of Route 66 (Central Ave.) cut it in half. In the 1960s, I-25 emerged on the eastern boundary, and liquor stores and cheap motels popped up near its intersection with Central Ave. The area was in rapid decline by the mid-1970s. Its first step toward recovery came in 1978, when the Huning Highland Historic District was added to the National Register of Historic Places. The rebound continued into the late 1990s and early 2000s with the city's initiative to redevelop east downtown, or EDo. The new name and gentrified urban face-lift is not without its critics, and there's still much room for improvement, but the push continues to restore and balance the celebrated characteristics of both the railroad era and the heyday of Route 66.

- **Start at the southeast corner of Central and Broadway. The enormous Gothic Revival complex to the north is the Old Albuquerque High School, which provided secondary education to local students as early as 1914 in the Old Main Building on Central. The Manual Arts addition on Arno St. was completed in 1927, and the gymnasium on Tijeras Ave. was added in 1938. Classes continued until the early 1970s. The building sat vacant until 2003, when renovations began to convert old classrooms into stylish apartments and commercial spaces. Visitors are not allowed to explore the interior** on their own, but EDo Spaces offers tours of The Lofts at Albuquerque High three times a week.

- Walk east on Central and follow the scent of comfort food to the Standard Diner. Housed in a 1930s gas station, the popular eatery is both nostalgic and contemporary in terms of both décor and cuisine. Bacon-wrapped meatloaf is a favorite. That and the country-fried tuna seemed to impress Guy Fieri when he stopped in on a 2013 episode of the TV series *Diners, Drive-Ins, and Dives.*

A three-story schoolhouse once stood on the northwest corner of Central and Edith Blvd. Originally it was the site of Albuquerque Academy, which became the Albuquerque Public School in 1891 and a public library and business college after 1900. The building was demolished in 1923 and replaced in 1925 with an excellent example of Pueblo Spanish–style architecture. It now houses the Special Collections Library, research collections on Albuquerque history and New Mexico history and culture, as well as The Center for the Book, a hands-on learning center about the history of printing.

Foodie alert on the southwest corner: Artichoke Cafe, an upscale New American cuisine establishment, earned its place on every local favorite list (along with the attention of a few national reviews) long before anyone else would've dared put a bistro in EDo. And, yes, they have artichoke on the menu.

- Turn right on Walter St. The restaurant on the east side of the parking lot should look familiar to fans of the TV series *Breaking Bad.* The Grove Cafe should also interest fans of breakfast and brunch. Go for the goat cheese burrito.

The McMillan House, at 119 Walter St., is the first of several unusual constructions you'll encounter in the next three blocks. Built for A. B. McMillan, a wealthy socialite in the 1890s, this chaotically designed house features a veranda that wraps around the east- and north-facing sides, along with gable trim that seems oddly reminiscent of Imperial Japan. The neighbor to the south seems even stranger, with its low-slope roof and widow's walk, details commonly associated with coastal housing, but you'll soon notice those are popular rooftops in this neighborhood. More seemingly coastal features can be found on the Cristy House, at 201 Walter St. Completed in 1897 the clapboard cottage is adorned with windows that resemble kisby rings.

The Learnard House, at 210 Walter St., rises from its stone foundation with an impressive three-story tower on its northwest corner. That and its complex mix of brick and shingles make it one of the finest Queen Anne houses in town. The Whitney House, at 302 Walter St., resembles a bank, but its Doric columns, metal cornice, and parapet roof are classical details popularized by "The White City" at the 1893 Chicago World's Fair. The cross-gabled house on the northwest corner of Walter St. and Lead Ave. is still known as Mrs. Hill's Boarding House, even though Mrs. Hill stopped taking in boarders way back in 1909. The eclectic mix of stylings, such as mismatched windows, suggests that the designer whimsically selected decorative features from a variety of builders' catalogs.

- Turn right on Lead Ave., the first of three one-way streets that divide the south side of the neighborhood and discourage pedestrian traffic. Walk three blocks west to Broadway Blvd.

- Turn left on Broadway and go south one block to Coal Ave. The Broadway Market, on the northwest corner of Broadway and Coal, was once a combined store and house known as the Vance Market. Dating back to 1910, this two-story redbrick structure was the childhood home of Vivian Vance, the actress best remembered for her role as Ethel Mertz on the 1950s sitcom *I Love Lucy.*

- Turn left on Coal and walk east. The urban decay that the Huning Highland Historic District Association has long fought persists along the fringes. (The original south boundary is Hazeldine Ave., but the current historic zone extends slightly past Iron Ave.) At the northeast corner of Coal and Walter is a former Conoco gas station built in the style of an

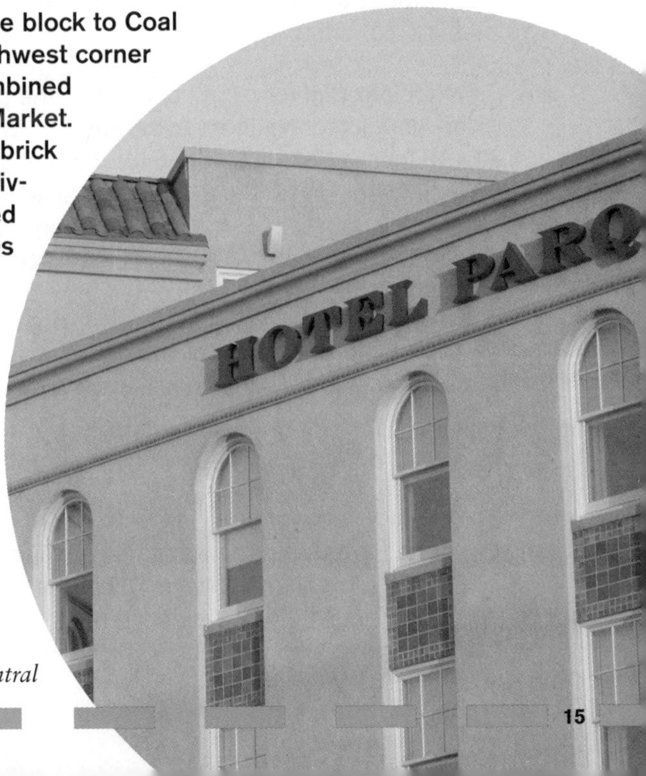

Hotel Parq Central

English cottage to fit into its residential surroundings. In 1997 it was dedicated as the H. B. and Lucille Horn Preservation Station and now serves as a meeting venue for The Albuquerque Conservation Association. A community garden with chicken coops is on the east side of the station.

- Turn left on High St. Two blocks north is St. George Greek Orthodox Church, site of a hugely popular Grecian Festival that falls on the first week of October. Across the street is a private residence converted from the old Albuquerque Fire Station 2, which sounds like an incredibly fun place to live until you consider that it's a single-story building, so it probably never had a fire pole.

- Turn right on Silver Ave. The Mary Strong House, on the corner of Elm St., was built in 1910 upon a foundation of cemented pebble stones native to the site. It's hard to imagine now that the city once ended here at the foot of barren sandhills, the same escarpment that runs east of Edith Blvd. all the way up to Rattlesnake Mesa (visited on Walk 13) and beyond.

- Turn left into Highland Park and follow the paved walkway to the top of the hill. The three-story log cabin there is the work of Charles Whittlesey, chief architect for the AT&SF Railway. His inspiration for the design was a Norwegian villa, which also influenced his design for the El Tovar Hotel at the Grand Canyon that same year. Whittlesey and his family lived in his dream home for a scant four years before his interest in peeled log cuts waned in favor of reinforced concrete. The cabin has a long and colorful history, though little is recorded about what happened within its walls from 1960 to 1966, when it served as a frat house. The building is plagued with paranormal activity, all of it harmless yet entirely inexplicable, even to jaded journalists who've witnessed the phenomena firsthand. Since 1973 it has been home to the Albuquerque Press Club. And like most press clubs, it's private, but you can probably talk your way in. Be warned, however, that it's not easy to leave the warm pub atmosphere once cozied up to the bar.

- Stagger down the driveway to Gold Ave. and continue straight on Elm. On your right is the Hotel Parq Central, which could easily qualify for the handsomest building in town despite its grim history. By the 1920s the AT&SF Railroad had well over 1,000 employees. Not surprisingly in this early era of heavy industry and huge machinery, work-related injuries were drastically high. Railroad execs responded by building the city's first medical facilities, collectively known as Santa Fe Hospital. The one on Elm was later renamed AT&SF Hospital. In the 1970s and early 1980s it served as a children's psychiatric ward known as Memorial Hospital. Spirits that allegedly circulate the building today are often described as the ghosts of children, though former patients attest the place was thoroughly haunted before they arrived. Best not to dwell on its grim past and instead enjoy another round of spirits in its hip rooftop lounge, the Apothecary.

- Continue straight on Elm to Dr. Martin Luther King Jr. Ave. The dark brick building is the Old St. Joseph's Hospital, completed in 1930—four years later than the hospital you last saw. This one is Romanesque in style, while the previous was distinctly Italianate. The difference in appearance from ground level is like night and day. Viewed from above, however, the size and shape of their diagonally winged designs are almost identical.

- Turn left on Dr. Martin Luther King Jr. Ave. and walk one block west.

- Turn left on High St. The establishment at 209 High St. was known as the Freeman Boarding House shortly after World War II. One of its first tenants was David Greenglass, a machinist assigned to the Manhattan Project in Los Alamos, New Mexico. On June 2, 1945, Greenglass sold diagrams for the atomic bomb to KGB operative Harry Gold for $500. The exchange occurred in room four of the boarding house. Later arrested by American counterintelligence, Gold ratted out Greenglass, who in turn ratted out his own sister, Ethel Rosenberg, and her husband, Julius. After refusing to testify to their alleged role in this plot of espionage, the Rosenbergs were executed on June 19, 1953. The Freeman Boarding House Apartments is now a quaint bed-and-breakfast known as the Downtown Historic Bed & Breakfast, featuring the Spy House and the Heritage House next door.

Across the street, Alhambra Apartments use porthole windows and arabesque designs as a playful reference to Alhambra, a palatial fortress complex 7 miles west of Santa Fe, Spain. The reference seems to end there, since the apartments' overall look is a mix of Pueblo and California Mission styles, and its interior living spaces were built on an absurdly dwarfish scale.

By contrast, the Mrs. T. I. Butts House, at 201 High St., is a robust, no-nonsense construction of wood and cast stone. Built in the late Queen Anne style, the house is named for a principal of the First Ward School in the early 20th century.

- Turn right on Copper Ave. Standing on the corner of Walter St., the McQuade House is a highly ornamented cottage with an octagonal gazebo porch. Its first resident, J. W. McQuade, was the architect for the John Milne House (visited on Walk 4).

- Turn right on Edith. The Mike Ehrmantraut House, residence for the badass hit man in the *Breaking Bad* series, is the third house on the right. (He doesn't live there anymore, so respect the privacy of the current residents.)

- Turn left on Tijeras Ave. and walk past the north end of the Old Albuquerque High School campus.

- Turn left on Broadway to return to the starting point.

  Notable architect and celebrated tubaist Mark Weaver fondly recalls his favorite features on the walk: "My mom graduated from Albuquerque High School in 1953. She used to hang out at the Highland Drugstore, which was on the southeast corner of Central and Broadway, and would frequent the library at Central and Edith, which at that time was the only public library in town. . . . There are so many fascinating houses in this neighborhood, but my particular favorite is the Cristy House with all its octagonal structural elements."

POINTS OF INTEREST

The Lofts at Albuquerque High (EDo Spaces) abqhigh.com, 401 Central Ave. NE, Suite D, 505-247-3935

Standard Diner standarddiner.com, 320 Central Ave. SE, 505-243-1440

Special Collections Library abclibrary.org/specialcollections, 423 Central Ave. NE, 505-848-1376

Artichoke Cafe artichokecafe.com, 424 Central Ave. SE, 505-243-0200

Grove Cafe & Market thegrovecafemarket.com, 600 Central Ave. SE, 505-248-9800

St. George Greek Orthodox Church stgeorgenm.org, 308 High St. SE, 505-247-9411

Albuquerque Press Club www.qpressclub.com, 201 Highland Park Cir. SE, 505-243-8476

Hotel Parq Central hotelparqcentral.com, 806 Central Ave. SE, 505-242-0040

Downtown Historic B&B downtownhistoric.com, 207 High St., 505-842-0223

route summary

1. Start at the southeast corner of Central Ave. and Broadway Blvd. and walk east on Central Ave.
2. Turn right on Walter St.
3. Turn right on Lead Ave.
4. Turn left on Broadway Blvd.
5. Turn left on Coal Ave.
6. Turn left on High St.
7. Turn right on Silver Ave.
8. Turn left into Highland Park and follow the paved walkway to the top of the hill; then follow the driveway down to Gold St.
9. Continue straight on Elm St.
10. Turn left on Dr. Martin Luther King Jr. Ave.
11. Turn left on High St.
12. Turn right on Copper Ave.
13. Turn right on Edith Blvd.
14. Turn left on Tijeras Ave.
15. Turn left on Broadway Blvd.

connecting the walks

Walk 1 begins at the southwest corner of Central and Broadway.

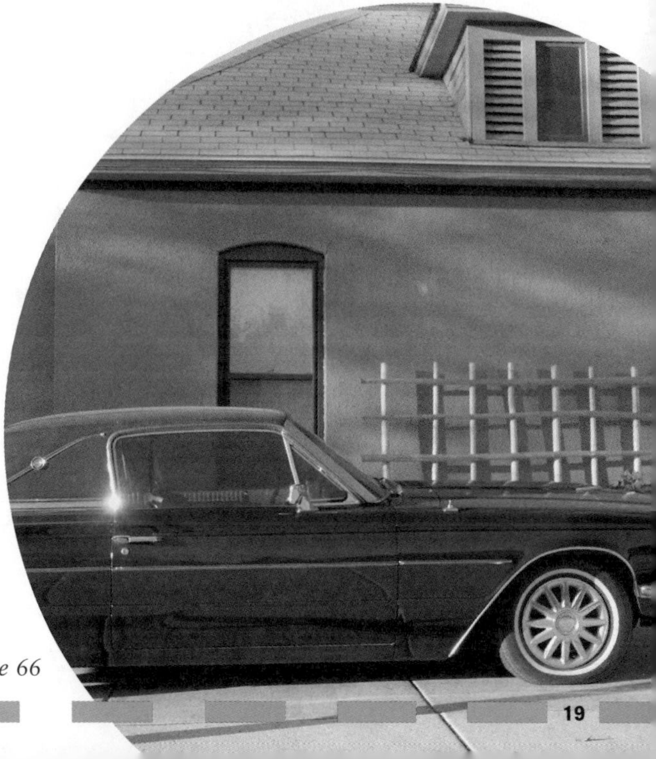

Ford Thunderbird, a classic for cruising Route 66

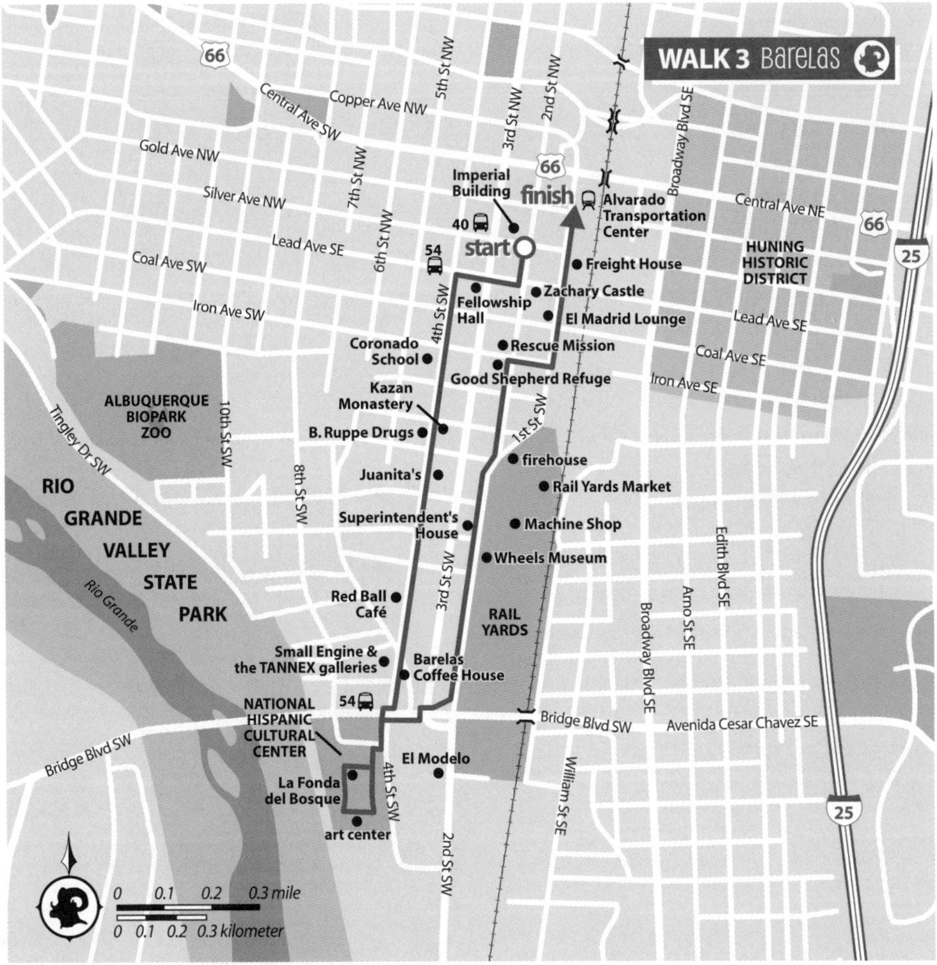
WALK 3 Barelas
Copper Ave NW
Central Ave SW
Gold Ave NW
Silver Ave NW
Lead Ave SE
Coal Ave SW
Iron Ave SW
5th St NW
3rd St NW
2nd St NW
7th St NW
6th St NW
4th St SW
Broadway Blvd SE
Central Ave NE
Imperial Building
finish
Alvarado Transportation Center
start
Freight House
Zachary Castle
Fellowship Hall
El Madrid Lounge
Rescue Mission
Good Shepherd Refuge
Coronado School
HUNING HISTORIC DISTRICT
Lead Ave SE
Coal Ave SE
Iron Ave SE
Kazan Monastery
B. Ruppe Drugs
ALBUQUERQUE BIOPARK ZOO
10th St SW
Tingley Dr SW
1st St SW
firehouse
Rail Yards Market
Juanita's
8th St SW
RIO GRANDE VALLEY STATE PARK
Superintendent's House
Machine Shop
Wheels Museum
Edith Blvd SE
Rio Grande
3rd St SW
Red Ball Café
RAIL YARDS
Broadway Blvd SE
Arno St SE
Small Engine & the TANNEX galleries
Barelas Coffee House
NATIONAL HISPANIC CULTURAL CENTER
Bridge Blvd SW
Avenida Cesar Chavez SE
Bridge Blvd SW
El Modelo
La Fonda del Bosque
4th St SW
William St SE
art center
2nd St SW
0 0.1 0.2 0.3 mile
0 0.1 0.2 0.3 kilometer

3 Barelas: Land of Mi Chante

BOUNDARIES: Gold Ave., 1st St., National Hispanic Cultural Center
DISTANCE: 2.5 miles
DIFFICULTY: Easy
PARKING: Street parking on Silver Ave. near 2nd St., parking garage on 2nd St. south of Gold Ave., ample free parking at National Hispanic Cultural Center
PUBLIC TRANSIT: Bus 40 on 3rd St. at Silver Ave. Buses 66, 766, 777, and many others stop at the Alvarado Transportation Center. Bus 54 travels 4th St. between Silver Ave. and the National Hispanic Cultural Center. Numerous other routes serve the area.

Barelas emerged in the 19th century as a farming village near a site where the Camino Real crossed the Rio Grande. With the arrival of the railroad in 1880, Barelas quickly grew from an agricultural community into an industrial neighborhood dominated by Atchison, Topeka, and Santa Fe Railway shops along 2nd St. Commerce increased when Route 66 coursed through the neighborhood in 1926, but its realignment in 1937 bypassed Barelas. The closure of the railroad shops in 1970 eliminated 1,500 jobs from the community. Adding insult to injury, the city disconnected the main route into Barelas to create Civic Plaza in 1974 (and reconnected it in 2014). Throughout the 1970s and 1980s, Barelas fostered a mean reputation as a crime-ridden barrio. Now with the National Hispanic Cultural Center well established and renovations of the Rail Yards moving full steam ahead, Barelas is making a phenomenal comeback.

- **Start at 2nd St. and Silver Ave. At the time of this writing (2014) plans for the northwest corner are underway for the construction of the Imperial Building, a mixed-use development with a 12,000-square-foot grocery store, which has downtown residents giddy with anticipation.**

- **Walk south one block to find Zachary Castle. In 1976 Gertrude Zachary opened a jewelry manufacturing operation on 2nd St. and soon came to be regarded as one of Albuquerque's most dynamic, if somewhat eccentric, business leaders. In 2006 construction began on her dream house, a Paris-inspired estate abutting an overpass just off Skid Row. The estimated cost: $2–$4 million. Zachary shared her estate with a Shih Tzu named Zipper until her death in 2013. The private compound includes a pool, a courtyard garden, and an 8,500-square-foot main house with four turrets, each** rising 50 feet. A separate tower stands directly in front of a billboard that advertises her wares. Gertrude Zachary's Castle Antiques, a quirky 12,000-foot showroom of American and European antiques, is directly south of the compound.

- Turn right on Lead Ave. and walk one block west. Reverend Nathaniel Gale, Albuquerque's first Methodist pastor, arrived from Silver City in 1879 and began holding services in a newly built adobe church on this site in 1880. His congregation outgrew the church by 1904, prompting the construction of a bigger one, which stands on the southwest corner of Lead Ave. and 3rd St. Dedicated in January 1905 the Gothic edifice is constructed of cast stone and concrete blocks. Its 24 stained glass windows show a mastery of the technique of Louis Tiffany, founder of the American stained glass style. This church building is listed as Fellowship Hall on the National Register of Historic Places. A newer, much bigger brick church stands on the corner ahead, indicating the congregation has continued to grow.

- Turn left on 4th St., which overlaps historical alignments of Highway 85, Route 66, and El Camino Real de Tierra Adentro (the Spanish Colonial "Royal Road" between Santa Fe and Chihuahua). Coal Ave. ahead designates the northern boundary of Barelas. A welcoming mosaic illustrates historic buildings in the neighborhood. Another block south, the Coronado School stands on the right. The Territorial-style structure was designed by Louis Hesselden in 1936 and completed in 1937 as a Public Works Administration project. It was an elementary school from 1937 to 1975. After 20 years of administrative use, it reopened as an elementary school in 2009.

  The Barelas–South Fourth Street Historic District begins at the next street ahead (Stover) and extends about eight blocks to Bridge Blvd. The corridor is characterized by vernacular interpretations of popular architectural styles. Along the way you'll find remnants of its eras—farming, railroad, and Route 66. Its decades of economic decline are still fairly evident, as are its recent years of recovery.

  On the southeast corner at Hazeldine Ave. is the Our Lady of Kazan Monastery. Its makeshift onion dome and Eastern Orthodox iconographic murals make it easy to spot. The local monastic community of Our Lady of Kazan began as a skete in the late 1970s. Initially established by Father Symeon Carmona, the skete has since grown into a small parish of about 30 converts. They observe Slavonic traditions but remain an independent Eastern Orthodox entity. Services are conducted in English, Slavonic, Greek, French, and Spanish. They also offer counseling services and iconography classes.

Similar iconography appears across the street on B. Ruppe Drugs, which opened here in 1964. Charles Bernard Ruppe opened his first drugstore in Old Town in 1883. The enterprise has evolved from a full-service pharmacy to a vendor of traditional Mexican *remedios.* The manager and master *curandera* (traditional healer) offers herbal consultations and gorgeous handmade rosaries.

However, one thing about Barelas will never change: The food is always phenomenal. Start with Juanita's Comida Mexicana. Slightly bigger than a taco stand, this family-run eatery serves up some fine home cooking. Catch a whiff of barbacoa and you'll know what to order before stepping through the door. Next, head down to Red Ball Café. Predating the original Route 66 by four years, this neighborhood hamburger stand was born in 1922, died in 1979, and was resurrected in 1998. The Red Ball Burger is arguably the best burger in town, but limit yourself to a slider-sized Wimpy Burger. There's lots more eating ahead.

Just past the X-shaped intersection of 4th St. and Barelas St. are a couple of unassuming noncommercial gallery spaces that operate sporadically. If you're lucky you'll find something artistic, musical, literary, or just wonderfully weird going on at either the Small Engine or TANNEX galleries.

Back to the food: The Barelas Coffee House menu touts Barelas as "Land of Mi Chante," *chante* being New Mexican slang derived from "shanty" as an endearing term for home. Aside from its souvenir shop, the restaurant does have a homey ambience. Founded on Valentine's Day 1978 by fourth-generation Bareleñas known as the Gonzales brothers, the BCH is famous for authentic New Mexican fare and the fat-cat politicos who come to feast on it.

The next restaurant is on the campus of the National Hispanic Cultural Center on the south side of Bridge St. Entering on the east side from 4th St., you'll first encounter the *torreón,* a tower housing a 4,000-square-foot concave fresco depicting more than 3,000 years of Hispanic history. Next is a renovated adobe Pueblo/Mission/Hacienda–style school formerly known as West San Jose School (aka River View Elementary) and built under the Works Progress Administration. La Fonda del Bosque opened here in 2000 and quickly garnered national praise. Dining in this stylish 280-seat restaurant is an elegant experience, and not as pricey as you might expect. (The NHCC is generously subsidized by the State of New Mexico.) Sunday brunch is especially popular. New management is expected to take over in 2015 with a greater variety of menu offerings.

The NHCC complex also features a stellar art museum with traveling exhibitions and permanent collections. Their events calendar is crammed with music and dance performances, film festivals, lectures, arts workshops, language classes, and more. Budget an hour minimum for a glimpse of it all. Perhaps the most interesting structure is the home of Adela Martinez, situated between the parking area and the main complex. The story behind it: Construction of the NHCC was ready to begin in the late 1990s. All that stood in the way was the humble abode where Martinez had lived since the 1920s. Problem was she refused to budge, despite a $200,000 offering for her homestead. It remains in place, front and center on the NHCC grounds, as an unintentional yet completely authentic sort of shrine to *mi chante*.

- Return to Bridge Blvd. and turn right.

Detour: If you haven't had enough to eat by now, take a short stroll to El Modelo. The take-out eatery with limited outdoor seating offers comfort food. Hot, heavy, messy, and delicious, it's indisputably the city's best Mexican dive. The red-chile spare ribs are perfectly spicy and savory. Gorge yourself, and then go north on 2nd St. to walk it off.

- If skipping the detour, turn left on 3rd and cross the dirt lot on the north side of the overpass (Guadalupe Bridge).

- Turn left on 2nd St. The neighborhood ahead fronts the rail yards, built between 1914 and 1924 and operated first by the Atchison, Topeka and Santa Fe Railway and later by Burlington Northern. (Since the merger in 1996, the rails have operated under the dominion of BNSF.) At their height in the early 20th century, the rail yards employed nearly a quarter of the city's workforce. Since their closure in the 1970s, the shops have been steadily falling into ruin. Recent drives to renovate the site into a commercial district have been enthusiastic, yet painfully slow. One theory on the delay involves the site's value in its current state of derelict. The massive industrial landscape is invaluable as a filming location. *The Avengers, Terminator Salvation,* and *Breaking Bad* are among the big-budget productions partially filmed here. In 2014, the blacksmith shop became the site for the Rail Yards Market, a highly popular Sunday event with local farmers, food trucks, healers, herbalists, artists, and entertainers.

The first structure you'll see behind the chain-link and barbed-wire fence is a narrow, single-story storehouse that covers nearly 19,000 square feet. Built in 1915, it's the oldest building still standing on the site. It currently houses the Wheels Museum, dedicated to preserving the history of transportation in the American West. To the immediate north, the machine shop, built in 1921, is the largest building, covering 165,000 square feet, or 3.8 acres. Its multicolored windows rival the stained glass on the Fellowship Hall.

On your left, the Railroad Superintendent's House at the corner of Pacific Ave. is one of the first and finest railroad buildings. Built in 1881 for Frank W. Smith, this Victorian Romantic cottage features three corbeled brick chimneys, a cross-gabled roof, finely carved sandstone lintels, carpenter Gothic pillars capped with arabesque corbels, and an open porch that wraps around the north and east sides of the house. The walls are red sandstone from a quarry near Laguna Pueblo.

A two-story firehouse built in 1920 stands near the Y where 1st St. begins. Entry to the Rail Yards Market is just ahead on the right. This route continues straight on 2nd St. The blocks ahead, particularly the one between Stover and Iron, showcase some fascinating architectural designs from the railroad era. The three-story Queen Anne–style house on the southwest corner of 2nd St. and Iron Ave., built in 1899, functioned as the American Hotel from 1910 to 1929 and later as rented apartments. In 1952 it became the founding site of the Brothers of the Good Shepherd and the first homeless refuge in Albuquerque. (See Walk 7 for more details.) The Albuquerque Rescue Mission is across the street on the northwest corner. As expected, this area draws transient crowds and tends to get a bit sketchy at times.

- Turn right on Iron Ave.

- Turn left on 1st St. On the left immediately after crossing beneath Coal, El Madrid Lounge is a drinking enterprise that has catered to the community in various incarnations since the mid-20th century. At last check, it was closed (hopefully a temporary status), but its murals and signage still hearken back to bygone eras of romantic lowriders and drive-thru liquor stores.

- After passing the grand east façade of Zachary Castle and beneath Lead, find the Santa Fe Freight House on your right near the south end of the Albuquerque depot complex. This two-story simplified Mission-style office, built in 1946, was one of the last AT&SF additions to the complex. Two more original buildings are still standing: a former telegraph office built in 1914 is directly behind the freight house, and the Indian Curio Store, built in 1912, stands to the north and now serves as an Amtrak office. The original AT&SF Depot, built in 1902, burned down in 1993. The Alvarado Hotel, also built in 1902, stood on the north end of the complex until 1970. In his 1963 reader's guide, *Southwestern Book Trails,* Lawrence Clark Powell described the Alvarado as "one of the last of the Harvey Houses, and the most beautiful of them all." The inexplicable demolition of the landmark hotel left the city scarred for decades. Much of the complex has been rebuilt (in a reinterpretation of the original California Mission style) as the Alvarado Transportation Center, the city's hub for Amtrak, Greyhound, and local mass transit. Locate historical markers along the sidewalk for additional information.

- To return to the starting point, go one block west on Gold Ave. and one block south on 2nd St.

Points of Interest

Gertrude Zachary's Castle Antiques gertrudezachary.com, 416 2nd St. SW, 505-244-1320

First United Methodist Church fumconline.org, 314 Lead Ave. SW, 505-243-5646

Our Lady of Kazan Monastery kazanmonastery.org, 324 Hazeldine Ave. SW, 505-242-6186

B. Ruppe Drugs facebook.com/bruppedrugsinc, 807 4th St. SW, 505-243-6719

Juanita's Comida Mexicana 910 4th St. SW, 505-843-9669

Red Ball Café redballcafe.com, 1301 4th St. SW, 505-247-9438

Small Engine Gallery smallenginegallery.com, 1413 4th St. SW

The TANNEX acebook.com/thetannex, 1417 4th St. SW

Barelas Coffee House 1502 4th St. SW, 505-843-7577

National Hispanic Cultural Center nhccnm.org, 1701 4th St. SW, 505-242-5289

La Fonda del Bosque lafondadelbosque.com, 1701 4th St. SW, 505-247-9480

El Modelo 1715 2nd St. SW, 505-242-1843

Wheels Museum wheelsmuseum.org, 1100 2nd St. SW, 505-243-6269

Rail Yards Market railyardsmarket.org, 777 1st St. SW, 505-203-6200

El Madrid Lounge 423 1st St. SW, 505-242-0829

Alvarado Transportation Center myabqride.com, 100 1st St. SW, 505-243-RIDE

route summary

1. Start at the corner of 2nd St. and Silver Ave. and walk south.
2. Turn right on Lead Ave.
3. Turn left on 4th St.
4. Cross Bridge Blvd. and enter the campus for the National Hispanic Cultural Center.
5. Explore the campus at your leisure and return to Bridge Blvd.
6. Turn right on Bridge Blvd.
7. Turn left on 3rd St. and cross the dirt lot on the north side of the overpass.
8. Turn left on 2nd St.
9. Turn right on Iron Ave.
10. Turn left on 1st St.

connecting the walks

Connect with Walk 1 at the corner of 2nd and Gold.

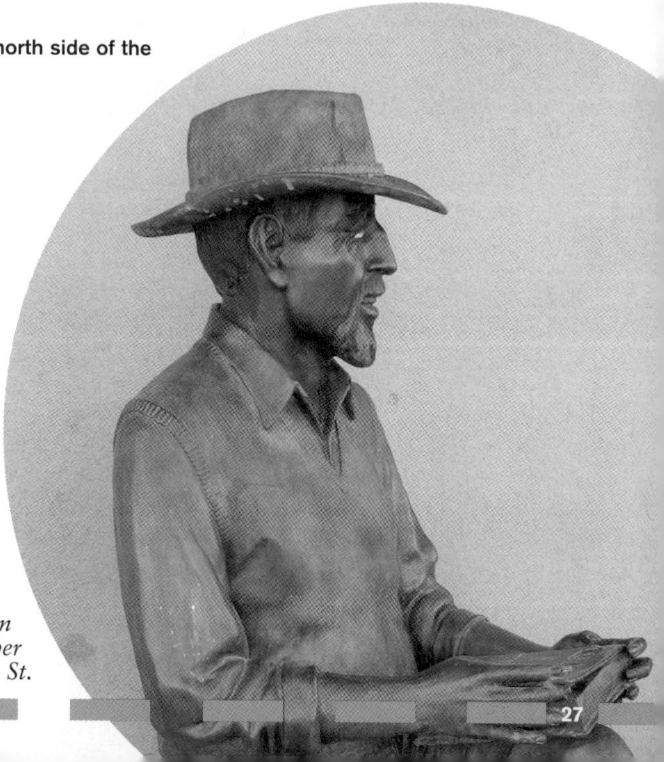

Bronze sculpture of Dr. John A. Aragón at the Albuquerque Hispano Chamber of Commerce on 4th St.

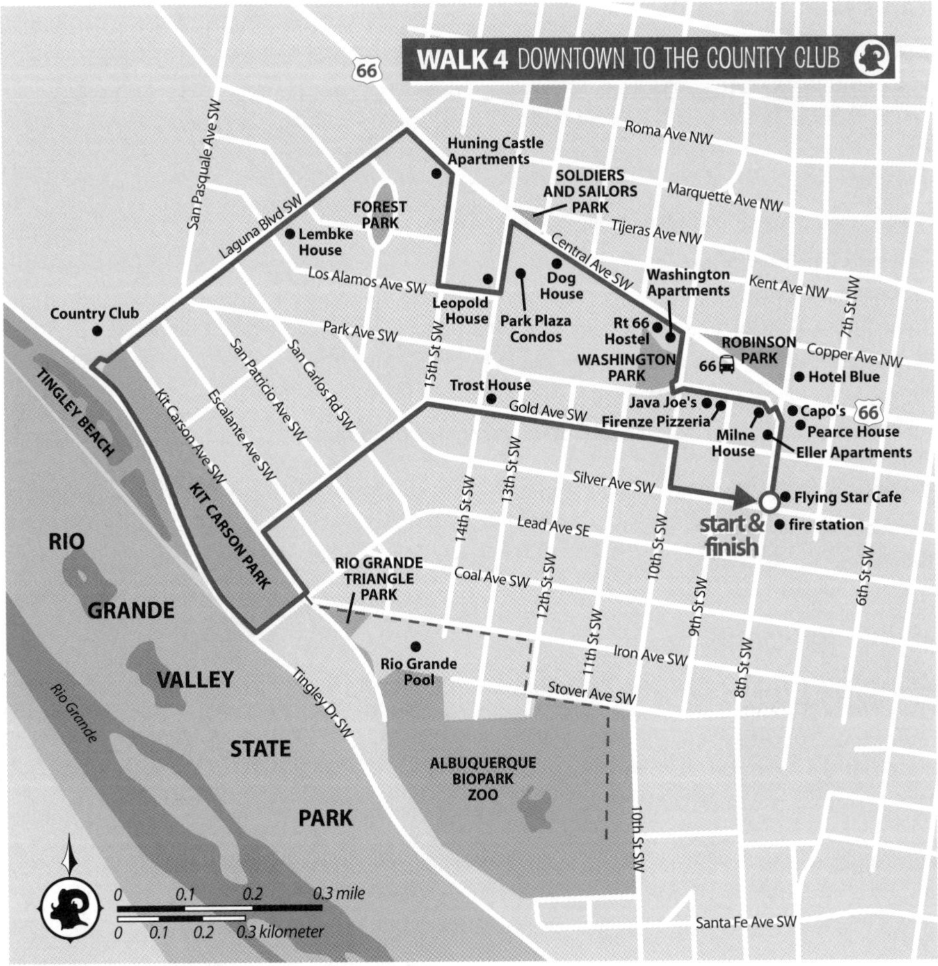

WALK 4 DOWNTOWN TO THE COUNTRY CLUB
66
Roma Ave NW
Marquette Ave NW
Tijeras Ave NW
Central Ave SW
Kent Ave NW
Copper Ave NW
Gold Ave SW
Silver Ave SW
Lead Ave SE
Coal Ave SW
Iron Ave SW
Stover Ave SW
Santa Fe Ave SW
Los Alamos Ave SW
Park Ave SW
Laguna Blvd SW
San Pasquale Ave SW
San Patricio Ave SW
San Carlos Rd SW
Escalante Ave SW
Kit Carson Ave SW
Tingley Dr SW
15th St SW
14th St SW
13th St SW
12th St SW
11th St SW
10th St SW
9th St SW
8th St SW
7th St NW
6th St SW
Huning Castle Apartments
SOLDIERS AND SAILORS PARK
FOREST PARK
Lembke House
Leopold House
Park Plaza Condos
Dog House
Washington Apartments
Rt 66 Hostel
WASHINGTON PARK
ROBINSON PARK
Hotel Blue
Trost House
Java Joe's
Firenze Pizzeria
Milne House
Capo's
Pearce House
Eller Apartments
Flying Star Cafe
fire station
start & finish
Country Club
TINGLEY BEACH
KIT CARSON PARK
RIO GRANDE TRIANGLE PARK
Rio Grande Pool
ALBUQUERQUE BIOPARK ZOO
RIO GRANDE VALLEY STATE PARK
Rio Grande
0 0.1 0.2 0.3 mile
0 0.1 0.2 0.3 kilometer

4 DOWNTOWN TO THE COUNTRY CLUB: MOVIN' ON UP

BOUNDARIES: 8th St., Central Ave., Laguna Blvd., Tingley Dr.
DISTANCE: 3 miles, 4.25 miles with detour
DIFFICULTY: Moderate (unpaved surfaces)
PARKING: Free street parking on Silver Ave. west of 8th St. and at Tingley Beach
PUBLIC TRANSIT: Bus 66 on Central Ave. at 10th St.; buses 53 and 54 on 6th St. at Silver Ave.

This walk shuttles between the west end of downtown's main drag and the south side of the Albuquerque Country Club. Though less than a mile apart, the two settings are nearly opposites in character. Along the way you'll encounter more contrasts as you explore two distinct neighborhoods. The Raynolds Addition, which spans 8th–17th Streets, was platted in 1912. The blocks gradually filled in with bungalows, Southwest-style houses, and some of the city's first apartment buildings. Some of the original structures were sacrificed in the "urban renewal" of the 1960s. Homes were razed to make way for businesses, and many of the lots sat empty for decades to follow. Recent efforts to revive neighborhood spirit include public art projects, xeric gardens, and tree sculpting. The Country Club area, spanning from 17th St. to Tingley Dr., was platted in 1928 as the Huning Castle Addition, named for the so-called castle built in the 1880s on an estate that spanned from Railroad (now Central) Ave. to the Rio Grande.

- **Start on the northeast corner of Silver and 8th. The former Southern Union Gas Company of New Mexico building was designed in the 1950s by quintessential Southwest architect John Gaw Meem, famed for concocting the "Sante Fe style" from a heady mix of Pueblo and Spanish Colonial architecture with a dash of modernism. Since 2005 the building has housed Flying Star Cafe, an extraordinarily popular local franchise. If you can't get a seat, get a couple of sandwiches to go for picnicking later on. As the bakery smell suggests, the pastries here are also phenomenal.**

  Across the street to the west is a relatively new development of four-story buildings with a classic live-work design. The sidewalk level accommodates office and retail space, while the upper floors are residential apartments.

- **Head north toward Central. Eller Apartments front the block north of Gold Ave. They were designed by Henry Trost for Dr. Charles Eller in 1922. Just ahead are the back** sides of two more historic structures. The smaller yet stately one on the right is the John Pearce House. On the left is the Skinner Building, longtime home to a popular Italian restaurant, Villa di Capo, or simply Capo's. Designed by former cabinetmaker A. W. Boehning and built in 1931 as a grocery store, the Art Deco building has been altered over the years, yet still retains many original features, such as the terra-cotta tile façade, green and black opalescent glass detailing, and, inside, a pressed metal ceiling.

- Turn left on Park Ave. and pause at 8 o'clock on the roundabout. At 3 o'clock, The Hotel Blue first opened as Downtowner Motor Inn in 1965 and was given its current name in the late 1990s, when it was renovated into a boutique hotel with an Art Deco theme. Across the street to the west is Robinson Park, the city's first outside of Old Town. A modest memorial in the park describes an incident involving former Indian scout John Braden. During a fiesta parade here in 1896, someone threw a firecracker into Braden's horse-drawn wagon, which was packed with ammunition. (To clarify: the "ammunition" was for a fireworks display.) As it detonated, he managed to steer his startled horses away from the crowd, sacrificing his life to save many others. He now rests in an unmarked grave in Fairview Cemetery (Walk 23). The park also hosts the Downtown Growers' Market on Saturday mornings, June–October. For more information, visit **downtowngrowers.com.**

- Continue west on Park Ave. The prairie-style home on the left is the Milne House, built in 1917. John Milne served as superintendent of Albuquerque public schools from 1911 until his death in 1956. The house is now headquarters for the Southwest Network for Environmental Justice.

  A pair of buildings ahead on the left have ground-floor business space and upstairs apartments. Firenze Pizzeria moved into 900 Park Ave. in 2011, after a successful run with a food truck and a mobile wood-fired oven. Next door is Java Joe's, a well-established yet funky café with a flashy mural, sidewalk seating, local ingredients on the menu, and handcrafted coffee. One wonders how the tenant in the apartment above could ever sleep with the invigorating aroma of high-octane morning brew permeating the walls.

- Continue straight to the southwest corner of Park Ave. and 10th St. Need a haircut? Check out the cute little *peluquería* to the south. On the northwest corner are three ceramic-tiled columns at the entry to Washington Park. Titled *Pillars of the Community,* this public artwork is a collaboration between artist Eddie Dominguez, students from Washington Middle School, and elders from the neighborhood.

- Turn right on 10th St. and head north to Central, passing the luxurious and stylish Silver Moon Lodge Apartments. The Pueblo Deco–style structure was built in 2014 on the site of the old Silver Moon Lodge, a classic Route 66 motel.

- Turn left on Central. Washington Apartments stand on the southwest corner. This pair of two-story buildings, formerly a children's hospital, was converted in 1917 to apartments. The floor plans for the 16 units are each unique. The building next door began as a single-family home in 1905. In 1930 the interior was divided into nine units, and it became the Colonial Arms Apartments. Additional units were added in the 1930s, bringing the total up to 16 by 1940. In the 1970s it became a youth hostel, and it's now known as the Route 66 Hostel. Nightly rates range from $20 to $35.

- Continue northwest on Central, noting the remains of its classic Route 66 motels and laundromats. Just past a minuscule brick duplex is the world-famous Dog House Drive In. The chili is lethally hot, so be sure to order it on everything, especially if you're a fan of *Breaking Bad*, which featured several scenes here.

  Ahead on the north side of Central Ave., Soldiers and Sailors Park is a triangular 0.15-acre military memorial that slumped into disrepair until local veterans banded together to fix it up in 2014.

- Turn left on 14th St. The first block of 14th St. constitutes the Aldo Leopold

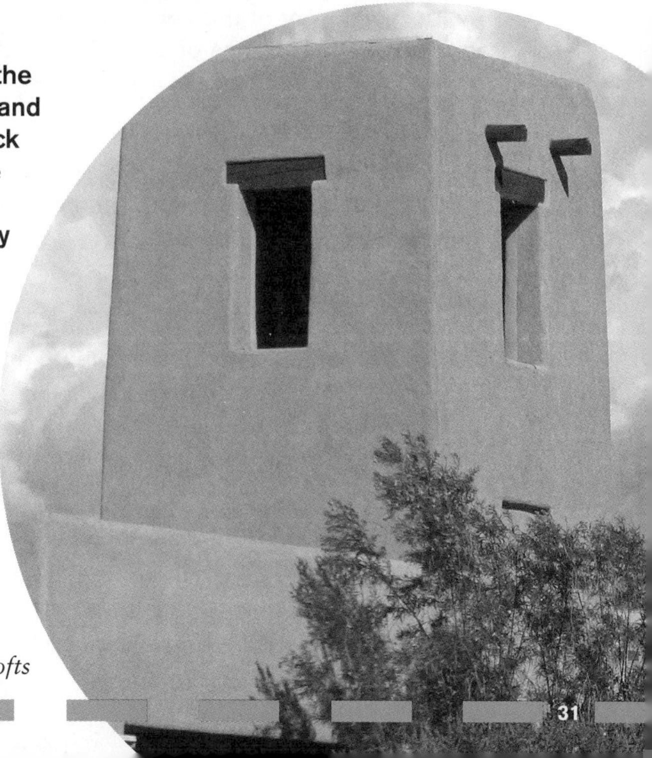

Bell Trading Post Lofts

Neighborhood Historic District. These eight bungalows were built between 1913 and 1920. The one at 135 14th St. was built for Aldo Leopold himself, who resided in Albuquerque from 1914 to 1924. Leopold is credited with establishing the nation's first federally protected wilderness area, and he's often lauded as the founder of the modern natural conservation movement. He was an avid outdoorsman who, according to his own obsessive records, somehow managed to shoot more than 2,000 wild animals during his decade in New Mexico. None shot back. Oh, and if you think you just heard a lion or an elephant, don't be alarmed. Though the city zoo is more than a half mile south, some animals' voices carry far.

Directly across the street are the massive Park Plaza Condos, the tallest residential building in New Mexico. Relative to the scale of things in its neighborhood, it somewhat resembles The Jeffersons' deluxe apartment in the sky. Built in 1964, it never interfered with the conservationist's view of the Sandia Mountains, yet one can't help but wonder if there was intentional irony in placing a 14-story luxury high-rise building directly in front of the Leopold House. The building is an all-welded structure, requiring about 700 tons of steel. The brick façade is simply decorative. The foundation is a reinforced concrete box 674 feet long, 202 feet wide, and 8 feet deep.

- Turn right on Los Alamos Ave. Note the traditional alley ahead on the right. Older neighborhoods like this were designed with backyard parking for carriages and cars so that streets and sidewalks would remain clear. This sensible layout fell out of fashion in favor of a trend for displaying vehicles in front of houses.

- Turn right on 15th St.

- Turn left on Central. Castle Apartments once stood here on the southeast corner. In 2009 fiery debris from an airline collision rained down upon the historic apartments. Or at least that's how it went down in a popular TV show. Actual news footage of the apartment fire was repurposed for the third season of *Breaking Bad.* No one was injured in the blaze, but the building was a loss. A bank has since been constructed on the lot.

Still standing unscathed, Huning Castle Apartments occupy the 1500 block of Central Ave. SW, the same site as the old Huning Castle. Constructed in 1880, the stately manor fell into disrepair faster than most traditional castles. It was offered to the city, but the city declined, citing the $400,000 restoration estimate. The notable landmark was demolished in 1955, and the land sat vacant until construction of the apartments began in the early 1990s. Architect Dekker Perich Sabatini intended to invoke the style of the original structure, which bore a closer resemblance to the Bates residence in *Psycho* than thc upbeat complex standing here today.

- Turn left on Laguna Blvd. and brace yourself for a completely different world. The divided boulevard and its broad median and sidewalks were completely treeless when the neighborhood was first platted. Large architect-designed homes began filling in this neighborhood in the 1920s and continued at a slower rate throughout the 1930s. The prevalence of California Mission, Mediterranean, and Pueblo Revival styles echoes the ambience of the adjacent Albuquerque Country Club. One exception is the Lembke House on the east corner at Los Alamos Ave. Adopting characteristics of both International and Streamline Moderne styles, contractor Charles Lembke took bold risks when he constructed it at the height of the Depression in 1937. Few other houses were built in the neighborhood at the time, and membership at the country club had already plummeted.

  The country club is at the end of the boulevard. Inside are elegant ballrooms, dining rooms, a pro shop, a fitness center, and card rooms for men and women. The construction of its 18-hole golf course, one of the first in the state, required draining about 100 acres of wetlands. The greens and fairways extend north to Central Ave. and west to Tingley Dr.

- Continue straight on the sidewalk to cross the Albuquerque Riverside Drain. Tingley Beach is one of four attractions in the ABQ BioPark. This walk comes closest to the beach and the zoo, while Walk 8 passes near the botanic garden and aquarium. (See the Back Story in Walk 8 on pages 62–63 for detailed information on all BioPark attractions.)

- Turn left on the ditch trail and follow it south to the first paved cross street. The narrow, well-shaded green on your left is Kit Carson Park, named for the legendary frontiersman, Union soldier, genocidal henchman, or Disney hero, depending on your view of history. (See the Back Story in Walk 30 on page 214 for more details.)

- Turn left on Alcade Pl. and go one block northeast.

Detour: On the right is Rio Grande Triangle Park, which sits next to the 25-meter outdoor Rio Grande Pool, open to the public daily Memorial Day weekend–mid-August. Directly southeast of the pool is the aforementioned ABQ BioPark Zoo. To visit all three sites, turn right on Iron Ave., right on 12th, and left on Stover; then follow the zoo fence around to the front entrance, which faces 10th St. The detour runs about 1.25 miles round-trip. Add another mile or so for wandering the zoo.

- Otherwise, turn left on Kit Carson Ave.
- Turn right on Raynolds Ave.
- Bear right at the Y onto Gold. Ahead on the southwest corner at 14th St., the cottage-style apartments were built in 1939. On the northeast corner is the Pueblo Revival house that Henry C. Trost built for himself in 1925. Trost designed many notable buildings in town, including Albuquerque High School, the Sunshine Theater, and the Occidental Life Insurance Building.
- Turn right on 10th St.
- Turn left on Silver. The 900 block is a showcase of charming houses from the early 20th century. The Craftsman bungalow at 918 Silver was built in 1915. A unique and award-winning brick house stands next door. The white house at 904 Silver makes a statement with pink stairs, gutters, and trim. Next door, at the end of the block, is a Spanish Pueblo Revival house with wavy parapets. It was built in 1924. Continue straight to return to the corner of Silver and 8th. One last detail: On a west-facing wall in back of the fire station is the mural *More than a Firefighter* by local artist PAZ. It's worth checking out if you can manage the half-block detour.

Points of Interest

Flying Star Cafe flyingstarcafe.com, 723 Silver Ave. SW, 505-244-8099

Villa di Capo villadicapo.com, 722 Central Ave. SW, 505-242-2006

The Hotel Blue thehotelblue.com, 717 Central Ave. NW, 505-924-2400

Firenze Pizzeria firenzepizzeria.com, 900 Park Ave., 505-242-2939

Java Joe's downtownjavajoes.com, 906 Park Ave. SW, 505-765-1514

Route 66 Hostel rt66hostel.com, 1012 Central Ave. SW, 505-247-1813

Dog House Drive In 1216 Central Ave. NW, 505-243-1019

Albuquerque Country Club albuquerquecountryclub.org, 601 Laguna Blvd. SW, 505-247-4111

Rio Grande Pool cabq.gov/parksandrecreation, 1410 Iron Ave. SW, 505-848-1397

ABQ BioPark cabq.gov/culturalservices/biopark; Aquarium and Botanic Garden, 2601 Central Ave. NW; Tingley Beach, 1800 Tingley Dr.; Zoo, 903 10th St. SW; 505-764-6200

route summary

1. Start at the corner of Silver Ave. and 8th St. and walk north.
2. Turn left on Park Ave.
3. Turn right on 10th St.
4. Turn left on Central Ave.
5. Turn left on 14th St.
6. Turn right on Los Alamos Ave.
7. Turn right on 15th St.
8. Turn left on Central Ave.
9. Turn left on Laguna Blvd., follow it to its end, and then continue straight on the walkway that crosses the ditch.
10. Turn left on the ditch trail.
11. Turn left on Alcade Pl.
12. Turn left on Kit Carson Ave.
13. Turn right on Raynolds Ave.
14. Bear right at the Y onto Gold Ave.
15. Turn right on 10th St.
16. Turn left on Silver St.

connecting the walks

Go one block east from Central and 8th St. to pick up Walk 1. Go two blocks north from Central and 14th St. to connect with Walk 5.

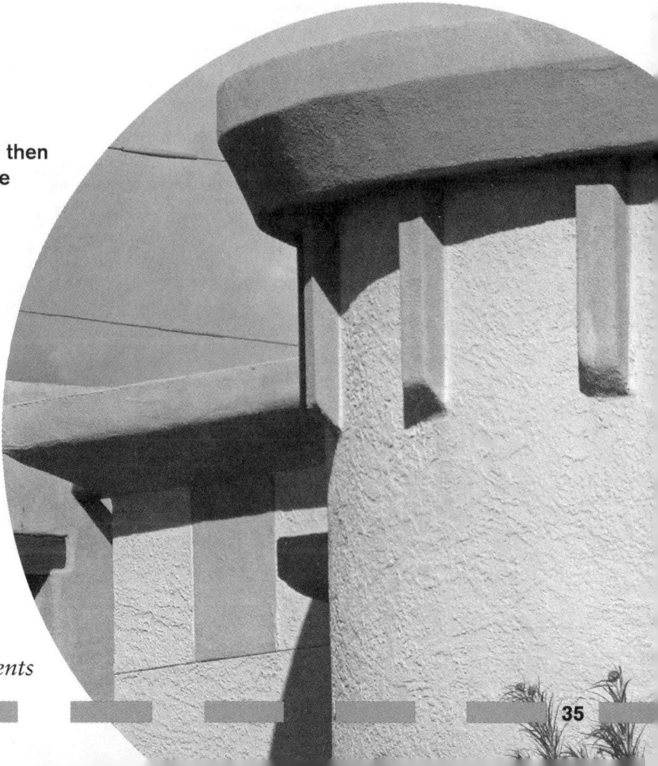

Huning Castle Apartments

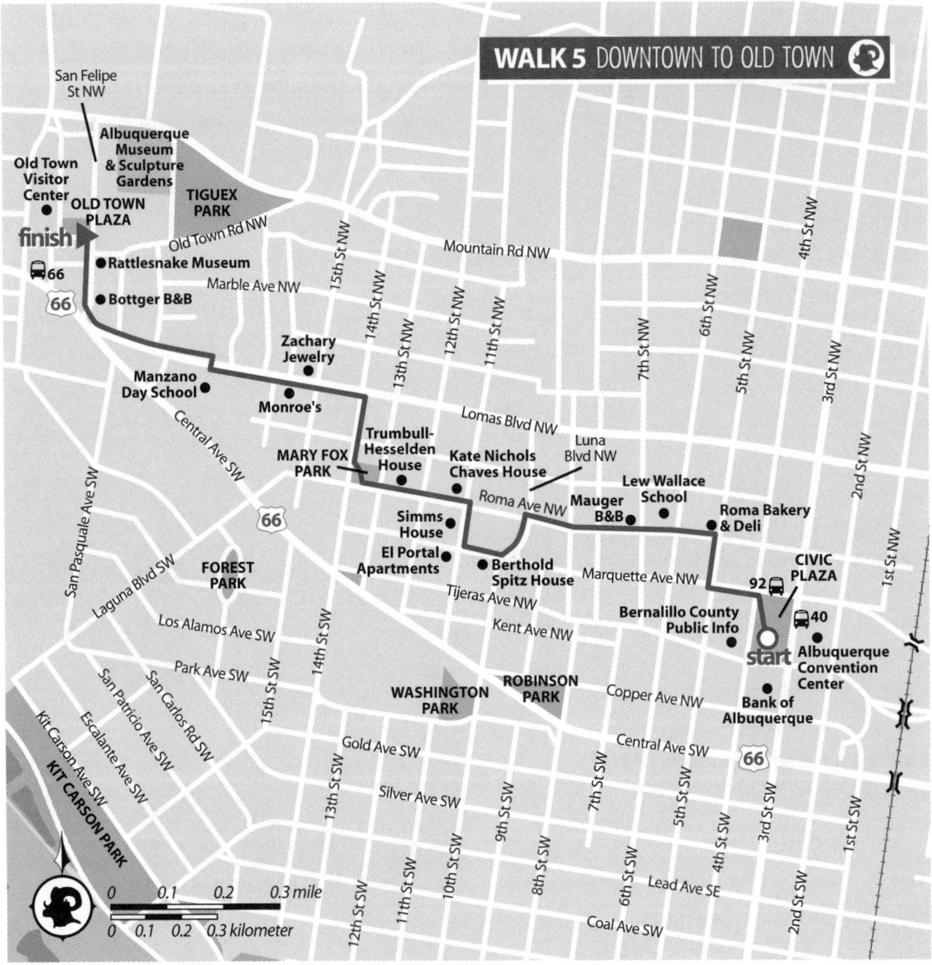
WALK 5 DOWNTOWN TO OLD TOWN
San Felipe St NW
Albuquerque Museum & Sculpture Gardens
Old Town Visitor Center
OLD TOWN PLAZA
TIGUEX PARK
finish
Old Town Rd NW
Mountain Rd NW
Rattlesnake Museum
66
Marble Ave NW
Bottger B&B
15th St NW
14th St NW
13th St NW
12th St NW
11th St NW
7th St NW
6th St NW
5th St NW
4th St NW
3rd St NW
2nd St NW
1st St NW
Zachary Jewelry
Manzano Day School
Monroe's
Central Ave SW
Lomas Blvd NW
Trumbull-Hesselden House
Kate Nichols Chaves House
Luna Blvd NW
MARY FOX PARK
Lew Wallace School
Roma Ave NW
Mauger B&B
Roma Bakery & Deli
Simms House
El Portal Apartments
Berthold Spitz House
Marquette Ave NW
CIVIC PLAZA
92
40
San Pasquale Ave SW
Laguna Blvd SW
FOREST PARK
Tijeras Ave NW
Kent Ave NW
Bernalillo County Public Info
start
Albuquerque Convention Center
Los Alamos Ave SW
Park Ave SW
15th St SW
14th St SW
WASHINGTON PARK
ROBINSON PARK
Copper Ave NW
Bank of Albuquerque
San Patricio Ave SW
San Carlos Rd SW
Escalante Ave SW
Kit Carson Ave SW
KIT CARSON PARK
Gold Ave SW
Central Ave SW
13th St SW
Silver Ave SW
7th St SW
5th St SW
4th St SW
3rd St SW
1st St SW
9th St SW
8th St SW
10th St SW
11th St SW
12th St SW
6th St SW
Lead Ave SE
2nd St SW
Coal Ave SW
0 0.1 0.2 0.3 mile
0 0.1 0.2 0.3 kilometer

5 DOWNTOWN TO OLD TOWN: FOLLOW THE BRASS

BOUNDARIES: Civic Plaza, Old Town Plaza
DISTANCE: 1.75 miles one way
DIFFICULTY: Easy
PARKING: Civic Plaza Parking Garage (Marquette Ave. west of 3rd St.); metered parking along Tijeras Ave. and 5th St.
PUBLIC TRANSIT: Bus 30 stops on the east side of Civic Plaza; bus 92 stops on the north side. Rail Runner Downtown Station is four blocks southeast of Civic Plaza.

In 1706 New Mexico Governor Francisco Cuervo y Valdes founded the Villa de Albuquerque on the site of what is now known as Old Town. Fast-forward to 1880: the railroad arrived about 2 miles east, encouraging commercial and residential development along its north–south tracks. The new town was called New Town and later New Albuquerque and was platted in a grid format—a pattern that sharply deviated from the plaza-oriented layout that was common to this Spanish Colonial region. Despite portents of the old-fashioned villa's imminent demise, the two towns maintained a tenuous connection via a streetcar system and a powerful political district known as the Fourth Ward. So the villa persisted, although not without a struggle, and in 1949 the city annexed Old Town without overwhelming its original character. This walk examines their remaining differences and the prominent neighborhood that developed to fill the space between them. The route mostly follows Albuquerque's official "Plaza to Plaza Tour," a trail marked with brass plaques embedded in the sidewalks. The corresponding brochure is recommended for supplemental coverage of sites along the way. It's available at visitor information centers located on both plazas.

- **Start anywhere in the Harry E. Kinney Civic Plaza. A statue of the former two-term mayor (striking a Captain Morgan pose) stands on the far northeast corner near Marquette Ave. and 3rd St. The plaza is big enough to accommodate 20,000 revelers during special events, typically on weekend evenings throughout summer. Prior to 1938 the original alignment of Route 66 ran through this space on its course between Santa Fe and Los Lunas. A later east–west alignment followed what is now Central Ave., two blocks south of the plaza. The intersection of 4th and Central (two blocks south) is the only place in America where historical alignments of Route 66 cross.**

On the south side of the plaza, a wrought iron column lit from within depicts 78 silhouettes ascending a smokestack. Five stone pillars surrounding it provide Holocaust memorial information. South of the sculpture, the Albuquerque Plaza building (aka the Bank of Albuquerque Tower) and its mini-me counterpart, the Hyatt Regency (aka Albuquerque Plaza II) are the two tallest buildings in town. Both were completed in 1990 on the site of what was a century earlier the heart of the red-light district. Built in the postmodern style, the pyramid-topped pair are the most recognizable features in the otherwise clunky skyline. Many of the larger structures nearby can be attributed to a decades-long infatuation with International-style architecture. Both Civic Plaza and the monstrous Convention Center on its east side were conceived in the height of the affliction and completed in 1972—more than 260 years after the plaza at the other end of this walk. At the time of this writing, the Civic Center was in the midst of an extensive and long-overdue makeover, 4th St. was reestablished between Marquette and Central, and plans were announced for additional renovations to the plaza.

Opposite the Civic Center, the mismatched trio of buildings is the City/County Complex, which includes the mayor's office and nearly 100 works from the Public Art Program collection. The old city hall building fronting Marquette Ave. appears to be the dullest on the block, but take a closer look at the polished limestone slabs facing the walkway and you'll find a variety of fossils, including clams and snails. Sea lilies (crinoids) are the easiest to spot. The limestone came from travertine quarries located approximately 40 miles southwest of Albuquerque.

- Walk west to the southwest corner of Marquette Ave. and 5th St., keeping an eye out for route markers. A mule cart indicates the direction to Old Town Plaza, and a locomotive to Civic Plaza. The pair of 14-foot Indians standing on the southwest corner is a masterpiece by Apache artist Allan Houser (1914–1994). Behind it is the 15-story Bank of the West, formerly the Albuquerque Petroleum Building. Dark red stone in the columns, walkways, benches, and entry is Carnelian granite from South Dakota, and the lighter stone is Radiant Red granite from Texas. The granites date back about 2.6 billion and 1.1 billion years, respectively.

- Turn north and cross Marquette Ave. The Compass Bank building on the northwest corner houses New Mexico's only Secret Service field office. Continue north, following the scent of fresh pastries, courtesy of Roma Bakery and Deli, ahead at the northwest corner of 5th and Roma. Directly across the street, narrow windows resembling embrasures are a security feature in the fortresslike Regional Correctional Center.

Turn west on Roma. A block ahead, Lew Wallace Elementary School stands on the west side of 6th St. While serving as governor of the New Mexico Territory from 1878 to 1881, Wallace also found time to finish his novel, *Ben-Hur*. The school building, completed in 1934, is Louis Hesselden's first project as Albuquerque Public Schools architect. Hesselden later designed Highland High School and the Nob Hill Shopping Center (Walk 26).

Just ahead on the northwest corner at 7th St. is the Brittania & W. E. Mauger Estate B&B Inn, a classic example of Queen Anne–style architecture. Maude Talbot ordered the construction of the brick house in 1897 for $1,600 on land she'd inherited from her father, W. E. Talbot, proprietor of the Montezuma Saloon on 2nd St. The popular saloon was the first in business in Albuquerque with electric lights. Likewise, Maude's house was outfitted with push-button switches. After an unhappy marriage, however, she left the house and returned to New York. In 1907 her mother sold the house to W. E. Mauger for $4,350. Mauger came to Albuquerque from Boston in the hopes that the sunny, dry climate would clear up his tuberculosis. He opened a hardware store on 1st St., amassed a small fortune in the wool trade, and died in 1923. His wife, Brittania, followed in 1970 at the age of 102. The Estate has since undergone a major restoration. It was listed on the National Register of Historic Places in 1985 and became a B&B in 1987.

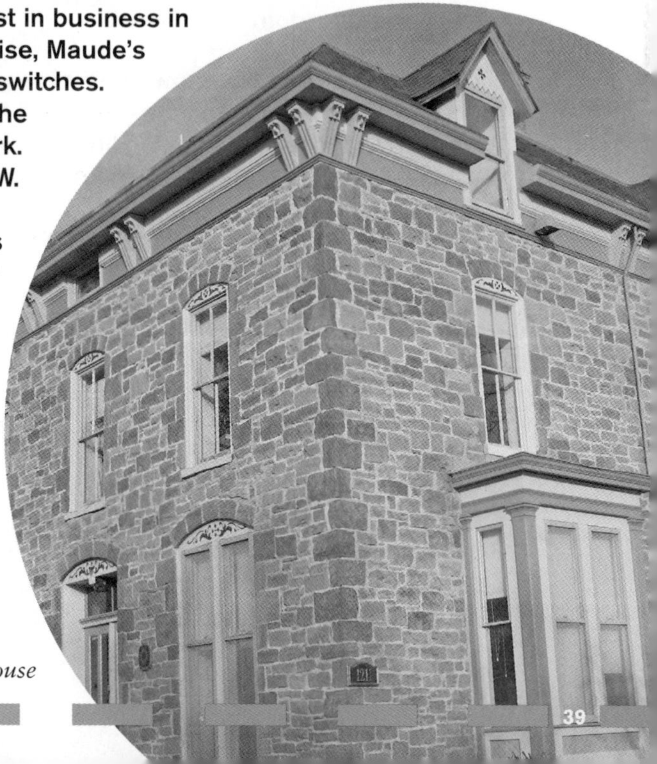

Trumbull-Hesselden House

A block ahead, 8th St. delineates the east boundary of the Fourth Ward District, one of the city's 14 historic districts listed on the National Register. The 1901 Albuquerque City Directory suggests that the Fourth Ward was a mix of middle class employers and laborers. However, it's better remembered today as the elite district during the railroad era. Only a few of the most opulent homes are intact today.

- Cross Luna Blvd. and turn south, deviating slightly from the official tour to see the best example of Prairie School–style architecture in Albuquerque. Located on the west corner of Marquette Ave. and 10th St., the Berthold Spitz House was named for one of the many German Jewish merchants who contributed to the early economic development of New Albuquerque.

- Turn west on Marquette Ave. and go one block to 11th St., also known as Judges' Row. Before turning up that street, note the neon sign on the historic El Portal Apartments on the southeast corner. The U-shaped single-story building has a courtyard, ten units, and seldom a vacancy.

- Turn north and head back toward Roma Ave. The house at 415 11th St. was home to John Simms when he served as a Justice for the New Mexico Supreme Court from 1929 to 1930. His sons John F. Simms Jr. and Albert G. Simms would later serve respectively as governor of New Mexico and a U.S. congressman.

- Turn west on Roma Ave. to rejoin the official route. The Tudor Revival home on the northwest corner of Roma and 11th was designed by Kate Nichols Chaves and completed in 1909. Daughter of architect Nicholas Nichols, she lived here with her husband, Amado Chaves, until her sudden death in the home in 1914.

At 1211 Roma, the Trumbull-Hesselden House has the distinction of being one of Albuquerque's few stone houses and possibly its first duplex. The mansard roof is another unique feature in this region known for flat rooftops, though at the time of its completion in 1882, not another structure stood near it. Its first owner, Walter Trumbull, died in 1891, and the house served for the next 11 years as the Goss Military Institute. The 1896 city directory mentions that the institute "furnishes for boys and young men, a training in military tactics as well as a mental training." Wallace Hesselden bought the duplex in 1902, using half for immediate family and the other half for other relatives.

- Veer northwest just past 13th St. for a quick stroll through Mary Fox Park.

- Turn north on 14th St. and enjoy this quiet stretch of cottages and bungalows before leaving the Fourth Ward.

- Turn west on Lomas. The sudden increase in traffic and nearby businesses—a smoke shop and a pawn shop—contributes to a dramatic shift in atmosphere. Gertrude Zachary Jewelry Etc., the indigo-tiled structure ahead, is hard to ignore (as is her castle in Walk 3). Pick up the scent of Monroe's Mexican Food and follow it down to its classic neon sign shaped like a heart and arrow. Customers have loved this restaurant since it opened in 1962 as a small drive-in.

- At the Manzano Day School, you might find it easier to use the crosswalk here to reach the north side of Lomas, then rejoin the marked route a quarter mile later at the west corner of Central and San Felipe. Or you can stay on course and negotiate the traffic at the Y-junction of Lomas and Central. The landscaped archipelago of traffic islands there, known as the Phil Chacon Transit-Pedestrianway, is maintained by the city's Park Management Division. On September 10, 1980, Albuquerque police officer Phil Chacon was volunteering at a shelter for battered women when two children who lived at the shelter alerted him to a robbery at the nearby Kinney shoe store. Unarmed and in civilian clothing, the off-duty officer chased a hooded bandit to a doughnut shop, where the suspect turned and gunned down Chacon. The murder remains unsolved. A city park and a police substation have also been named in his honor.

- Turn north on San Felipe St. The salmon-pink American Foursquare on the east side of the street is the Bottger Mansion. Completed in 1912, this Old Town home is relatively new. Charles Bottger demolished a 19th-century governor's mansion to make way for what would eventually become the bed-and-breakfast inn you see today.

  The portal-shaded walkways so characteristic of Old Town begin at the American International Rattlesnake Museum. You can earn a certificate of bravery just for going inside. Continue north to the intersection with S. Plaza St., where Old Town Plaza is in full view. Finish the walk at the gazebo and take a moment to rest in this arboreal oasis.

POINTS OF INTEREST

Roma Bakery and Deli romabakeryanddeli.com, 501 Roma Ave. NW, 505-843-9418

Mauger Estate B&B Inn maugerbb.com, 701 Roma Ave. NW, 800-719-9189

Gertrude Zachary Jewelry Etc. gertrudezachary.com, 1501 Lomas Blvd. NW, 505-247-4442

Monroe's Mexican Food monroeschile.com, 1520 Lomas Blvd. NW, 505-242-1111

Bottger Mansion of Old Town bottger.com, 110 San Felipe St. NW, 505-243-3639

American International Rattlesnake Museum rattlesnakes.com, 202 San Felipe St. NW, 505-242-6569

ROUTE SUMMARY

1. Start at Civic Plaza. Walk to the southwest corner of Marquette Ave. and 5th St.
2. Turn north and go to the northeast corner of 5th St. and Roma Ave.
3. Turn west and go to the northwest corner of Roma Ave. and Luna Blvd.
4. Turn south and go to Marquette Ave.
5. Turn west and go to 11th St.
6. Turn north and return to Roma Ave.
7. Turn west and go to Mary Fox Park.
8. Walk northwest through the park to 14th St.
9. Turn north and go to Lomas Blvd.
10. Turn west on Lomas Blvd. and go to the west corner of Central Ave. and San Felipe St.
11. Turn north and go to Old Town Plaza.

CONNECTING THE WALKS

Walk 1 crosses 4th St. 1.5 blocks south of Civic Plaza. Walk 6 begins on the west side of Old Town Plaza. You can return to Civic Plaza via Walk 7, which begins nearby on the west corner of 19th St. and Mountain Rd.

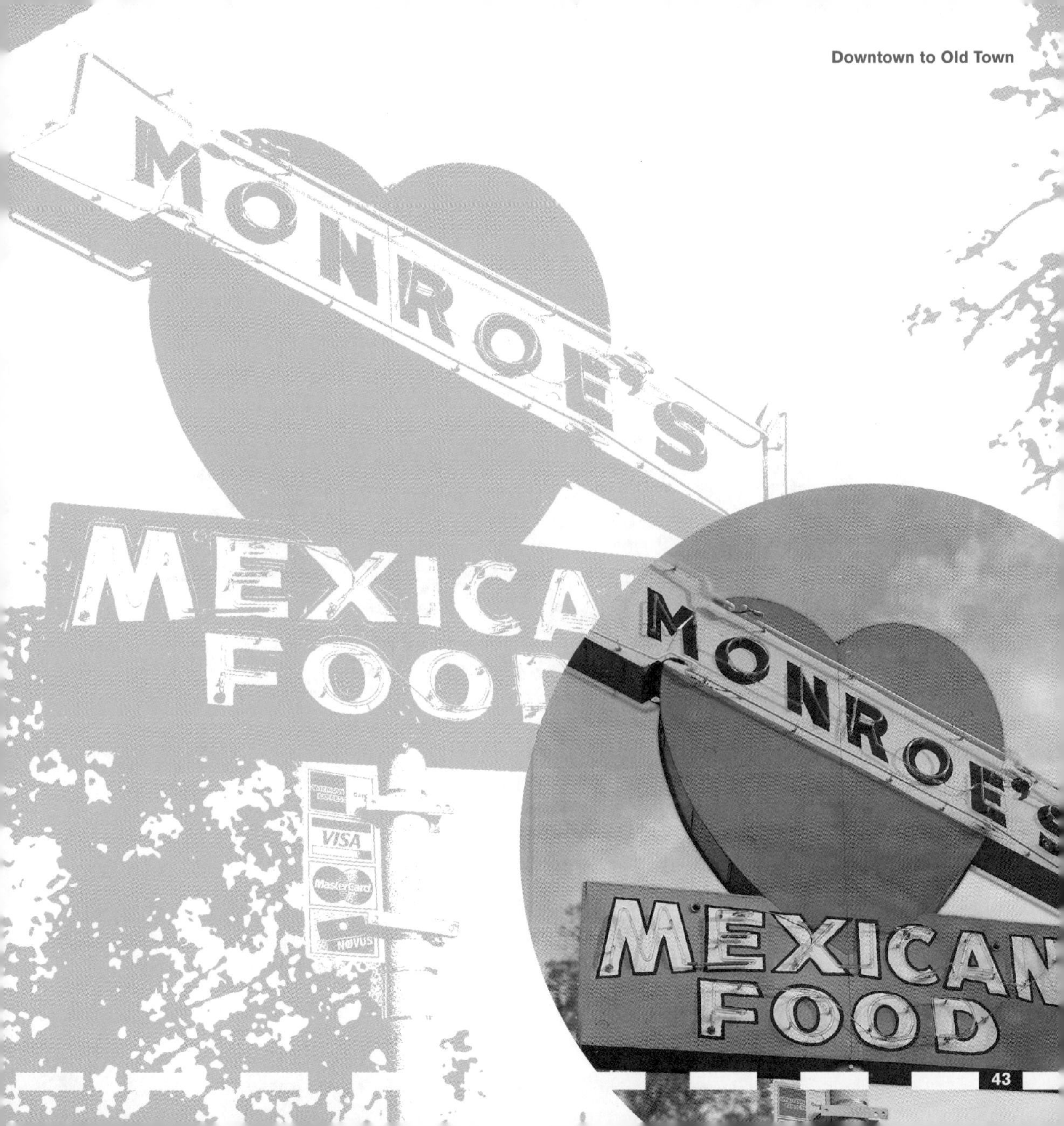
MONROE'S
MEXICAN FOOD
VISA
MasterCard
NOVUS
MONROE'S
MEXICAN FOOD

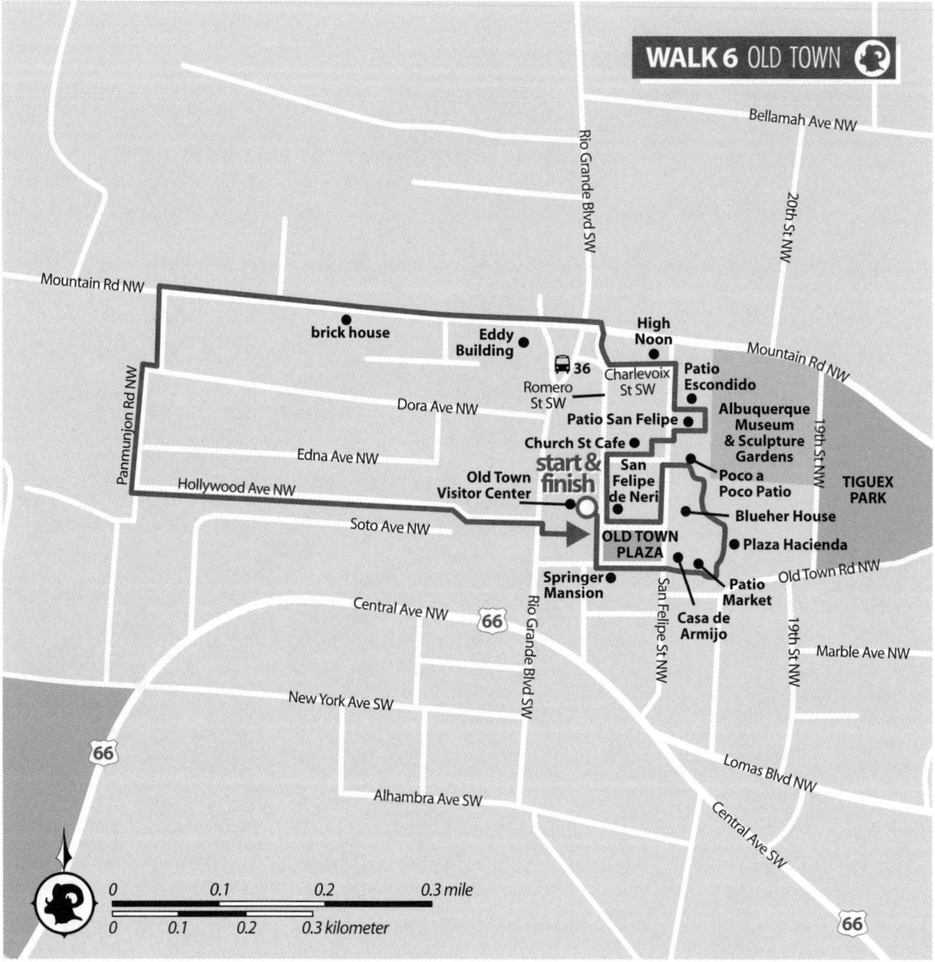

WALK 6 OLD TOWN
Bellamah Ave NW
Rio Grande Blvd SW
20th St NW
Mountain Rd NW
Mountain Rd NW
brick house
Eddy Building
High Noon
36
Charlevoix St SW
Patio Escondido
Romero St SW
Dora Ave NW
Patio San Felipe
Albuquerque Museum & Sculpture Gardens
19th St NW
Church St Cafe
Edna Ave NW
start & finish
San Felipe de Neri
Poco a Poco Patio
TIGUEX PARK
Panmunjon Rd NW
Hollywood Ave NW
Old Town Visitor Center
Blueher House
Soto Ave NW
OLD TOWN PLAZA
Plaza Hacienda
Old Town Rd NW
Springer Mansion
Patio Market
Central Ave NW
66
Rio Grande Blvd SW
San Felipe St NW
Casa de Armijo
19th St NW
Marble Ave NW
New York Ave SW
66
Lomas Blvd NW
Alhambra Ave SW
Central Ave SW
66
0
0.1
0.2
0.3 mile
0
0.1
0.2
0.3 kilometer

6 OLD TOWN: DON CUERVO'S ILLEGITIMATE VILLA

BOUNDARIES: **S. Plaza St., San Pasqua Ave., Mountain Rd., Panmunjon Rd.**
DISTANCE: **1.75 miles**
DIFFICULTY: **Easy**
PARKING: **Free parking on 20th St., north of Mountain Rd.**
PUBLIC TRANSIT: **Buses 66 and 766 on Central Ave. at Rio Grande Blvd.; bus 36 on Rio Grande Blvd. at Mountain Rd.**

In 1706 Don Francisco Cuervo y Valdes, acting governor of the Province of New Mexico, boldly announced the founding of the Villa of Albuquerque. It proved to be a poor decision. In his haste, he'd failed to ask permission from the viceroy and, through him, the King of Spain. He also neglected the paperwork necessary to obtain a land grant for the new villa. The oversight soon cost him his job, and the legitimacy of Albuquerque would be debated for centuries to follow, even in the New Mexico Supreme Court as late as 1959. Legitimate or not, what stands on the founding site today is Old Town, a former town center packed with hundreds of boutiques, galleries, museums, hotels, and historic sites. This walk winds through hidden alleys and patios, then strays west to explore an "authentic" residential area outside of the tourist zone.

- **Start at Plaza Don Luis, where you'll find the Old Town Visitor Center. Pick up a few brochures and maps to enhance the walk ahead. If you start out with an odd sensation of walking on somebody's grave, it's probably because this small brick plaza was built upon Albuquerque's first cemetery and the burials were supposedly left intact.**

  Construction on the first church of Old Town began in 1706 nearby on the west side of the main plaza, but the structure wasn't functional until 1718. It was originally named in honor of San Francisco Xavier but was renamed by decree of the Duke of Alburquerque to honor San Felipe, the patron saint of Spain's new sovereign, King Felipe V. The order went neglected for many years. In 1776 Fray Francisco Domínguez inspected the church and found a painting of the local favorite saint over the main altar. Outraged, he demanded an image of San Felipe de Neri to be installed in its place. The name stuck from then on. Domínguez also expressed disappointment in the overall gloomy aspect of the church. There were no pews. The congregation sat

on a dirt floor, women on the right side of the imaginary aisle, men on the left. It also lacked bell towers. A small arch held a pair of mismatched bells, both of them broken. He blamed the disorder on "lethargy and laziness."

In 1792 the alcalde mayor requested help from local residents to repair the distressed church, but the response was unenthusiastic. The structure continued to deteriorate until the following winter, when it completely collapsed. Rather than clear the rubble and rebuild on the original site, construction of the present San Felipe de Neri Church began on the north side of the plaza. The Folk Gothic spires were added in response to French Bishop (later Archbishop) Lamy's 1851 reformation of New Mexico missions. The church remains active today and stands as one of Albuquerque's most stunning landmarks. It's open to the public daily. Masses are held on Saturday and Sunday.

- Go south on Romero St. On your left, five flags fly over the main plaza, each representing a governing entity that ruled here: Spain (1598–1821); Mexico (1821–1846); USA (1846–present); New Mexico (1912–present); and the Confederate States (1862) represented by the First Confederate National Flag (not the Stars and Bars).

Somewhere within the Territorial-style souvenir shop ahead is a Queen Anne home known as the Henry Springer House. One of Albuquerque's first German immigrants, Springer ran his hardware store into bankruptcy in the 1870s but later amassed a fortune in the saloon business. His house, built in 1890, is allegedly haunted by a harlot named Scarlett.

- Turn left on S. Plaza St. and walk along the stuccoed façade of storefronts and restaurants. On your left, a plaque on the Old Town Gazebo explains the Skirmish of Albuquerque. On April 8–9, 1862, shortly after the Union victory at Glorieta Pass near Santa Fe, Union troops positioned in Barelas (Walk 3) exchanged cannon fire with Confederates positioned in Old Town. Often exaggerated as "The Battle of Albuquerque," the skirmish ended when a group of concerned citizens asked Major Canby to stop lobbing cannonballs at Old Town.

On the east side of the plaza are replicas of Mountain Howitzers, the smallest cannon used in the Civil War. As Confederate forces continued their retreat to Texas, Confederate artillery commander Major Trevanion T. Teel secretly buried eight cannon barrels to prevent their capture by pursuing Union forces. He returned in 1889 to reveal the location: A chile pepper patch 500 feet northeast of San Felipe de Neri Church. If Teel had kept his secret, they'd be beneath the Albuquerque Museum. Instead, two of the eight original cannons are on display there.

Signage on the adobe complex ahead claims that Casa de Armijo was built in 1706, though it's more likely that the earliest construction began in the 1820s. It's a classic *placita* (little plaza), developed for defense against Navajo and Apache raiders. Ironically one of the resident ghosts wears a gown with elaborate Navajo beadwork. The red and black pattern is based on the whirling log symbol, which traditionally denotes abundance, prosperity, healing, and luck. Visitors unfamiliar with native iconography occasionally mistake it for a swastika and describe the Armijo apparition in some variation of "the Mexican Nazi girl."

- Continue straight down the *zaguán* (carriageway) to Patio Market. A branded board on the ceiling of the gateway seems to authenticate the property as belonging to Ambrosia Armijo. The fountain in this *placita* originally supplied the home with water. The buildings around you were the servants quarters for the Armijo Hacienda. Rooms were later converted into a schoolhouse, and later still into a boutique and photo gallery. Exit the patio on the east side.

- Turn left and walk through Plaza Hacienda. This secluded plaza with an outdoor kiva fireplace previously served as a hot spot for romantic rendezvous and thus became colloquially known as Honeymoon Row. The buildings also used to be the stables for the Armijo Hacienda and the Blueher House, which stands to the immediate northwest of Plaza Hacienda. German immigrant Herman

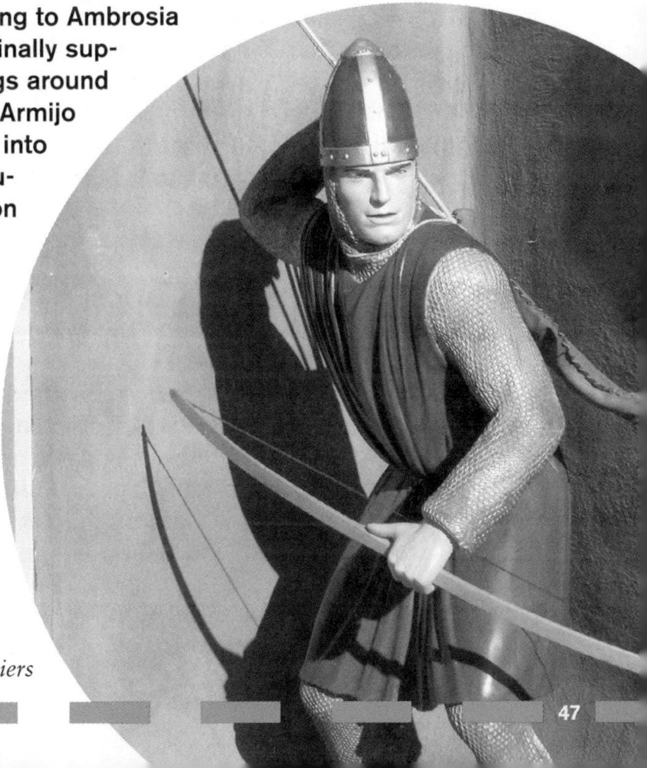

Steadfast Soldiers

Blueher introduced draft horses to Albuquerque in the early 1900s. His house was intact as recently as 1950, but soon after was "pueblo-ized" for its conversion to La Hacienda Restaurant. However, from this vantage point behind the restaurant, traces of the original Italianate style are evident.

- Walk to the northwest corner of the parking lot, where you'll find two gates. The one on the right goes to the Albuquerque Museum patio, which is not accessible after 4:30 p.m. Go through the gate on the left for a walk through Poco a Poco Patio. A recent addition to this eclectic collection of cafés and stores, Steadfast Soldiers specializes in hand-painted, expertly crafted, metal toy soldiers. So if you're in the market for, say, a 1/32-scale Shogun warrior or miniature Panzerfaust gunners, don't miss this place. Otherwise, exit the patio on the west side.

- Turn left on San Felipe St., and go south to N. Plaza St . Hidden in the trunk of a centuries-old cottonwood is the likeness of Our Lady of Guadalupe, her head adorned with a royal-yellow crown atop an azure mantilla. Toby Avila, one of only 26 Albuquerque men to return from the Korean War, began work on this unusual masterpiece in 1958. Using only a kitchen knife, a sharpening stone, and a mallet, he completed the carving in 1959 and died a week later with paint still on his fingertips. The tree itself survived another 55 years on an obscure corner of the parking lot behind the church. Church officials relocated the trunk to its current location after a storm toppled it in 2014.

- Stroll west on N. Plaza for a closer look at San Felipe de Neri Church.

- Turn right on Romero. At the end of the block, consider exploring well-hidden galleries and gift shops in Plazuela Sombra on your left. Otherwise…

- Turn right on Church St. About halfway down this block you'll find Casa Ruiz, supposedly the oldest residence still standing in Albuquerque. Possibly (though unlikely) built in the early 1700s, the hacienda remained in the Ruiz family until 1991, when it was sold and converted into Church Street Cafe. It looks tiny from the outside, but it's a surprisingly long walk through to the patio out back. Keep an eye out for Sarah Ruiz, an alleged witch who still haunts the joint.

- Continue east on Church St. Turn left into the alley after Blue Portal; then go down the first alley on your right to return to San Felipe St.

- Turn left on San Felipe St. and take a quick right into Patio San Felipe. The exotic cuisine you smell is La Crêpe Michel. Born in Lebanon and educated in Paris, owner Claudie Zamet-Wilcox opened the café nearly 25 years ago. Over the years since, her gourmet establishment has often been rated as Albuquerque's best French restaurant. It might be more accurate to say it's the best restaurant, period.

- Exit Patio San Felipe through the rear gate, turn left, and enter the first gate on your left for a walk through Patio Escondido—the secret patio. The Chapel of Our Lady of Guadalupe, which is more on the scale of a grotto shrine, was built for the students of Sagrada Art Studios. The chapel and its gorgeous patio are open to visitors daily, though you might stumble upon a wedding ceremony. Continue straight to San Felipe St. On your right is Routes Rentals & Tours, which offers bike rentals and themed tours throughout Albuquerque. The winery and brewery bike tours are particularly popular.

- Turn right on San Felipe St. The Chavez House on the north corner of Charlevoix St. dates back to 1785 and has housed the High Noon Restaurant & Saloon since 1974. The ghost who inhabits this place seems to favor the Santo Room. Her interests include rearranging furniture and starting fires.

- Turn left on Charlevoix St. Probably named for Jesuit missionary and French explorer Pierre Francois Xavier de Charlevoix, this seldom-traveled backstreet mysteriously appeared on maps sometime in the late 20th century. It's lined with small homes, quiet gardens, and a gallery. At the end of this street you have a choice: You can turn left to stay within the historic district or stick to the route for a 1-mile detour through the residential area of West Old Town. If choosing the latter . . .

- Turn right on Romero St.

- Turn left on Mountain Rd. Built in the rare Quonset Triplex style, Jerome O. Eddy Memorial Building on the southwest corner opened in 1954 as the Albuquerque Boys Club. The remaining area west of Rio Grande Blvd. was originally farmland for Old Town residents. Traces of its agricultural past remain, but mostly what remains today is a mixed-income neighborhood of eclectic homes built over the past century or so. At 2406 Mountain Rd., a brick cottage is hidden in a cluster of trees. The segmental arched windows and pitched roof are unusual features in this neighborhood but are commonly found on houses near the railroad line. The house was probably built shortly after the railroad arrived in 1880.

Just over a quarter mile west of Rio Grande Blvd., the Alameda Lateral crosses beneath Mountain Rd. Ideally you would follow it a short distance north for a look at fascinating homes along Carson Rd. and Zearing Ave. However, the public right-of-way is well secured behind chain-link fence and padlocks.

- Turn left on Panmunjon Rd., named for the borderland village where the 1953 Korean Armistice Agreement was signed.
- Turn left on Hollywood Ave. This narrow street is a showcase of yard cars, coyote fences, wrought iron, quirky outdoor ornamentation, cinder block gardens, adobe walls in various states of decay and restoration, and a surplus of chain-link fence. Aside from the bustle of Central Ave. (one block south) it's a fairly quiet street that carries a bouquet of car fresheners and patchouli.
- Cross Rio Grande Blvd. and return to Old Town Plaza via the alley on your right.

POINTS OF INTEREST

Old Town Visitor Center albuquerqueoldtown.com, 303 Romero St. NW, 505-243-3215

San Felipe de Neri Parish sanfelipedeneri.org, 2005 N. Plaza St. NW, 505-243-4628

La Hacienda Restaurant haciendadelriocantina.com, 302 San Felipe St. NW, 505-243-3131

Steadfast Soldiers steadfastsoldiers.com, 328 San Felipe St. NW, 505-247-2310

Church Street Cafe churchstreetcafe.com, 2111 Church St. NW, 505-247-8522

La Crêpe Michel lacrepemichel.com, 400 San Felipe St. NW, 505-242-1251

Routes Rentals & Tours routesrental.com, 404 San Felipe St. NW, 505-933-5667

High Noon Restaurant & Saloon highnoonrestaurant.com, 425 San Felipe St. NW, 505-765-1455

route summary

1. Start at Plaza Don Luis on Romero St. and walk south.
2. Turn left on S. Plaza St.
3. Continue straight through Patio Market.
4. Turn left and walk through Plaza Hacienda.
5. Walk to the northwest corner of the parking lot.
6. Turn left and walk through Poco a Poco Patio.
7. Turn left on San Felipe St.
8. Turn right on N. Plaza St.
9. Turn right on Church St.
10. Turn left into the alley after Blue Portal.
11. Turn down the first alley on your right.
12. Turn left on San Felipe St.
13. Turn right into Patio San Felipe.
14. Exit through the rear gate and turn left.
15. Enter the first gate on your left and walk through Patio Escondido.
16. Turn right on San Felipe St.
17. Turn left on Charlevoix St.
18. Turn right on Romero St.
19. Turn left on Mountain Rd.
20. Turn left on Panmunjon Rd.
21. Turn left on Hollywood Ave.
22. Cross Rio Grande Blvd. and return to Old Town Plaza via the alley on your right.

connecting the walks

Walk 5 ends at Old Town Plaza. Walk 7 begins on the northwest corner of the Albuquerque Museum grounds.

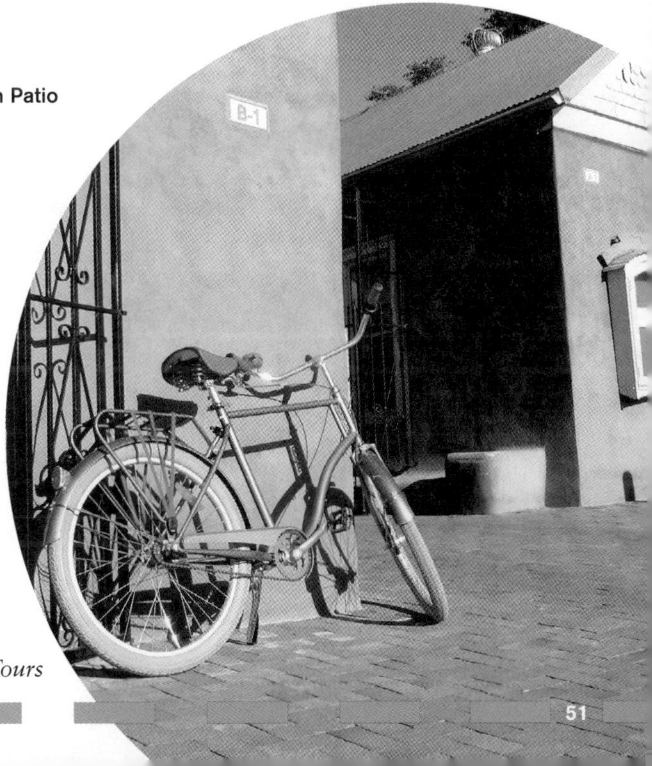

Routes Rentals & Tours

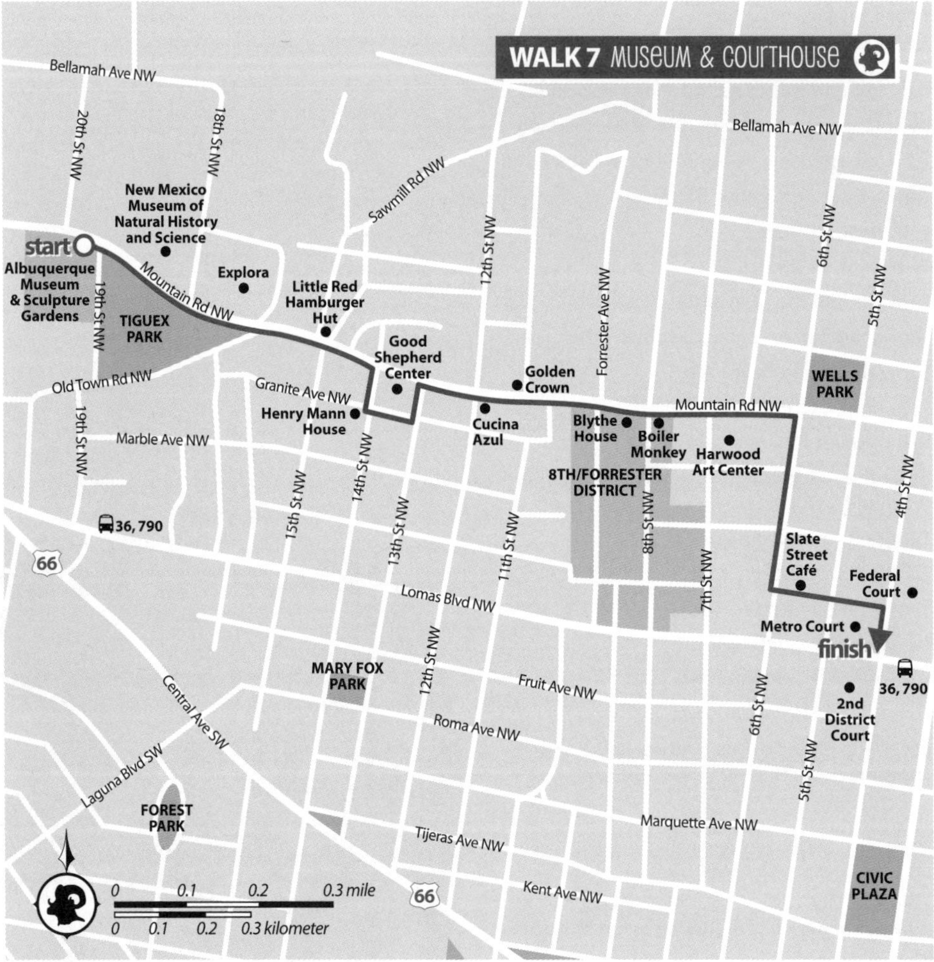
WALK 7 MUSEUM & COURTHOUSE
Bellamah Ave NW
20th St NW
18th St NW
Sawmill Rd NW
12th St NW
Forrester Ave NW
6th St NW
5th St NW
New Mexico Museum of Natural History and Science
start
Albuquerque Museum & Sculpture Gardens
19th St NW
TIGUEX PARK
Mountain Rd NW
Explora
Little Red Hamburger Hut
Good Shepherd Center
Golden Crown
Old Town Rd NW
Granite Ave NW
Henry Mann House
Cucina Azul
Blythe House
Boiler Monkey
Harwood Art Center
Mountain Rd NW
WELLS PARK
Marble Ave NW
8TH/FORRESTER DISTRICT
15th St NW
14th St NW
13th St NW
11th St NW
8th St NW
7th St NW
4th St NW
36, 790
66
Slate Street Café
Federal Court
Lomas Blvd NW
Metro Court
finish
36, 790
MARY FOX PARK
12th St NW
Fruit Ave NW
2nd District Court
Central Ave SW
Roma Ave NW
6th St NW
5th St NW
Laguna Blvd SW
FOREST PARK
Marquette Ave NW
Tijeras Ave NW
0 0.1 0.2 0.3 mile
0 0.1 0.2 0.3 kilometer
66
Kent Ave NW
CIVIC PLAZA

7 Museum and Courthouse: Better Know the Districts

BOUNDARIES: **19th St., Mountain Rd., Marble Ave., Broadway Blvd.**
DISTANCE: **1.25 miles one way**
DIFFICULTY: **Easy**
PARKING: **Free parking on 20th St., 1 block north of Mountain Rd.**
PUBLIC TRANSIT: **Bus 36 on Rio Grande Blvd. at Mountain Rd.; buses 36, 66, 766, 790 on Central Ave. at Rio Grande Blvd.**

Most of this route follows Mountain Road, one of Albuquerque's first thoroughfares. Formerly known as Carnuel Road, it once connected the plaza of what is now Old Town to the villages of the Cañón de Carnué Land Grant. Cañón de Carnué later became known as Tijeras ("scissors") Canyon, a rechristening that may refer to the two major roads that came together here like scissor blades. Residents of Carnuel used the road to bring chopped piñon and juniper to Albuquerque. The trade likely began in the mid-19th century. The last delivery via horse-drawn wagon arrived in 1937. The trek on that approximately 15-mile dirt road took a full day. The Mountain Rd. route described below is mercifully shorter, a mere stroll through revitalized areas east of Old Town, starting from the Museum District and taking a short detour south to finish at the Courthouse District. Three museums stand at one end, three courthouses at the other. The districts are only a mile apart, as the crow flies, yet feel like separate cities. And with galleries, shops, eateries, and side streets to explore along the way, just this short walk could take a full day.

- **Start at the west corner of Mountain Rd. and 19th St. The assembly of bronze sculptures here is *La Jornada*. Installed in 2005 the monument depicts in life-size form the "Epic Journey of the First European Colonists to the Southwest." It's just one of about two dozen works that grace the grounds on the north and east sides of the Albuquerque Museum of Art and History. (The sculpture garden proper is on the west side.) In 2015 the museum opened the $8 million, 9,338-square-foot exhibition "Only in Albuquerque," which tells the city's history through ancient artifacts and high-tech displays. Also worth checking out: Slate at the Museum, which serves up a modest sample from the menu at Slate Street Café, which you'll encounter near the end of** this walk. So you might want to save your appetite for that, particularly if somebody else is buying.

- Go east on Mountain Rd., crossing 19th St., to the north corner of Tiguex Park. In 1883 land in this area was leased to the Mann Blueher Gardeners. By the mid-1890s Herman Blueher had a truck farm on the south side of the road, while John and Henry Mann's market gardens were on the north side. Herman Blueher and the Mann brothers were German immigrants who arrived in Albuquerque in 1882. Now Tiguex Park occupies the site of Blueher Farm, with ball courts, playing fields, and nearly a mile of graded walking paths that are suitable for wheelchairs. The park also serves as a venue for city events, including the annual Carnuel Road Parade and Fiesta. Directly north of the park, the New Mexico Museum of Natural History and Science houses a planetarium, an observatory, and the Lockheed Martin DynaTheater, which features the world's first 2-D/3-D digital 4K dual projection system. (You really have to see a movie here to fully appreciate what that means.)

- Continue east on Mountain past 18th. The building with the geodesic dome is Explora! This interactive science museum is a great place to bring the kids, or release your inner one. The hands-on displays are designed to nurture the mad scientist in all of us.

  Just past Explora! is a welcome sign for the Sawmill District. The neighborhood sprang up around the American Lumber Company sawmill, built nearby in 1903. By 1908 it was the largest manufacturing company in the Southwest, with more than 1,000 employees. At the time, Mountain Rd. delineated the northern city limits. By the 1970s Sawmill and neighboring Wells Park had succumbed to urban blight and industrial pollution. However, restoration plans began in 1991 and have materialized steadily since 2008. Innovative efforts have revitalized the area without sacrificing the low-key character of Mountain Rd. Note the posted speed limit: 18 miles per hour. That oddity, along with purple street signs, is part of a 7-mile crosstown "bicycle boulevard."

- Ahead at 15th St., burgers at the Little Red Hamburger Hut are indeed little, but not at all red—unless ordered with red chile, which is highly recommended. Stop in for a snack, keeping in mind that several more opportunities for snack breaks remain ahead.

- Turn south on 14th St. for a quick detour to the Henry Mann House. This Queen Anne–style residence on the southwest corner of 14th and Granite is listed on the

National Register of Historic Places. On the northeast corner is the Good Shepherd Center, which claims to be the city's first homeless refuge. The Congregation of the Little Brothers of the Good Shepherd was founded in Albuquerque in 1951 by Irish-born aspirant Brother Mathias Barrett. (See Walk 3 for the founding site.)

- Go one block east on Granite to Brother Mathias Pl. Note along the way how the Good Shepherd Villa adds to the eclectic architectural styles of its neighborhood.

- Turn north on Brother Mathias Pl. and return to Mountain Rd.

- Turn east on Mountain. Cocina Azul is a block ahead on the right. If arriving during breakfast hours, get the French-toasted waffles, or "wa'toffle's". The café is a renovated 1920s grocery store. The commercial development that houses Zimmerman Photography and the New Mexico Tea Company on the north side of Mountain is a recent addition designed to emulate the style and massing of the grocery store.

  The alluring bakery smell comes from the Golden Crown Panaderia, ahead on the left. Its claim to fame is pizza with green chile crust. Kids are rewarded with a free *biscochito,* New Mexico's official state cookie. Everybody is a kid here, so go in and grab a free cookie.

- After another block, look south for a peek into the Eighth and Forrester Historic District. This neighborhood, added to the National Register of Historic Places in 1980, contains numerous homes built between the 1880s and the 1920s, along with several post-WWII residences. Architectural styles vary from Queen Anne

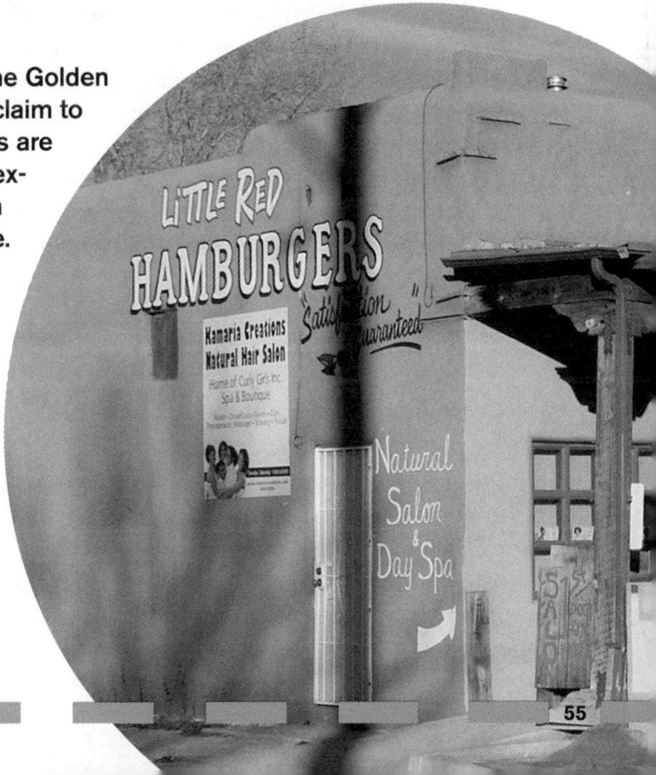

to Spanish Revival to Bungalow/Craftsman. Numerous white picket fences enhance curb appeal throughout the area.

- Ahead at the southwest corner of 8th St. is the Blythe House, added to the State Register of Historic Places in 1979. The structure on the southeast corner originally functioned as a gas station. Tiles de Santa Fe, a custom tile business, opened here in 1971 and added a hip little coffee shop to its showroom in 2009. Albuquerque's first food truck, the Boiler Monkey, took over in 2014 and added a crêperie. Landscape art and occasional music acts liven this cozy bistro.

- At the southeast corner of 7th St. is Cassandra Reid's contribution to the Albuquerque Public Art Program. Her creation, *Poets Plaza,* includes four benches made from a mosaic of ceramic tiles depicting spirals and other celestial patterns. Each bench represents one of the four seasons, compass directions, and universal elements. Take a closer look to find the tiles stamped with lines from various poems. The work was installed here on the northwest corner of the Escuela del Sol Montessori campus in 2005. Founded in 1968, Escuela del Sol is an independent primary and elementary school that emphasizes a holistic approach to education.

  The brick building nearby is the Harwood Art Center. Built in the Neoclassical Revival style in 1925, it served as the Harwood Girls School until 1976. In 1985, Escuela del Sol acquired the abandoned building to create studios and exhibition space for a community of artists. The Harwood now also offers art classes for all ages, as well as after-school programs and summer art camps for kids. Feel free to drop in to see what's on display in its galleries.

- Continue east along the north side of the campus to the old adobe church that now serves as the Harwood Art Center's 6th Street Studio on the southwest corner. On the northeast corner, Wells Park has a spray pad on the playground for cooling down in summer, as well as a community center equipped with a computer lab and a game room. In 2013, the gym at Wells Park was renamed in honor of boxing legend Johnny "Mi Vida Loca" Tapia, who trained there in his formative years. The five-time world champion died of heart failure at home in Albuquerque in 2012 at the age of 45.

- Turn south on 6th St. and follow it three blocks to Slate Ave. The subtle transition from small city ambience to urban vibe occurs somewhere along this stretch. Bail bond companies and law offices along the way hint that the Courthouse District isn't far.

- Turn east on Slate Ave., home of the aforementioned Slate Street Café, a contemporary gourmet eatery with shaded patio dining and a wine loft. Elegant yet informal, it scores high on the list of places to take someone you need to impress. Just a snack? Ahi tuna nachos.

- Continue east on Slate, passing by what just might be the world's cutest bail bond storefront. ABC Bail Bonds is a 300-square-foot bundle of adobe and neon with a solid A+ rating from the BBB. By contrast, the Bernalillo County Metropolitan Courthouse, to its immediate south, is a 244,000-square-foot structure with nine floors, a contemporary Art Deco style, and a history of scandal. The Metro Courthouse was completed in 2003 to the tune of $46 million. In 2005, the FBI began investigating a $4.3 million conspiracy in the form of bribes and kickbacks. The case ended in 2009 with the sentencing of a former city mayor and several other high-profile figures. One of New Mexico's most powerful politicos, Manny Aragon, was sentenced to 67 months at the Federal Correction Complex in Florence, Colorado, sharing the supermax security facility with such distinguished guests as Ted Kaczynski (the "Unabomber") and Richard Reid (the "Shoe Bomber"). Aragon was released in 2013.

  The seven-story domed building straight ahead is the Pete V. Domenici United States Courthouse. Completed in 1998 at $43 million, this 311,000-square-foot federal courthouse stands at 176 feet, making it the tenth tallest building in town. Its construction controversy involves allegations that the federal government illegally obtained and demolished a historic site, McClellan Park, to make way for the courthouse. The U.S. General Services Administration eventually restored the park's central feature, the *Madonna of the Trail* statue, to an obscure location on the northwest corner of the courthouse grounds.

- Turn south on 4th St. and walk one block to Lomas Blvd. On the southeast corner stands a Pepto-pink, turquoise-topped trinket shop. Architect J. O. Zucal designed the structure before 1940 as an automotive service station. Since 1970 it has housed a 5,000-square-foot showroom for Sunwest Silver, "the largest supplier and manufacturer of charms and findings in the USA." On the northwest corner, the 36-foot-tall brass and copper sculptural fountain by Evelyn Rosenbergh is confirmed as the world's largest scales of justice. On the southwest corner, the eight-story building is the turquoise-topped Bernalillo County Courthouse. Home of New Mexico's Second Judicial District Court, this 272,000-square-foot courthouse was completed in 2001 for $34 million. The controversy here is relatively minor: Judges often complain that its courtrooms are too small to be of any use. De facto, they are absurdly tiny, which is hard to imagine while gazing upon its palatial exterior and postmodern references to the Italian Renaissance.

Remembering where this walk began and considering the three majestic institutions of justice at its end, is it absurd to dream of a day when our Museum District rivals the grandeur of the Courthouse District and, in lieu of bail bondsmen and law offices, the streets are lined with curators and art studios? You be the judge.

● The quickest way back to the starting point is by going west on Lomas. The walk to 19th St. is 1 mile. Or walk half a block east to the bus stop in front of the federal courthouse and catch bus 36 or 790 to Old Town. See Connecting the Walks below for more options.

Cycling/pedestrian/transit advocate Bob Tilley recounts his favorite feature on this route: "I travel Mountain Road fairly often. It's a pretty funky road. So many great places to choose from, but for me, the Boiler Monkey Bistro is a real standout. I had passed the ancient abandoned gas station that the café is located in for years. So sad, just yearning to be saved. I was ecstatic when a little coffee shop finally materialized in the beautifully renovated station, but even happier when the little coffee shop far exceeded my expectations with amazing homemade pies and quiches. We have lost so much of our history in America to bulldozers and neglect, so it really makes me happy to see an old building repurposed, and done so well."

POINTS OF INTEREST

Albuquerque Museum of Art and History cabq.gov/culturalservices/albuquerque-museum, 2000 Mountain Rd. NW, 505-242-4600

New Mexico Museum of Natural History and Science nmnaturalhistory.org, 1801 Mountain Rd. NW, 505-841-2800

Explora! explora.us, 1701 Mountain Rd. NW, 505-224-8300

Little Red Hamburger Hut littleredsburgers.tripod.com, 1501 Mountain Rd. NW, 505-304-1819

Cocina Azul cafeazul.com, 1134 Mountain Rd. NW, 505-831-2500

Golden Crown goldencrown.biz, 1103 Mountain Rd. NW, 505-243-2424

Routes Bicycle Rentals & Tours routesrentals.com, 1102 Mountain Rd. NW,

Boiler Monkey Bistro boilermonkeybistro.com, 724 Mountain Rd. NW, 505-315-0567

Harwood Art Center harwoodartcenter.org, 1114 7th St. NW, 505-242-6367

Slate Street Café slatestreetcafe.com, 515 Slate Ave. NW, 505-243-2210

Sunwest Silver sunwestsilver.com, 324 Lomas Blvd. NW, 505-243-3781

route summary

1. Start at the west corner of Mountain Rd. and 19th St. Walk east to 14th St.
2. Turn south on 14th St. and go to Granite Ave.
3. Turn east and go to Brother Mathias Pl.
4. Turn north and return to Mountain Rd.
5. Turn east and walk to 6th St.
6. Turn south and walk to Slate St.
7. Turn east and walk to 4th St.
8. Turn south and finish at Lomas Blvd.

CONNECTING THE WALKS

You can return to Old Town via Walk 5, which begins three blocks south at Civic Plaza.

Walk 6 begins at Old Town Plaza.

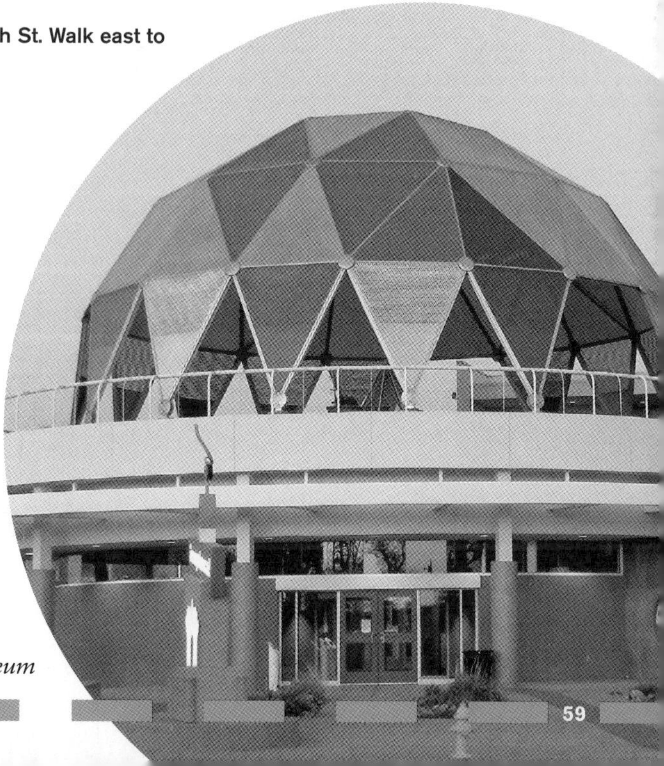

¡Explora! Science Center and Children's Museum

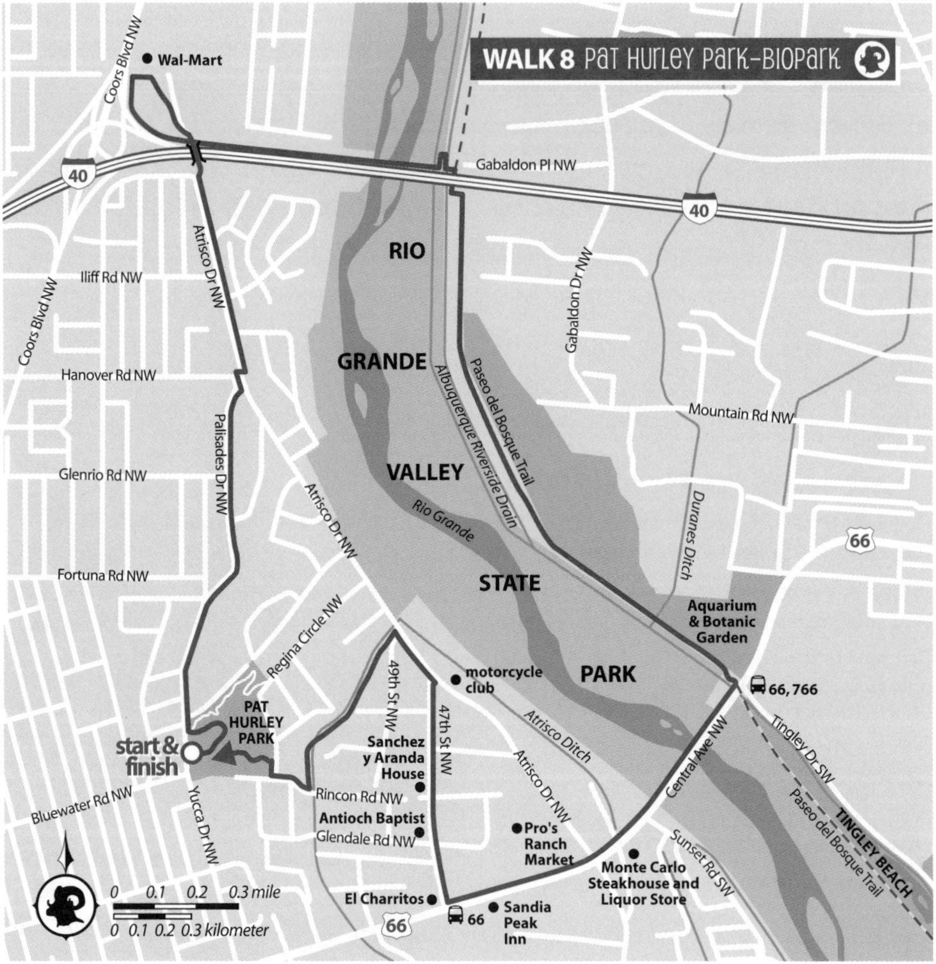
WALK 8 Pat Hurley Park–BioPark
Wal-Mart
Coors Blvd NW
40
Gabaldon Pl NW
Atrisco Dr NW
Iliff Rd NW
Coors Blvd NW
Hanover Rd NW
Palisades Dr NW
Glenrio Rd NW
Fortuna Rd NW
RIO
GRANDE
VALLEY
STATE
PARK
Albuquerque Riverside Drain
Paseo del Bosque Trail
Gabaldon Dr NW
Mountain Rd NW
Duranes Ditch
Rio Grande
66
Aquarium & Botanic Garden
66, 766
Regina Circle NW
49th St NW
47th St NW
motorcycle club
Atrisco Ditch
PAT HURLEY PARK
start & finish
Sanchez y Aranda House
Rincon Rd NW
Bluewater Rd NW
Yucca Dr NW
Antioch Baptist
Glendale Rd NW
Pro's Ranch Market
Central Ave NW
Tingley Dr SW
Paseo del Bosque Trail
TINGLEY BEACH
Sunset Rd SW
Monte Carlo Steakhouse and Liquor Store
El Charritos
66
Sandia Peak Inn
0 0.1 0.2 0.3 mile
0 0.1 0.2 0.3 kilometer

8 Pat Hurley Park–BioPark: The Mother Road Loop

BOUNDARIES: **Coors Blvd., Miami Rd., Paseo del Bosque, Central Ave.**
DISTANCE: **6 miles; 8–10+ miles with a BioPark tour**
DIFFICULTY: **Difficult (steep terrain, unpaved surfaces)**
PARKING: **Free parking at Pat Hurley Park, Walmart on Coors Blvd., west end of Gabaldon Pl., and Tingley Dr. west of Central Ave.**
PUBLIC TRANSIT: **Buses 66 and 766 on Central Ave. at Tingley Dr.; bus 66 on Central Ave. at 47th St.**

Both the interstate and the river harbor interesting corridors built exclusively for pedestrians and bicyclists, but because they also pose significant barriers to local traffic, you may likely find other points on the loop that are more convenient to access than the designated starting point, Pat Hurley Park. The loop begins (and ends) here because you can get a helpful preview of the environs from the overlook. But wherever you choose to start, you'll eventually find a unique neighborhood on the cusp of the West Mesa, a riverside woodland known as the bosque, a brief stretch of a transcontinental interstate, and a struggling remnant of historic Route 66. It also crosses four bridges, two of them relatively high. Gephyrophobiacs and acrophobiacs alike are advised to preview the I-40 segment of the route before committing to the walk. And if these 6 miles aren't enough, you can tack on many more with optional detours through the ABQ BioPark.

- **Start on the west side of Pat Hurley Park. The overlook ahead is on the edge of an escarpment that rises 135 feet from the playgrounds, ball courts, and community center on the east side of the park. Few places afford such a commanding view of the city. Downtown Albuquerque is the cluster of modest skyscrapers about 2.5 miles east. About 13 miles farther east and slightly to the north, South Peak rises to 9,782 feet. From there, the Sandia Mountains stretch another 13 miles north. To the south, the Manzanita, Manzano, and Pino ranges are in full view. On a clear day you can pick out Whiteface Mountain 50 miles south-southeast.**

  Impressions of the immediate environs may vary. Autumn foliage paints the valley in fiery hues. Springtime brings a tranquil sea of green, while winter may reveal a hollow

Back Story: Albuquerque Biological Park

ABQ BioPark Aquarium: Opened in 1996, the aquarium illustrates the journey of the Rio Grande from its headwaters in the Rocky Mountains to its destination in the Gulf of Mexico. Highlights include a 285,000-gallon shark tank, a walk-through eel tunnel, and jellyfish tubes.

ABQ BioPark Botanic Garden: Located on 52 acres next to the aquarium, the Botanic Garden is actually a series of themed gardens. Highlights include a 10,000-square-foot glass conservatory, the 10-acre Heritage Farm, the Butterfly Pavilion, and the Sasebo Japanese Garden.

Tingley Beach: Developed in the late 1920s on the site of a riverside dump, Conservancy Beach was an artificial lake filled with water diverted from the Rio Grande. Later renamed for Mayor Clyde Tingley, it was once a popular destination for swimming, waterskiing, and swimsuit pageants. The city closed the facility in 1951 due to the polio scare. The area then deteriorated for decades until extensive renovations in 2004 restored it to its current state. Tingley Beach now features three fishing ponds and a model boat pond. Ponds are stocked by the New Mexico Department of Game and Fish with catfish in the summer and rainbow trout in the winter. Fishing is free, but a state fishing license is required. Paddle boats are available for rent in the summer. Riverside viewing platforms are west of the north pond. Two more ponds with wildlife blinds are located in the bosque west of the South Pond. With paved paths around the pond and a web of trails spun between the ponds and river, a tour of Tingley Beach can amount to a substantial walk on its own.

landscape echoing with distant gunshots and police sirens. Incidentally, the ever-changing influence of time and season is a recurring theme in the work of prominent Southwestern painter Wilson Hurley, son of the park's namesake. Patrick J. Hurley served as President Herbert Hoover's secretary of war, and the park named in his honor long held a reputation as a battlefield in the city's ongoing gang wars. A $3 million face-lift in 2009 has since softened its image. (Unfortunately, there's still an issue with unleashed dogs.) Among the most impressive improvements are the winding paths and stairs that zigzag up and down the escarpment. Tempting as it is to run down to explore the lower elevations, this walk starts in the opposite direction. So for now take

ABQ BioPark Zoo: Established in 1927 and incorporated into the Albuquerque Biological Park in 1996, the Rio Grande Zoo (as it was formerly known) shelters more than 250 species from all continents in its 64-acre facility. A thorough tour of the zoo runs about 2.25 miles. Highlights include African painted dogs, polar bears, and snow leopards. It's also one of only two facilities in the U.S. that house Tasmanian devils.

The Aquarium and Botanic Garden are located at 2601 Central Ave NW. The Zoo is at 903 10th St. SW. All three are open daily 9 a.m.–5 p.m. Admission fees vary. Tingley Beach, which spans between them, does not charge admission and is open sunrise–sunset. A narrow-gauge train stops at all attractions. A round-trip journey takes about an hour and requires BioPark admission.

For more BioPark info: 505-764-6200, **cabq.gov/culturalservices/biopark**

advantage of this aerial view of the neighborhood below (also named for Pat Hurley) to familiarize yourself with all that awaits you at the end of the loop.

- Follow the overlook path back to Yucca Dr. and turn right. The street name changes to Palisades Dr. somewhere north of Cloudcroft Rd. Continue north through this diverse residential area to Atrisco Dr.

- Turn left on Atrisco and continue north to the bridge ahead. This span crosses six lanes of interstate traffic, plus another six lanes spooling off the tangle of exchanges with Coors Blvd. to the immediate west. Wave hello to I-40, the behemoth that killed the Mother Road and every small-town economy that relied on it. Tall fences adorned with oxidized steel sculptures enclose this overpass. Its wide column caps extend west, indicating that lanes for vehicles will be added someday. For now, the bridge is exclusively for bicycles and pedestrians. However, the exchange to the I-40 Trail doesn't show much thought for the latter. What could've been accomplished with a gate and a few stairs instead takes a half-mile loop. (Look closely for a well-worn footpath in the steep embankment below and a hole in the chain-link fence ahead for a tempting, albeit illegal shortcut.)

- Follow the sidewalks counterclockwise around a vacant dirt lot, and in 10 minutes or so you'll be directly beneath the bridge you just crossed. Continue straight to the next bridge. Again, footpaths and damaged chain-link in the vicinity reveal shortcuts to the neighborhood on the south side of the interstate, and to riverside trails below. Straight ahead, the Gail Ryba Memorial Bridge is a 1,100-foot crossing completed in 2010 for $6.9 million. It's named for the founder of Bike ABQ, the city's first bicycle advocacy group. Ryba died of cancer three months before the official opening. The bridge provides an essential link in the city's 400-mile walking/biking network. (ABQ The Plan, the current blueprint for the city's next renaissance, calls for a 1,000-mile network. We shall see.) Functionality aside, it's decked out with marvelous details: Two viewing platforms overlook the Rio Grande. Sculptures of river animals—a turtle, a frog, and a heron—adorn the archways. The concrete surface is inlaid with brass fish, paw prints, and tree leaves. Oxidized steel cottonwood leaves are set in mesh fencing. The scale of some details—too small to notice at the speed of bikes—indicates special consideration for pedestrians.

- Cross the Rio Grande and follow the ramp down to the nearest bridge. For this next 1.3-mile bosque segment, you have several choices. Two dirt roads run along the west side of the Atrisco Feeder Canal. The paved Paseo del Bosque Trail (signed at the bridge as Bosque Trail South) runs along the east side of the Albuquerque Riverside Drain. Two more dirt roads run between the ditches. There's also a network of shaded trails closer to the river. Take your pick. The paved route soon runs along the northern reaches of the Albuquerque BioPark. This research section, devoted in large part to breeding the endangered Silvery Minnow, is not open to the public. Soon after rounding the eastward bends, you might see the BioPark Train, also known as the Rio Line, which travels 1.5 miles with stops at the Aquarium & Botanic Garden, Tingley Beach, and the BioPark Zoo. If you timed your walk right, you can catch it right off the Bosque Trail. If not, visit the botanic garden and aquarium first, since they're both just north of the station. (See the Back Story on pages 62–63 for more info on BioPark attractions.)

  West of the crossroads of Central and Tingley, Rotary River Park is a picnic area in a small corner of Rio Grande Valley State Park, which isn't really a state park, but rather a wildlife preserve managed by the city of Albuquerque's Open Space Division and the Middle Rio Grande Conservancy District. A chapter in The Plan titled "The Rio Grande Vision" would bring boardwalks, boutiques, cafés, condos, and other enhancements to the wildlife preserve—but in such a manner that wouldn't disrupt the natural wildlife aspect of it. We shall see. Renovations and restorations to the 4,300-acre state park are slated to begin here on the north side of Central in Spring 2015. Once that's done, you're likely to find much more here than a little choo-choo train.

- Turn right on Central (historic Route 66) and cross the bridge. Artwork and interpretive plaques transform the railings and viewing platforms into a timeline that illustrates the multimillion-year saga of the region. (Look out for the plesiosaur.) Meanwhile, the river courses southeast as though heading toward the Manzano Mountains. Mosca Peak rises to 9,509 feet exactly 25 miles from the bridge.

Central Ave. west of the bridge is in an area historically known as Atrisco. According to one version of local history, Nahuatl Indians later referred to the area of settlements on the west bank of the Rio Grande as Atlixo, meaning "across the water." The earliest known record of its name comes from a 1662 government document that describes the valley of Atrisco as "the best site in all New Mexico." In 1692 the Spanish crown awarded the 41,000-acre Atrisco Land Grant to Fernando Durán y Chávez for his services in the reconquest of New Mexico. It would be the first of 300 such grants in the province. By 1896, heirs of the grant successfully petitioned to incorporate additional lands, expanding the Atrisco Land Grant to nearly 83,000 acres. The community maintained its agrarian character well into the 20th century. Its small farm economy boomed during World War II, but began to falter in the following decades. The Atrisco neighborhood, with its proximity to Route 66, was among the first to experience the ensuing pressures for rapid development and the consequences of it. The interstate arrived in the late 1960s to relieve it of its traffic and prosperity. It hasn't quite recovered, and proposals for redevelopment tend to falter.

But initial appearances can be deceiving. Monte Carlo Steakhouse, for example, rightfully boasts the best steaks in Albuquerque. Don't let the dodgy package store that fronts the joint deter you. The Katsaros family has been running the restaurant since 1972. They know their T-bones from their kebabs. A block ahead on the right, at the far side of a massive parking lot, Pro's Ranch Market is a megastore of Mexican food. Inside you'll find a *panadería, tortilleria, carnicería,* and more. Its cafeteria-style *cocina* is your best fast-food option in the area.

Ahead at the southeast corner at 47th, Sandia Peak Inn is a classic Route 66 motel that received extensive makeovers in recent years. The elegant sculptures in the parking lot (by artist/co-owner Kim Young) set the tone for this well-appointed motel. Directly across the street, El Charritos is a family-run restaurant with a pleasant atmosphere, friendly service, and excellent *carne adovada.* Both the red and green chile here have serious bite, and the place is packed during Sunday brunch.

- Turn right on 47th. On the corner at Glendale Rd., Antioch Baptist Church stands and testifies to the diversity of the community. The church was organized under Reverend James A. Hopkins in 1958 and moved to this brick and stucco building in 1970. A block farther on the northwest corner at Rincon Rd., the Spanish Vernacular farmhouse crouching behind a coyote fence is the Manuel Sanchez y Aranda House. It has a linear construction with 20-inch-thick *terrón* walls and a stone rubble foundation. It was built in 1895 on a 28-acre farm that has since vanished. Most of the community's agricultural fields have been converted into residential lots, but a few remain ahead.

  When you reach the end of the road, look east across Atrisco Dr. for a Southwestern Vernacular–style house with dark *vigas* poking through its volcanic-stone façade. Carved letters in the beam above its blue frames identify the house as the Albuquerque Motorcycle Club. Completed in 1940, the clubhouse is now a private residence.

- Turn left on Atrisco Dr.

- Turn left on the sandy ditch road and follow the Arenal Canal down the next crossroad, Rincon Rd. It's a pleasant stroll when the water is running. Backyard animals—dogs and horses, mostly—take interest in passing strangers. (To avoid gathering soles full of thorny goat heads, go two blocks past the ditch and take Regina Cir. back to the park.)

- Turn right on Rincon Rd.

- Turn right on Regina Dr. Your options for the ascent to the overlook are clear. Choose the most meandering route up the escarpment.

POINTS OF INTEREST

Pat Hurley Park cabq.gov, 350 Yucca Dr. NW, 505-768-2000

Monte Carlo Steakhouse and Liquor Store 3916 Central Ave. SW, 505-831-2444

Pro's Ranch Market prosranch.com, 4201 Central Ave. NW, 505-833-1765

Sandia Peak Inn sandiapeakinnmotel.com, 4614 Central Ave. SW, 505-831-5036

El Charritos Mexican Restaurant 4703 Central Ave. NW, 505-836-2464

Antioch Baptist Church antiochbc-abq.cwwsites.com, 305 47th St. NW, 505-831-2088

route summary

1. Start at the overlook on the west side of Pat Hurley Park.
2. Walk north on Yucca Dr./Palisades Dr. to its end.
3. Turn left on Atrisco Dr. and continue north to its end, just past the bridge over I-40.
4. Turn left on Miami Rd.
5. Turn left on I-40 Trail East.
6. Cross the Rio Grande and follow the ramp down to the nearest bridge.
7. Turn right on Bosque Trail South.
8. Turn right on Central Ave.
9. Turn right on 47th St.
10. Turn left on Atrisco Dr.
11. Turn left on the ditch road.
12. Turn right on Rincon Rd.
13. Turn right on Regina Rd.
14. Return to the overlook via the paths and stairways.

connecting the walks

Switch to Walk 4 by continuing southeast on Tingley Dr. about half a mile from the corner of Central. Connect with Walk 9 by continuing east through the parking area on the north side of I-40. Follow Gabaldon Pl. about a quarter mile to Gabaldon Dr. Turn left and go a block north to Duranes Rd.

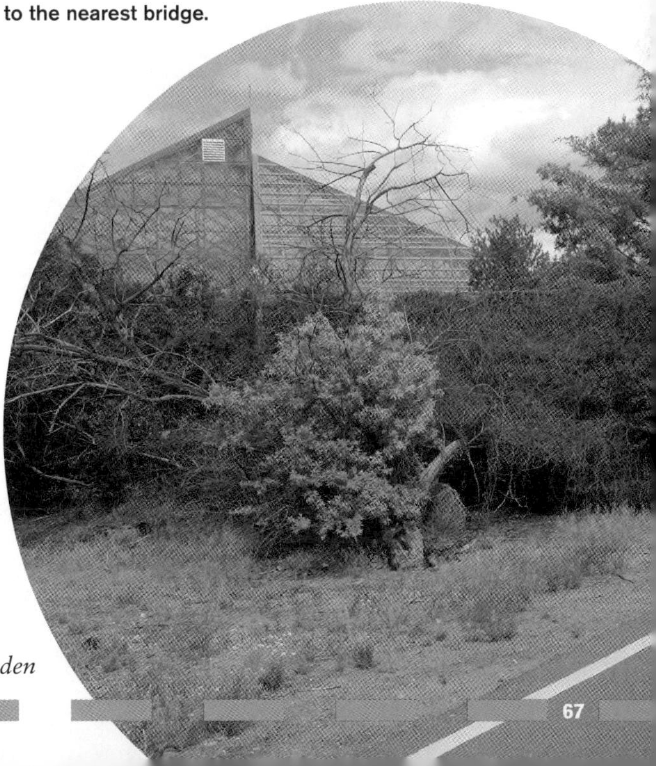

Conservatories in the Botanic Garden

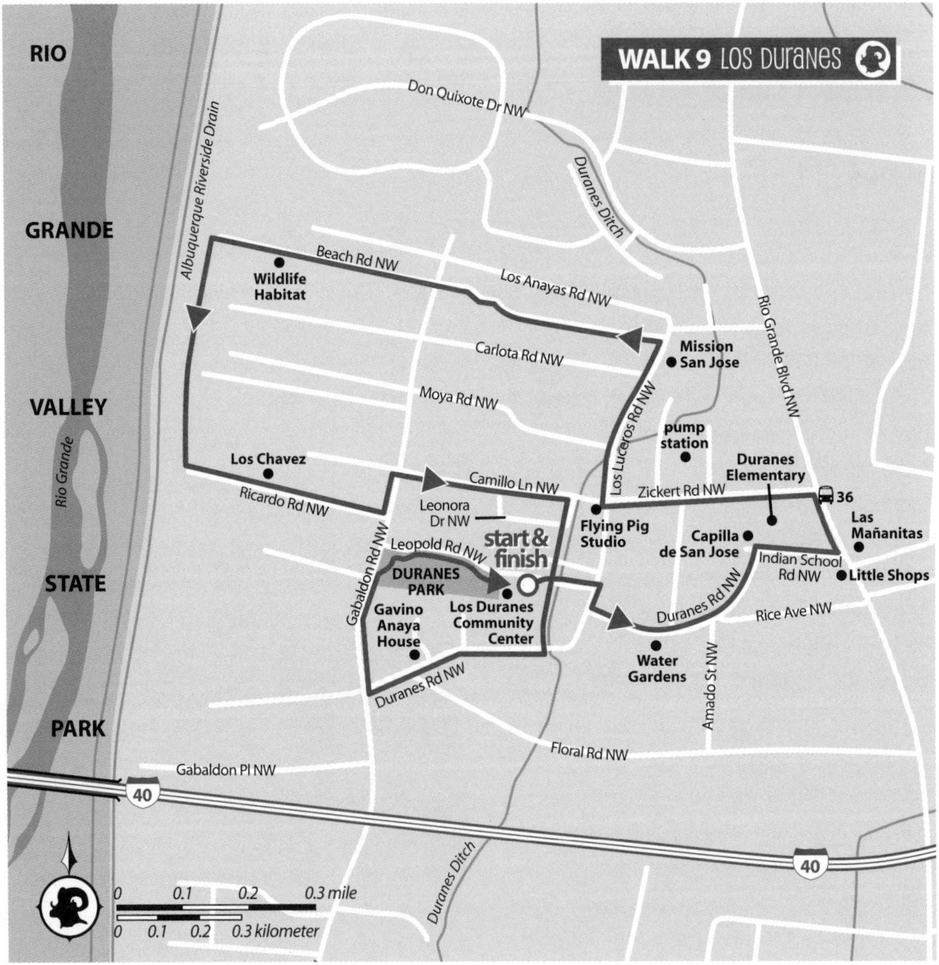
WALK 9 LOS DURANES
RIO GRANDE VALLEY STATE PARK
Rio Grande
Albuquerque Riverside Drain
Don Quixote Dr NW
Duranes Ditch
Beach Rd NW
Los Anayas Rd NW
Carlota Rd NW
Moya Rd NW
Camillo Ln NW
Ricardo Rd NW
Leonora Dr NW
Leopold Rd NW
Gabaldon Rd NW
Los Luceros Rd NW
Zickert Rd NW
Rio Grande Blvd NW
Indian School Rd NW
Duranes Rd NW
Rice Ave NW
Amado St NW
Floral Rd NW
Gabaldon Pl NW
Wildlife Habitat
Mission San Jose
pump station
Los Chavez
Duranes Elementary
36
Flying Pig Studio
Capilla de San Jose
Las Mañanitas
Little Shops
start & finish
DURANES PARK
Gavino Anaya House
Los Duranes Community Center
Water Gardens
40
0 0.1 0.2 0.3 mile
0 0.1 0.2 0.3 kilometer

9 LOS DURANES: SOMETHING OLD, SOMETHING NEW

BOUNDARIES: **Rio Grande Blvd., Beach Rd., Paseo del Bosque, Duranes Rd.**
DISTANCE: **3.5 miles; optional 1.5-mile detour**
DIFFICULTY: **Moderate (unpaved surfaces, narrow streets)**
PARKING: **Los Duranes Community Center**
PUBLIC TRANSIT: **Bus 36 on Rio Grande Blvd. at Zickert Rd.**

Los Duranes claims to be Albuquerque's second oldest neighborhood. The Duranes *acequia madre,* or mother ditch, was established in 1706. In the mid-1790s, La Plaza de Señor San Jose de Los Duranes was the first of several small plazas along the Rio Grande north of Old Town. As with the other plazas, the proximity to the river was both a blessing and a curse. The flood of 1870 was exceptionally devastating. Yet the rural, agricultural character of the neighborhood remains today, and traditional settlement patterns persist, with multiple generations living in family compounds. A rapid influx of new residents and upscale developments don't always fit the old patterns, but nonetheless seem reverent to the community's traditional values. The route below winds along the narrow roads and ditch trails for a glimpse of what's new and old in this dynamic, multifaceted community.

- **Start, appropriately enough, at Los Duranes Community Center. The $5 million, 19,000-square-foot facility, completed in 2013, has two large meeting rooms, an arts and crafts room, a game room, a computer lab, an activity room, a fitness center, and a full-size gymnasium.**

- **Head to the east end of Leopoldo Rd., crossing the Duranes Ditch along the way. You'll get a chance to stroll along this fine acequia later in the walk. The steady roar of traffic from nearby I-40 might be distracting at first, but it soon fades into the background.**

- **Turn right on Los Luceros Rd.; then make a quick left on Duranes Rd. As you pass the intersection with Duranes Dr., note the unusual undulating wall near the east corner. Close ahead on the right is Albuquerque Water Gardens, a unique garden center specializing in aquatic plants. This at-home business has been growing steadily since it started in 1994. Four ponds near the back of the property serve as the main**

Back Story: Indian Pueblo Cultural Center

August 1976 saw the opening of the Indian Pueblo Cultural Center, the official cultural interpretive center for New Mexico's 19 Pueblo tribes. Since then it has grown into one of Albuquerque's top attractions. The award-winning, 10,000-square-foot centerpiece museum illustrates the culture and history of the Pueblo people from pre-Columbian time to present day through its permanent collections, changing exhibitions, and cultural education programs. A restaurant, gift shop, and travel center are also on-site. To visit it on this walk, take a 0.75-mile detour east on Indian School Rd. from Rio Grande Blvd.

For more information: **indianpueblo.org,** 2401 12th St. NW, 505-843-7270

showroom, but the most creative display is the "sunken garden," which resembles a small swimming pool filled with perennials.

- Bear left at the Y ahead to stay on Duranes Rd. The street narrows and loses its sidewalks, and its centerline becomes a gutter. The old chapel at the end of the road, constructed in 1890 on land donated by Maria Jaramillo, Capilla de San Jose is one of five largely unaltered late-19th-century chapels remaining in the city. The wooden steeple and a pitched tin roof atop stuccoed *terrón* and adobe exemplify New Mexico's Vernacular style. A fiesta is held annually in March in honor of the church's patron saint and intercessor.

- Turn right on Indian School Rd. Toward the end of the 19th century, the federal government contracted Protestant churches to educate Indian children. On behalf of the Presbyterians, Dr. Sheldon Jackson founded the U.S. Indian Training School in a rented house in Los Duranes in 1881. In 1882 the campus was relocated to a 60-acre farm less than a mile east of Duranes, near where the Indian Pueblo Cultural Center stands today. (See the Back Story above for more details.)

On the southwest corner ahead, Little Shops on Rio Grande sports pastoral Southwestern murals on its cinderblock walls, and a curious assortment of vendors and wares inside. On the northeast corner, the sprawling adobe complex allegedly dates back 300 years. On its long resume are a stagecoach stop, a saloon, a brothel, a blacksmith shop, and Las Mañanitas (1985–2011). Named for the traditional Mexican birthday song, the restaurant was a local favorite with a memorable atmosphere that included 11 rooms decked out in Talavera tiles, kiva fireplaces, and a stately patio shaded under a venerable cottonwood with low-slung limbs that made it irresistible to climb after a few margaritas. The building remains, but the restaurant is sorely missed.

- Turn left on Rio Grande Blvd.

- Turn left on Zickert Rd. On the left is Duranes Elementary School, originally built in 1919. In 2008, Baker A+D overhauled and expanded the school to meet Leadership in Energy and Environmental Design (LEED) standards. The stylish, sustainable new design scored an AIA award.

  The massive concrete dome on your right is the Duranes Pump Station, built in the 1950s to boost the delivery of city water. On the southwest corner ahead is Flying Pig Studio. Proclaiming itself as "Albuquerque's Smallest Gallery," it includes a freestanding wall with a door, a framed picture, and not much else. You'll have to cross the street and look for it. (Hint: It faces north.)

- Go north on Los Luceros Rd. to the Mission San Jose, which bears no resemblance to the *capilla,* namely because of the successor's Mission style. The walls look like traditional stuccoed adobe. Contours in the façade create the appearance of weathered stucco over adobe brick. However, cracks in the veneer expose the illusion. And craters in the church hall behind the mission reveal cinder block coated in an exterior insulation finishing system, or EIFS—plastic foam cladding concealed beneath a wafer-thin synthetic stucco shell. Apparently it doesn't hold up as well as the old stuff.

- Turn left on Beach Rd. Yards along this narrow stretch range from salvage lots to immaculate gardens, with the latter gaining ground. Rusted farm equipment is often scavenged from one to be quaintly displayed in the other. Near the west end of the road, a hexagonal watchtower rises from a xeric garden. The property is certified by the National Wildlife Federation as Wildlife Habitat for providing four basic elements needed for wildlife to thrive. Paths wind throughout a densely vegetated landscape of drought-tolerant plants, including chamisa, Apache plume, rugosa rose, snakeweed, and Russian sage. Nightshade, larkspur, and iris are also abundant. Continue straight to the west end of Beach Rd. and go through the pedestrian access gateway.

- Turn left onto the ditch road. This sandy trail runs parallel to the paved recreational trail, Paseo del Bosque. Approximately 200 feet down on the left is a tree stump adorned with found objects—broken ceramics, weather-worn glass, plastic toys, stray bits of wire, string, and rope. It's unclear how it started or why it continues, but chances are you'll find something colorful nearby to contribute to the menagerie. Continue on the ditch road another quarter mile or so.

- Turn left through a gap in the cement barriers to reach the west end of Ricardo Rd. The barrier is obscured by a two-story house. (If you see a bridge, you've gone just over a quarter mile too far.) Ahead on the left side of Ricardo Rd., Los Chavez is an agricultural compound populated with amusing animals, mostly goats. Tempting as it is to pet them, heed the stern warnings against trespassing. Continue to the east end of the road, where you'll see the charter school, Montessori of the Rio Grande.

- Turn left on Gabaldon Rd.

- Turn right on Camillo Ln., keeping in mind that narrow roads are part of the traditional character this community has struggled to preserve.

- Turn right on Leonora St., which looks more like a sidewalk. As the street bends west, continue straight on the path alongside Duranes Ditch. This will soon return you to the entrance to the community center parking lot, but there's another 0.75-mile loop left to this route, so continue straight on the shaded ditch path to the next paved road.

- Turn right on Duranes Rd. The road bends south to reveal a modest complex that exemplifies the agricultural ideals of the neighborhood. The one-story house and outbuilding to its east likely date to the 1940s and feature stucco exteriors, large metal casement windows, wood trim, and gabled roofs. Horses and goats roam the surrounding green pasture. Across the street on the west corner of Delta Rd. is the

Gavino Anaya House, built in the early 19th century and added to the National Register of Historic Places in 1984. Recently added exterior decorations include folksy artworks depicting American patriotism and Mexican stereotypes.

- Turn right on Gabaldon Rd. With trees lining both sides to form a canopy over the narrow road, the stretch ahead just might be one of the shadiest streets in Albuquerque. Just past the trailer park on the left is a one-story pitched-roof building with a wood-framed porch and a wood-paneled façade. The rest of the house is stuccoed. It was likely a motel or boardinghouse at one time.

- Turn right into Los Duranes Park and follow the paved walkway back to the parking lot.

Points of Interest

Los Duranes Community Center cabq.gov, 2920 Leopoldo Rd. NW, 505-848-1338

Albuquerque Water Gardens albuquerquewatergardens.com, 2704 Duranes Rd. NW, 505-246-8278

Little Shops on Rio Grande littleshopsonriogrande.com, 1507 Rio Grande Blvd. NW, 505-765-5489

Mission San Jose de los Duranes 2110 Los Luceros Rd. NW, 505-243-4628

Route Summary

1. Start at the Los Duranes Community Center.
2. Walk to the east end of Leopoldo Rd.
3. Turn right on Los Luceros Rd.
4. Take the first left, Duranes Rd.
5. Bear left at the Y to stay on Duranes Rd.
6. Turn right on Indian School Rd.
7. Turn left on Rio Grande Blvd.
8. Turn left on Zickert Rd.
9. Turn right on Los Luceros Rd.

10. Turn left on Beach Rd. and follow it to its west end.
11. Turn left onto the ditch road.
12. Turn left through the gap in the concrete barriers and follow Ricardo Rd. to its east end.
13. Turn left on Gabaldon Rd.
14. Turn right on Camillo Ln.
15. Turn right on Leonora St. and follow the ditch trail south to Duranes Rd.
16. Turn right on Duranes Rd.
17. Turn right on Gabaldon Rd.
18. Turn right into Los Duranes Park and follow the walkway back to the parking lot.

Connecting the Walks

Continue south on the ditch road to I-40 to connect with Walk 8.

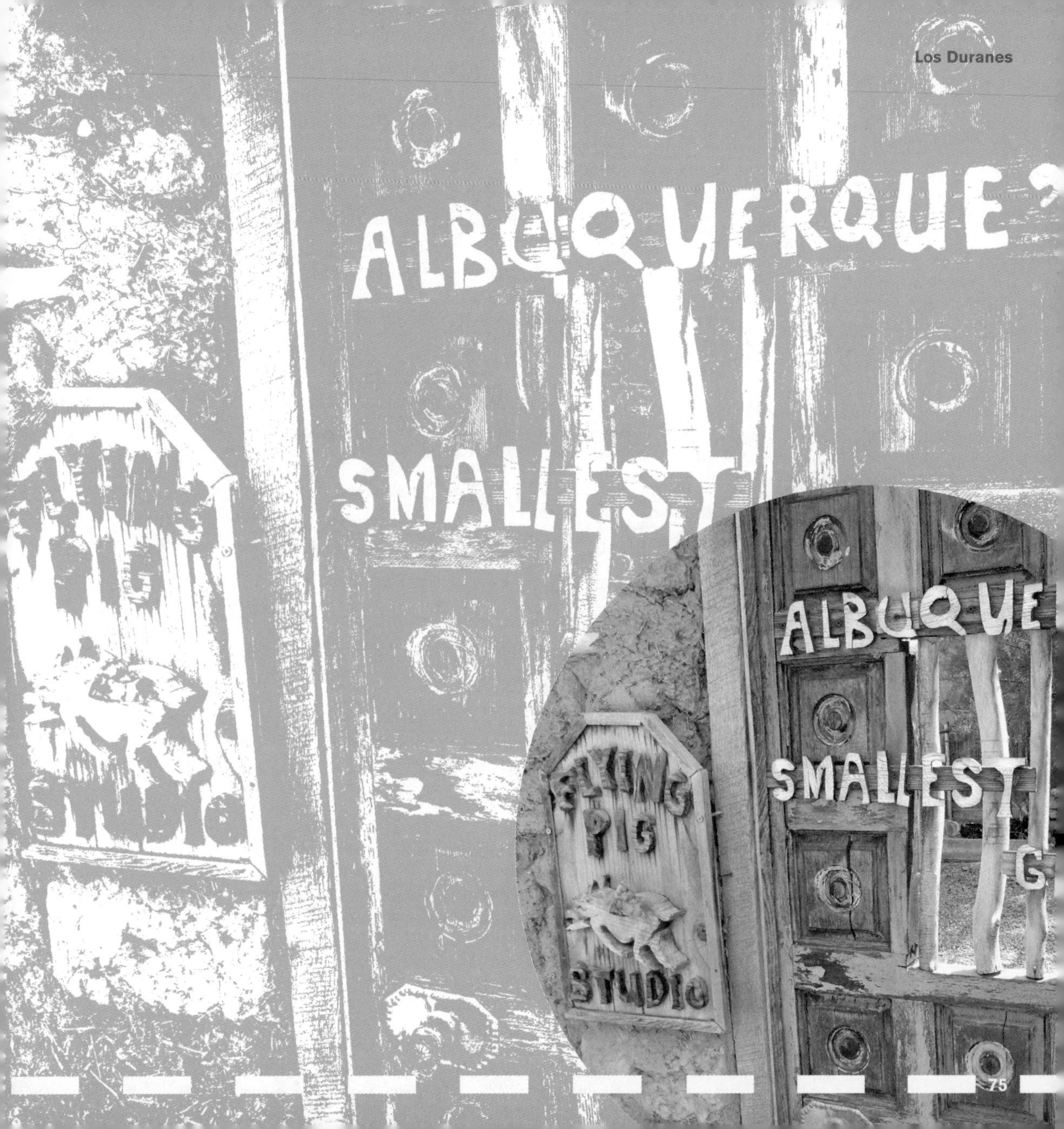
ALBUQUERQUE
SMALLEST
FLYING PIG STUDIO

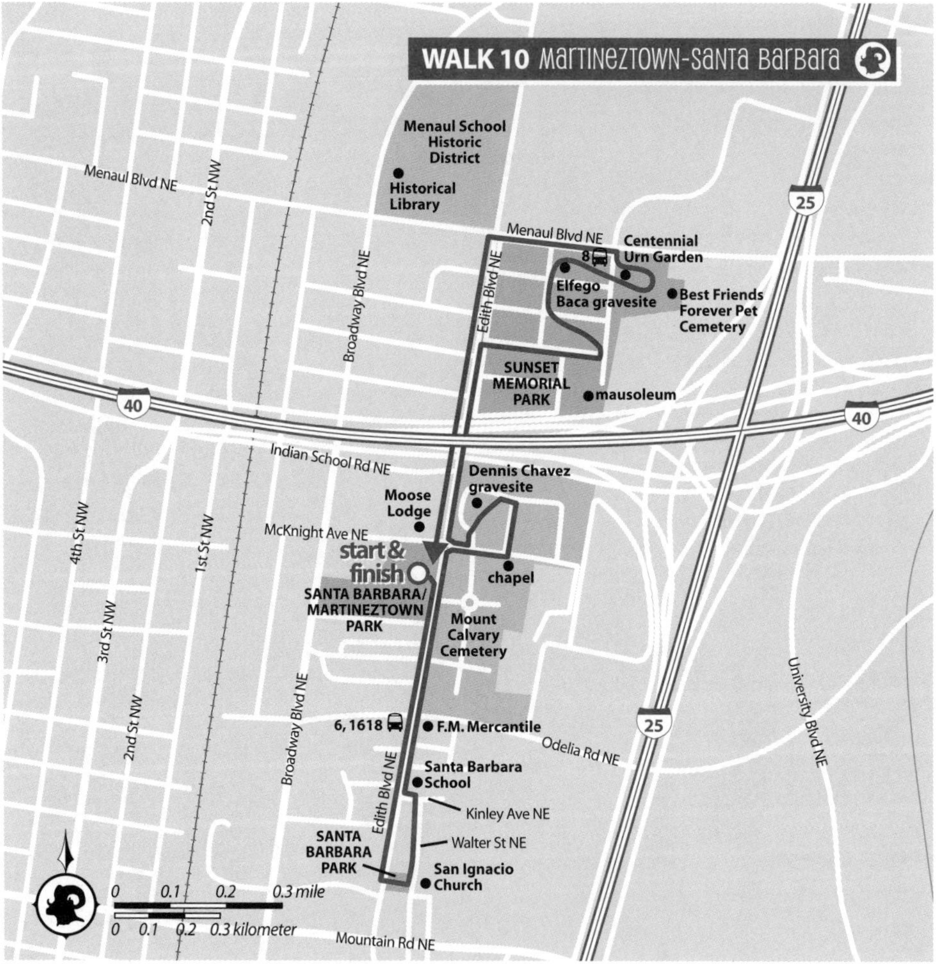
WALK 10 Martineztown-Santa Barbara
Menaul School Historic District
Historical Library
Menaul Blvd NE
2nd St NW
Broadway Blvd NE
Edith Blvd NE
Menaul Blvd NE
8
Centennial Urn Garden
Elfego Baca gravesite
Best Friends Forever Pet Cemetery
25
SUNSET MEMORIAL PARK
mausoleum
40
40
Indian School Rd NE
Dennis Chavez gravesite
Moose Lodge
McKnight Ave NE
start & finish
chapel
SANTA BARBARA/ MARTINEZTOWN PARK
Mount Calvary Cemetery
4th St NW
1st St NW
3rd St NW
2nd St NW
Broadway Blvd NE
6, 1618
F.M. Mercantile
Odelia Rd NE
25
University Blvd NE
Santa Barbara School
Kinley Ave NE
Walter St NE
SANTA BARBARA PARK
San Ignacio Church
0 0.1 0.2 0.3 mile
0 0.1 0.2 0.3 kilometer
Mountain Rd NE

10 Martineztown–Santa Barbara: The Quick and the Dead

BOUNDARIES: **Edith Blvd., Mountain Blvd., Locust Pl., Menaul Blvd.**
DISTANCE: **3 miles**
DIFFICULTY: **Moderate (hilly terrain)**
PARKING: **Free parking at Santa Barbara/Martineztown Park**
PUBLIC TRANSIT: **Buses 6 and 1618 on Odelia Rd. at Edith Blvd.; bus 8 on Menaul Blvd. at Broadbent Pkwy.**

Martineztown–Santa Barbara is an old neighborhood that stretches north from Dr. Martin Luther King Jr. Ave. to Menaul Blvd. Despite its proximity to downtown Albuquerque and the University of New Mexico North Campus, it's an isolated community squeezed between the industrial railroad corridor and the tangle of interstate exchanges known as the Big I. Though the area has suffered disinvestment and decline, signs of improvement are starting to show in the early stages of redevelopment projects focused on cultural and historic preservation and commercial revitalization. This walk visits historic schools, chapels, and two large cemeteries on opposite sides of I-40.

- **Start at Santa Barbara/Martineztown Park (listed as Martineztown–Santa Barbara Park in the city's recreation directory), a 10-acre site equipped with basketball courts, picnic tables, a soccer field, and a lighted softball field. The nearby mural reflects the history of the barrio. (For murals with more pop, go to the southwest corner of the park and look across Hannet Ave.)**

- **Walk south on Edith Blvd., locally known as El Camino del Lado (The Road along the Edge, in reference to an ancient trade route that squeezed between what was then sandhills and marsh). The private residence on the southeast corner at Odelia Rd. previously housed a general store, a blacksmith shop, a wood yard, and the headquarters of the Martineztown Bridge Club. It's listed as F.M. Mercantile on the New Mexico Register of Cultural Properties. Close ahead, a mysterious dragon-boat mosaic adorns the wall across the street from Cordero Ave.**

San Ignacio Catholic Church crowns the hill behind Santa Barbara Park. The Santa Barbara community grew up around this handsome white adobe church in the early 1900s. By contrast, Martineztown grew in part from the Second Presbyterian Church, about a quarter mile south on Edith. Manuel and Anna María Martín, founders of Martineztown in 1850, broke with the Catholic church in the 1880s and helped establish the Presbyterian church in 1889. Portions of Martineztown were annexed by the city of Albuquerque in 1898, Santa Barbara in 1948. The two communities were united in their common economic despair that followed World War II.

- Cross Santa Barbara Park and go up the stairs for a closer look at San Ignacio. Community members did most of the adobe brick construction in 1916. The year on the arch (1926) refers to when it was given official parish status.

- Turn left on Walter St. The old Santa Barbara School ahead was originally two adobe-walled rooms built around 1908 as part of the county school system. It expanded in stages until the 1930s, when Albuquerque Public Schools acquired it. It functioned as an elementary school until the 1970s, then as a Special Services Annex until 1986. In 1991, the city of Albuquerque converted it to the Santa Barbara Apartments for senior citizens. Newer structures behind the Mission-style building house a community learning center. Historic photographs and manuscripts adorn the walls of the main hallway inside the center. On its grounds are murals depicting the community's agriculture-to-urban evolution. *Zia,* a Corten steel sculpture of a Zia symbol by William Goodman, stands nearby.

- Turn left on Kinley Ave.

- Turn right on Edith and go north to cross back over Odelia. The southern part of Mount Calvary Cemetery was established in 1870 as Santa Barbara Cemetery to handle the overflow of internments from San Felipe de Neri Church (Walk 6). Jesuit Father Donato Gasparri selected this distant site, favoring its barren hills over the swampy lowlands then surrounding Old Town. Efforts to beautify the grounds began in 1936. Trees were planted, a stone wall was erected along Edith Blvd., and a new chapel was dedicated on the grounds by 1938. Though several impressive memorials with prominent family names remain today, many other monuments have been vandalized or destroyed, and the chapel is in ruins. Water rights were lost, the trees are dead, and the ground has long since reverted to its natural state—so, naturally, goat heads dominate the gravelly landscape. (My first bike ride in New Mexico began in the apartment complex to the immediate east and ended moments later with two flat tires.) If you happen to find the gate at Exculpating Rd. unlocked, please take a moment to visit the lonely souls in this neglected *camposanto.* Otherwise . . .

- Turn right into the main gate, opposite McKight Ave., and walk east into the modern section of Mount Calvary Cemetery. Metalheads should *quietly* visit the chapel ahead and locate the crypt on the top row in the northwest corner to pay tribute to Randy Castillo, legendary drummer for The Motels, Mötley Crüe, and Ozzy Osbourne.

- Go north on Malthusian Way, then west at the T-junction ahead. Locate row 16 in section 615 on your left, and then walk south while counting off 60 headstones. There you'll find a large marker for Dennis Chavez, who served in the U.S. House of Representatives from 1931 to 1935, and in the United States Senate from 1935 to 1962. The nearby interstate is imposing, but local wildlife doesn't seem to mind. Stellar's jays in particular are drawn to this part of the cemetery. More commonly found near forest campgrounds, they dominate this nook with their scolding calls, sheen crests, bouncy gait, and graceful flight.

- Wander southwest to locate an unlocked exit; then turn right to continue north on Edith Blvd. Cross beneath I-40 and locate the gate on the west side of Sunset Memorial Park. To enjoy a walk on grounds this green anywhere else in Albuquerque, you'd have to dodge golf balls. Diverse trees shade the verdant rolling hills. The presence of cypress, juniper, mulberry, and elm—all restricted under a city ordinance to control allergenic pollen—may help explain why the bereaved here can seem excessively weepy. Other trees on-site include Bartlett pear, willow, and blue spruce, which park founder Chester T. French had transplanted from the Jemez Mountains. The Chester T. French Memorial Mausoleum dominates the southeast corner of the park and contains 3,000 crypts. Built in 1954, the structure features marble corridors accented with walnut paneling and stained glass windows. Outside the mausoleum are marble-faced crypts, niches, and the Old Town Columbarium, with a mosaic mural created by Italian artisans. U.S. Olympian Pat Porter is buried on the west side of the mausoleum. Tucked behind the east side, the Scattering Rose Garden provides a serene setting with 50 rose bushes and ornamental trees where families can scatter the remains of loved ones.

The northwest corner is the oldest part of the park, which opened in 1929. Legendary lawman Elfego Baca (1865–1945) is buried in block 11, section 41, grave 1. He's best remembered for The Frisco Shootout, his solitary standoff against 80 Texas cattlemen in 1884. The gunfight lasted nearly 40 hours, with more than 4,000 rounds fired at the self-appointed deputy sheriff. Buried nearby (block 9, section 57, grave 1) is Medal of Honor recipient Harold H. Moon (1921–1944). Private Moon found himself in a situation similar to Baca's when his foxhole became the target for a concentration of mortar and machine-gun fire during the Battle of Leyte on a Filipino beach in World War II. He was posthumously awarded the U.S. military's highest decoration for his heroic stand against enemy attack. The citation credits him for killing nearly 200 Japanese soldiers.

- Wander the grounds at your leisure, and then aim for the northeast corner. The Centennial Urn Garden is a secluded pavilion with elegant fountains and a kiva fireplace. Directly behind it is the Best Friends Forever Pet Cemetery, where dead pets and their deceased owners can rest together eternally.

- Exit through the north gate and turn left on Menaul Blvd. to return to Edith, where you'll see Menaul School, an independent day and boarding school for grades 6–12. In 1896, Rev. James A. Menaul secured funding for a boarding school that would serve Spanish-speaking boys from New Mexico, primarily from the northern portion of the territory. The first class graduated in 1906. The Menaul School Historic District contains 17 significant buildings. Architectural styles include Queen Anne and Mission/Spanish Revival. Campus tours start at 8 a.m. on Tuesday and Thursday, October 15–March 15. Menaul Historical Library, a repository on the history of Presbyterians in the Southwest, is open Tuesday–Friday, 10 a.m.–4 p.m., and is located in Bennett Hall on the west side of campus.

- Go south on Edith Blvd. past the Moose Lodge to return to Santa Barbara/Martineztown Park.

POINTS OF INTEREST

Martineztown–Santa Barbara Park cabq.gov/parksandrecreation, 1825 Edith Blvd. NE

San Ignacio Catholic Church 1300 Walter St. NE, 505-243-4287

Mount Calvary Cemetery archdiocesesantafe.org , 1900 Edith Blvd. NE, 505-243-0218

Sunset Memorial Park sunset-memorial.com, 924 Menaul Blvd. NE, 505-345-3536

Menaul School menaulschool.com, 301 Menaul Blvd. NE, 505-345-7727

ROUTE SUMMARY

1. Start at Santa Barbara/Martineztown Park and walk south on Edith Blvd.
2. Turn left to cross Santa Barbara Park.
3. Turn left on Walter St.
4. Turn left on Kinley Ave.
5. Turn right on Edith Blvd.
6. Turn right to enter Mount Calvary Cemetery.
7. Exit the cemetery and turn right to continue north on Edith Blvd.
8. Turn right to enter the gate on the west side of Sunset Memorial Park.
9. Exit through the north gate.
10. Turn left on Menaul Blvd. to return to Edith Blvd.
11. Turn left on Edith Blvd. to return to Santa Barbara/Martineztown Park.

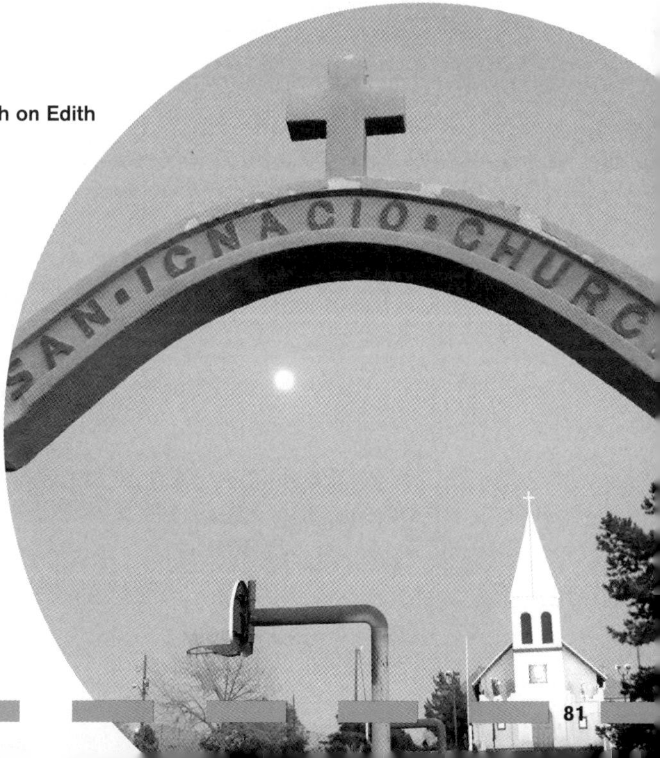

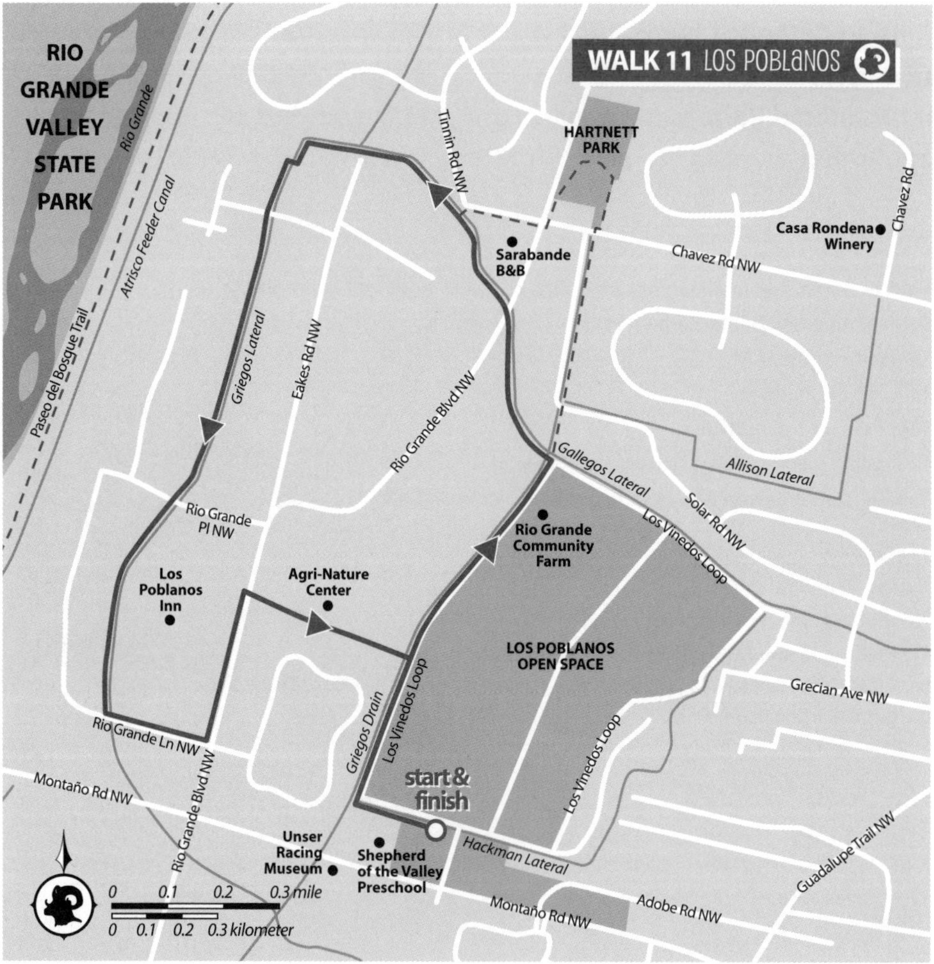
WALK 11 LOS POBLANOS
RIO GRANDE VALLEY STATE PARK
Rio Grande
Atrisco Feeder Canal
Paseo del Bosque Trail
Griegos Lateral
Eakes Rd NW
Tinnin Rd NW
HARTNETT PARK
Sarabande B&B
Chavez Rd NW
Casa Rondena Winery
Chavez Rd
Rio Grande Blvd NW
Gallegos Lateral
Allison Lateral
Solar Rd NW
Los Vinedos Loop
Rio Grande Community Farm
Rio Grande Pl NW
Los Poblanos Inn
Agri-Nature Center
LOS POBLANOS OPEN SPACE
Grecian Ave NW
Rio Grande Ln NW
Griegos Drain
start & finish
Montaño Rd NW
Unser Racing Museum
Shepherd of the Valley Preschool
Hackman Lateral
Adobe Rd NW
Guadalupe Trail NW
0 0.1 0.2 0.3 mile
0 0.1 0.2 0.3 kilometer

11 LOS POBLANOS: WINE COUNTRY

BOUNDARIES: Montaño Rd., Los Poblanos Open Space, Chavez Rd., Rio Grande
DISTANCE: 4.5 miles, 4.75 with detour
DIFFICULTY: Moderate (unpaved surfaces)
PARKING: Free parking at Los Poblanos Open Space
PUBLIC TRANSIT: Bus 157 on Montano Rd. at Poblanos Ct.

Before and after the founding of the Villa of Albuquerque in what is now better known as Old Town, numerous farming and ranching communities were established along the Rio Grande. Spanish for "the Pueblans," Los Poblanos was supposedly named for settlers originally from Puebla, Mexico. A 1790 census shows six settlements in Albuquerque's North Valley, including La Plaza de Señor de San Jose de Los Ranchos and La Plaza de San Antonio de Los Poblanos. Ambrosio and Juan Cristobal Armijo owned the 500-acre Los Poblanos Ranch throughout most of the 19th century. An 1860 census suggests Los Poblanos was one of several farms in the expanding Los Ranchos de Albuquerque community. Recurring floods in the late 1800s and early 1900s destroyed most of the early settlements in the North Valley, making it difficult to determine the locations of the original plazas. Agriculture and other developments returned in the 1920s when the Middle Rio Grande Conservancy District was formed to mitigate flooding with a vast system of levees, ditches, laterals, drains, and canals. The name "Los Poblanos" later resurfaced in the 1930s in reference to a ranching estate owned by former U.S. Representative Albert G. Simms. Since then the name has been readily applied to everything in the vicinity, including a National Historic District. True to history, it's once again a wealthy settlement on the south end of Los Ranchos; or to put it in modern terms, it's an upscale subdivision in The Village of Los Ranchos de Albuquerque, an incorporated municipality since 1958.

- **Start at the Los Poblanos Open Space parking lot and walk west. The ditch on your right is the Hackman Lateral. Shepherd of the Valley Preschool, with its tiny gardens and whimsical folk art, is on your left.**

- **Turn right, go through the gate, and follow the dirt road (Los Vinedos Loop) alongside the Griegos Drain. The land here has been continuously farmed for centuries and remains one of the largest pieces of agricultural land in Albuquerque. About 25 percent of the crops are grown to attract birds. Sandhill cranes flock here for the** sorghum in November. It's not uncommon to see hawks pouncing on pigeons or coyotes stalking Canada geese. In October, a giant labyrinth is blazed through the cornfields. Navigating the maize maze can add miles to your walk.

Rio Grande Community Garden is in the northwest corner of Los Poblanos Open Space. Aspiring gardeners can rent garden rows to grow and harvest their own crops. The project is part of Rio Grande Community Farm, a 50-acre, nonprofit urban farm that grows organic food for local schools, restaurants, and stores.

Detour: At the junction of the Griegos Drain and the Gallegos Lateral, you can continue about half a mile straight ahead to visit Hartnett Park. Named for the first mayor of Los Ranchos, the 4-acre facility includes a playground, tennis and racquetball/handball courts, and the Alfredo Garcia Community Barn. Also named for a former mayor, the barn is the site of the Growers' Market & Arts and Crafts Fair, held Saturday mornings throughout the year. Prior to park construction in 1997 excavations on the site revealed archaeological remains from La Plaza de Señor de San Jose de Los Ranchos, the center of a village established in 1750. From 1851 to 1854, Los Ranchos was designated the Bernalillo County seat. At that time it was a wealthy community of haciendas with well-cultivated vineyards. The flood of 1904 was the last in a catastrophic series that led to its desertion. In the 1930s the highway department cleared off the last of the ruins and used the old adobe to set the roadbed for Rio Grande Blvd., which you'll find on the west side of the park. Follow it south back to Chavez Rd. Turn right and walk to Tinnin Rd. Turn left through the pedestrian access to rejoin the route on the Gallegos Lateral near the Griegos Lateral.

- If skipping the detour, turn left at the Gallegos Lateral and go north to Rio Grande Blvd. Use care crossing this moderately busy road and continue north/northwest to the Griegos Lateral. Not all homes along the ditches make use of the irrigation ditches. Many have sold off their water rights. But agriculture persists throughout Los Poblanos Estates, despite the rapid development of supersized residences. Some homes resemble resorts; others are harder to define in terms of style and purpose. Towers and domes are not uncommon, nor are five-digit monthly mortgages. It gets stranger: You might hear the occasional cries of peacocks and the mournful drones of bagpipes, but you're unlikely to encounter another soul. In all the times I've walked in this neighborhood, I've never seen a person outside a passing vehicle. Nor have I ever seen a roadrunner here. Seems that common creature has been replaced with pheasants. And in lieu of tumbleweeds, windblown boxes bearing the label for Gruet sparkling wines gather in the corners of luscious green lawns. (The Gruet family, originally from Champagne, France, recently established a crushing, aging, and bottling facility 4 miles east of Los Poblanos.)

Follow the Griegos Lateral south to Rio Grande Ln., the third paved road that crosses the ditch. Here you might detect the rumble of traffic on Montaño Bridge, about a quarter mile southwest. Most North Valley residents, particularly those in the Los Poblanos Historic District, vehemently opposed construction of the bridge for nearly 30 years. When the project was finally completed in 1996, they managed to forestall motor-vehicle access another year, during which time it served as the biggest and most expensive bicycle/pedestrian bridge ever to span the Rio Grande.

- Turn left on Rio Grande Ln.

- Turn left on Rio Grande Blvd. Less than a quarter mile on your left is the entrance to Los Poblanos Historic Inn and Organic Farm, located at the former headquarters for a vast ranch. In the early 1930s, owner Albert Simms hired the architect John Gaw Meem, aka Father of Santa Fe Style, to take charge of remodeling the ranch house and designing La Quinta Cultural Center. The ranch house now serves as the inn and La Quinta functions as a conference center. Both are listed on the National Register of Historic Places. Nestled on 25 acres, the luxurious compound also features a B&B, agricultural fields, historic gardens, and walking paths. Unfortunately only guests are permitted to walk on the property except during public events such as the annual Lavender Festival. However, you can enjoy a view of the barns and silos—remnants of the original Creamland Dairies complex—from the shoulder of Rio Grande Blvd. Or you can get a closer look by returning in your vehicle and driving up to the Farm Shop, which sells gourmet treats, garden tools, kitchen cutlery, folksy ornaments, and a wide assortment of lavender-based products.

- Turn right on the driveway that leads to Los Ranchos Agri-Nature Center. This site was formerly home to Anderson Valley Vineyards, founded in 1973 by Maxie Anderson. (See Walk 13 for the balloon museum that bears his name.) In 2009, the Village of Los Ranchos purchased 19 acres of the winery, including an 11,000-square-foot building once used for winemaking, for a mere $5.9 million. The Agri-Nature Center serves as a venue for community events and a "Farm Camp" for kids.

- Turn right on Los Vinedos Loop and follow it back to the parking lot.

Nearby attractions not directly on the route but well worth mentioning include the Unser Racing Museum. High-tech interactive exhibits and loads of automotive memorabilia celebrate New Mexico's racing family. True, a museum dedicated to cars might be an inappropriate recommendation for a walking guidebook, but check it out anyway since it's just across the street.

In the 1880s, New Mexico produced nearly a million gallons of wine annually. The flood years that followed reduced the output to less than 2,000 gallons by 1910. A state-imposed prohibition nearly killed the industry soon after, but winemaking in the Land of Enchantment bounced back in 1978. Resembling a Tuscan villa and vineyard, Casa Rondeña Winery opened in 1997 and soon proved to be the most essential stop on New Mexico's wine tour. The tasting room is open to the public daily noon–7 p.m. Or join them for Pilates+Wine on weekend mornings.

POINTS OF INTEREST

Los Poblanos Open Space cabq.gov/parksandrecreation, 1701 Montaño Rd. NW, 505-768-5353

Rio Grande Community Farm riograndefarm.org, 1701 Montaño Rd. NW, 505-510-1837

Hartnett Park losranchosnm.gov/services, 6718 Rio Grande Blvd., 505-344-6582

Los Poblanos Inn lospoblanos.com, 4803 Rio Grande Blvd. NW, 505-344-9297

Los Ranchos Agri-Nature Center losranchosnm.gov, 4920 Rio Grande Blvd. NW, 505-344-9426

Unser Racing Museum unserracingmuseum.com, 1776 Montaño Rd. NW, 505-341-1776

Casa Rondeña Winery casarondena.com, 733 Chavez Rd. NW, 505-344-5911

Sarabande Bed and Breakfast sarabandebnb.com, 5637 Rio Grande Blvd. NW, 888-506-4923

route summary

1. Start at the Poblanos Open Space parking lot and walk west.
2. Turn right on Los Vinedos Loop.
3. Turn left at the Gallegos Lateral and go north to Rio Grande Blvd.
4. Cross Rio Grande Blvd. and continue north/northwest to the Griegos Lateral.
5. Follow the Griegos Lateral south to Rio Grande Ln.
6. Turn left on Rio Grande Ln.
7. Turn left on Rio Grande Blvd.
8. Turn right on the driveway to the Los Ranchos Agri-Nature Center.
9. Turn right on Los Vinedos Loop and follow it back the parking lot.

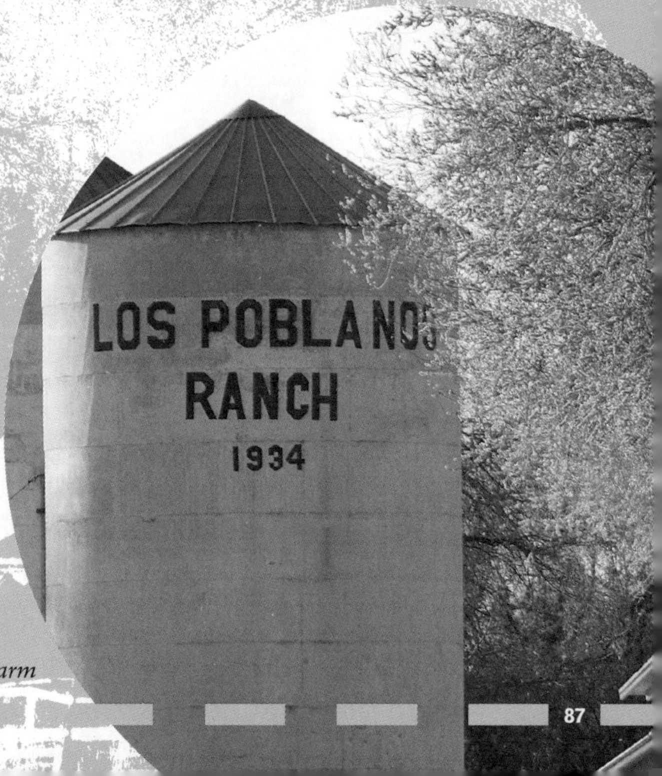

Silos at Los Poblanos Historic Inn and Organic Farm

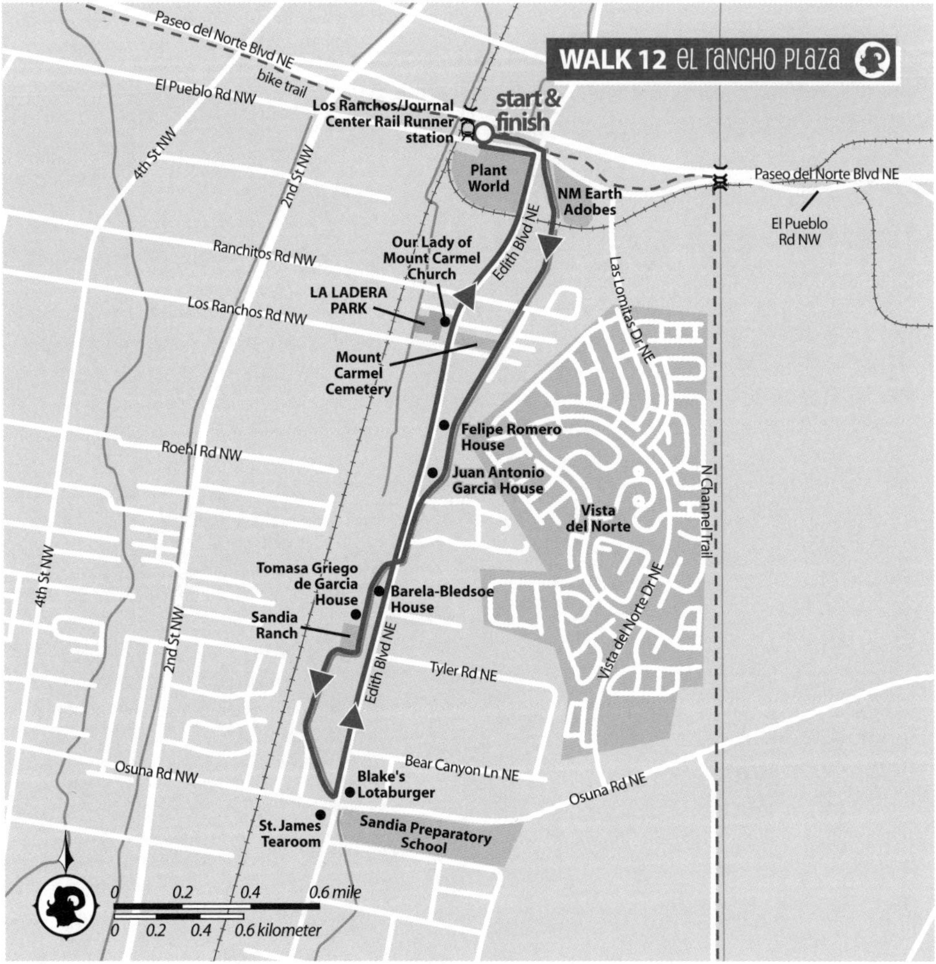
WALK 12 el rancho plaza
start & finish
Los Ranchos/Journal Center Rail Runner station
Paseo del Norte Blvd NE
bike trail
El Pueblo Rd NW
4th St NW
2nd St NW
Plant World
NM Earth Adobes
Paseo del Norte Blvd NE
El Pueblo Rd NW
Our Lady of Mount Carmel Church
Edith Blvd NE
Ranchitos Rd NW
LA LADERA PARK
Los Ranchos Rd NW
Las Lomitas Dr NE
Mount Carmel Cemetery
Felipe Romero House
Roehl Rd NW
Juan Antonio Garcia House
N Channel Trail
Vista del Norte
Tomasa Griego de Garcia House
Barela-Bledsoe House
Sandia Ranch
Vista del Norte Dr NE
Tyler Rd NE
Bear Canyon Ln NE
Osuna Rd NW
Blake's Lotaburger
Osuna Rd NE
St. James Tearoom
Sandia Preparatory School
0 0.2 0.4 0.6 mile
0 0.2 0.4 0.6 kilometer

12 El Rancho Plaza: Life on the High Road

BOUNDARIES: **Paseo del Norte, Alameda Lateral, Osuna Rd.**
DISTANCE: **4 miles**
DIFFICULTY: **Moderate (sandy, possibly muddy paths; few paved surfaces)**
PARKING: **Free parking at Rail Runner station on El Pueblo Rd., west of Edith Blvd.**
PUBLIC TRANSIT: **Bus 251 at the Rail Runner station**

Edith Boulevard has gone by many names: Camino de Bernalillo, Camino de la Ladera, and Highland Road, to name a few. It emerged as an alternate route during times when mud and floods overwhelmed the Camino Real, the primary route between Santa Fe and Chihuahua in the Spanish Colonial era. The old high road was the borderline between arable and arid land, a middle ground between the floodplain to the west and dry barren hills to the east. Divided evenly between ditch roads and the main boulevard, this walk revisits a stretch historically known as El Rancho Plaza. Several structures on this route date back to the early Territorial Period (1850–1912) and have since been listed on the National Register of Historic Places. It also passes near the haunted ruins of an insane asylum. Both the houses and the hospital are privately owned, so don't stray from public right-of-ways described below.

- **Start at the Los Ranchos/Journal Center Rail Runner station. The paved path on the north side of the parking lot is the Paseo del Norte Bicycle Trail. This multiuse trail, inaccessible to motorized vehicles, runs between the west side of the Rio Grande and the North Diversion Channel.**

- **Walk a quarter mile east to the southeast corner of Edith and El Pueblo Rd. Turn south and follow the dirt road on the near side of the ditch known as the Alameda Lateral. This weedy and usually dry channel runs along the west side of the manufacturing yard for New Mexico Earth Adobes, which produces nearly half a million adobes annually. The yard is often filled with mud bricks drying in the sun. Check their website for adobe-related classes, events, and art exhibitions.**

  Continue south across the tracks, a railroad spur that connects numerous nearby factories and industries to the main line. Just shy of a block past Ranchitos Rd. is the back side of Mount Carmel Cemetery. The lot—about 50 by 200 yards—gives a general idea of

the size and shape of a parcel in this neighborhood a century ago. By Spanish custom, land was divided in strips so that each piece would have access to both a water source and a common road. In the early 19th century, parcels tended to run about 15–20 yards wide and a mile or more in length. Family plots continued to divide with each new generation, while roads and acequias proliferated. Hence, the narrow form persisted, and the "plaza" communities of the North Valley tended to develop in a linear form rather than the defensive square formation typically found elsewhere in the Spanish colonies. These long, narrow lot configurations are sometimes referred to as *lineas* or *tripas*.

As demand for real estate increased and farming declined, water rights were sold and the long parcels were cut into patterns common to contemporary residential development. Most yards in this neighborhood fit that pattern. Directly north of the cemetery, about a dozen square plots crowd what was previously a single parcel. Note however that as the ditch angles closer to the road, parcels tend to be wider. Old acequias, now lined with concrete, still provide irrigation to small holdings of agriculture and livestock that remain in the area. Well-tended barns, corrals, and stables are difficult to spot through the trees on the left. Old-growth cottonwoods are common, though many of the ancient ones have died off in recent years. Close ahead, a creaky wooden staircase mysteriously descends to the bed of the lateral. To the east, the walled subdivision on the hill is Vista del Norte. Real estate analysts describe its 3,700 inhabitants as "Striving Immigrant Families," and the Department of the Interior's 2010 Surface Management map labels the decade-old neighborhood as "Gravel Pits." Both descriptions seem somewhat inaccurate. In reality the majority of residents are American-born, and in 2000 the gravel pits began filling with a thousand homes on a hundred streets and cul-de-sacs, all packed into a labyrinth with only two points of entry/escape. My house is in there somewhere.

Just past Tornaso Ln., the Alameda Lateral runs parallel to Edith for less than a quarter mile before crossing beneath it. Firmly planted posts and tangles of barbed wire prevent vehicles from accessing the traces of ditch roads that remain on either side of the lateral ahead.

- Cross Edith and pick up the path on the north side of the lateral. It soon curves south and the view opens to reveal farm fields on the near side of the railroad tracks and heavy industry farther west. Just ahead, the lateral passes behind the Barela de

Bledsoe House. Originally built as a U-shaped hacienda around 1840 for El Rancho Plaza's leading *patrón,* the house is named for the widow who inherited it (Abundia Barela) and the gambler she later married (Horace Bledsoe). The present house is now L-shaped, with only the east end remaining from the original structure. Restorations include Greek Revival window and door frames. Four boxcar-sized shipping containers are parked in its weedy field. About 100 yards ahead, you'll pass the Tomasa Griego de Garcia House, which is well concealed from Edith Blvd. It was originally built as an L-shaped *terrón* (similar to adobe) building in 1855, and later owners added two more wings and then covered the central *placita*. This Spanish Revival–style home is also known as the Koeber House.

The next 150 yards of ditch road run along the east side of Sandia Ranch. It started as one adobe structure—allegedly a stagecoach stop—in the 1860s. Three more cinder block buildings were added, framing a central courtyard, and in the 1920s or (more likely) 1930s, the complex became the Sandia Ranch Sanitarium. Dr. John Meyers arrived in 1935 to serve as medical director. Throughout the 1960s, this private facility was embroiled in litigation, but operations didn't cease until 1969, shortly after Meyers' death. Ghost stories about the asylum often refer to torturous experimental practices that are too grim to repeat here. The complex soon became a nursing home. Reports of appalling conditions, along with repeated failures to meet fire code and licensing requirements, led to its final closure in 1998. Over the next five years or so, the abandoned structure served as a gang lair, meth lab, and crack den. Repeated incidents of arson and vandalism have since rendered it unsuitable for crackhead habitation.

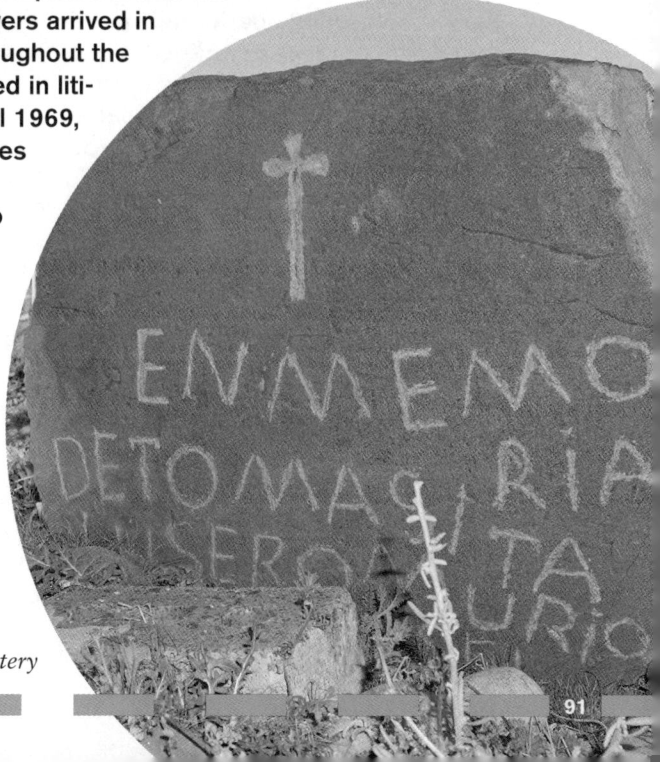

Homemade tombstone in Mt. Carmel Cemetery

With a history that reads like *One Flew Over the Cuckoo's Nest* and *Breaking Bad* rolled into one horrific script, this haunted insane asylum has achieved epic notoriety. The building is condemned, and the owner has announced his intentions to raze it to make room for a cemetery. However, that was several years ago, and the obscure ruins still stand, albeit barely, in a dense cluster of trees. Its morbid allure begs for exploration, but beware that the owner lives on the ramshackle compound just across the ditch. Rumor has it he's armed, ornery, and justifiably intolerant of trespassers.

- The ditch road turns west, passing near the sanitarium's south wing, which collapsed sometime during the monsoon season of 2014. From here the lateral and road turn south again. You're a safe distance from the hospital, but you're not entirely in the clear: A gate ahead was designed to block access for both pedestrians and unauthorized vehicles. However, at last check, it was damaged well beyond its function. "No Dumping" signs appeared on the fence sometime around 2012, shortly after the body of a teenager was found in the ditch here, but there's nothing posted about trespassing. The remaining quarter mile of ditch road is an unobstructed escape route to the northwest corner of Edith Blvd. and Osuna Rd.

If by now you need assurance that a civilized world still exists, take heart in the immediate proximity of both a tearoom and a prep school. The St. James Tearoom stands on the southwest corner. Formal tea here is a luxurious experience in a vintage atmosphere with elegant cuisine. On the southwest corner is the Sandia Prep campus. Catch a soccer match if you can. The boys' team took the 4-1A state title 17 times in 28 years (1985–2013).

Blake's Lotaburger, a local franchise that began in 1952, stands on the northeast corner. *National Geographic*'s *The 10 Best of Everything* ranks Blake's at number four on the hamburger list and goes on to contentiously claim, "Their green chile cheeseburger is the best in the world."

- Turn left and walk north on Edith. The Barela de Bledsoe House mentioned earlier is a half mile up on the left at 7017 Edith. At 7442 Edith is the Juan Antonio Garcia House, sometimes referred to as the Ranchos House or the Tappan House. Originally built as yet another stagecoach stop circa 1865, this private residence reportedly preserves the only known oxblood-cured mud floor in the Albuquerque area. A vintage pickup truck permanently parked in the yard adds a certain charm.

The Felipe Romero House, at 7522 Edith, is a modest adobe Territorial-style home built around 1904 and added (along with the other houses mentioned) to the National Register of Historic Places in 1984. The blue door and window frames are meant to indicate hospitality or keep out evil spirits, depending on whom you ask. The tradition dates back to the Spanish Colonial era and is more common in northern New Mexico.

- Continue north another quarter mile or so to find the aforementioned cemetery on the right and Our Lady of Mount Carmel Church slightly farther up on the left. The latter was built sometime between 1870 and 1890 as the Candelaria family's private chapel. When the 1903 flood destroyed the plaza of Los Ranchos and its chapel, along with the Alameda Church, services for those communities were held here. Renovations in 1940 included a proper floor to cover the original packed dirt floor, the addition of a pitched tin roof, and a reorientation to face east rather than west. The National Register of Historic Places notes, "Its remodeling is an outstanding example of a vernacular interpretation of the Pueblo Revival style." That relates to the New Mexico Vernacular style, which combines traditional building styles with new or recycled materials that were not widely available in the region prior to the arrival of the railroad in the 1880s.

- Another quarter mile or so north brings you to the southeast corner of Plant World, the largest wholesale nursery in the state. It's a great place to browse for landscaping ideas, but you must be a registered member to buy anything. Its entrance is on El Pueblo Rd., directly south of the Rail Runner parking lot.

POINTS OF INTEREST

New Mexico Earth Adobes newmexicoearth.com, 310 El Pueblo Rd. NE, 505-898-1271

St. James Tearoom stjamestearoom.com, 320 Osuna Rd. NE, Suite D, 505-242-3752

Blake's Lotaburger lotaburger.com, 6600 Edith Blvd. NE, 505-344-7105

Our Lady of Mount Carmel Church 7813 Edith Blvd. NE

Plant World plantworldinc.com, 250 El Pueblo Rd. NE, 505-898-9627

route summary

1. Start at the Los Ranchos/Journal Center Rail Runner station and walk a quarter mile east to the southeast corner of Edith Blvd. and El Pueblo Rd.
2. Turn south and follow the dirt road on the near side of the ditch.
3. Turn right to cross Edith Blvd. and pick up the path on the north side of the ditch.
4. Turn left and walk north on Edith Blvd.
5. Turn left on El Pueblo Rd. to return to the Rail Runner station.

connecting the walks

Pick up Walk 13 by going 0.75 mile north on Edith to Alameda.

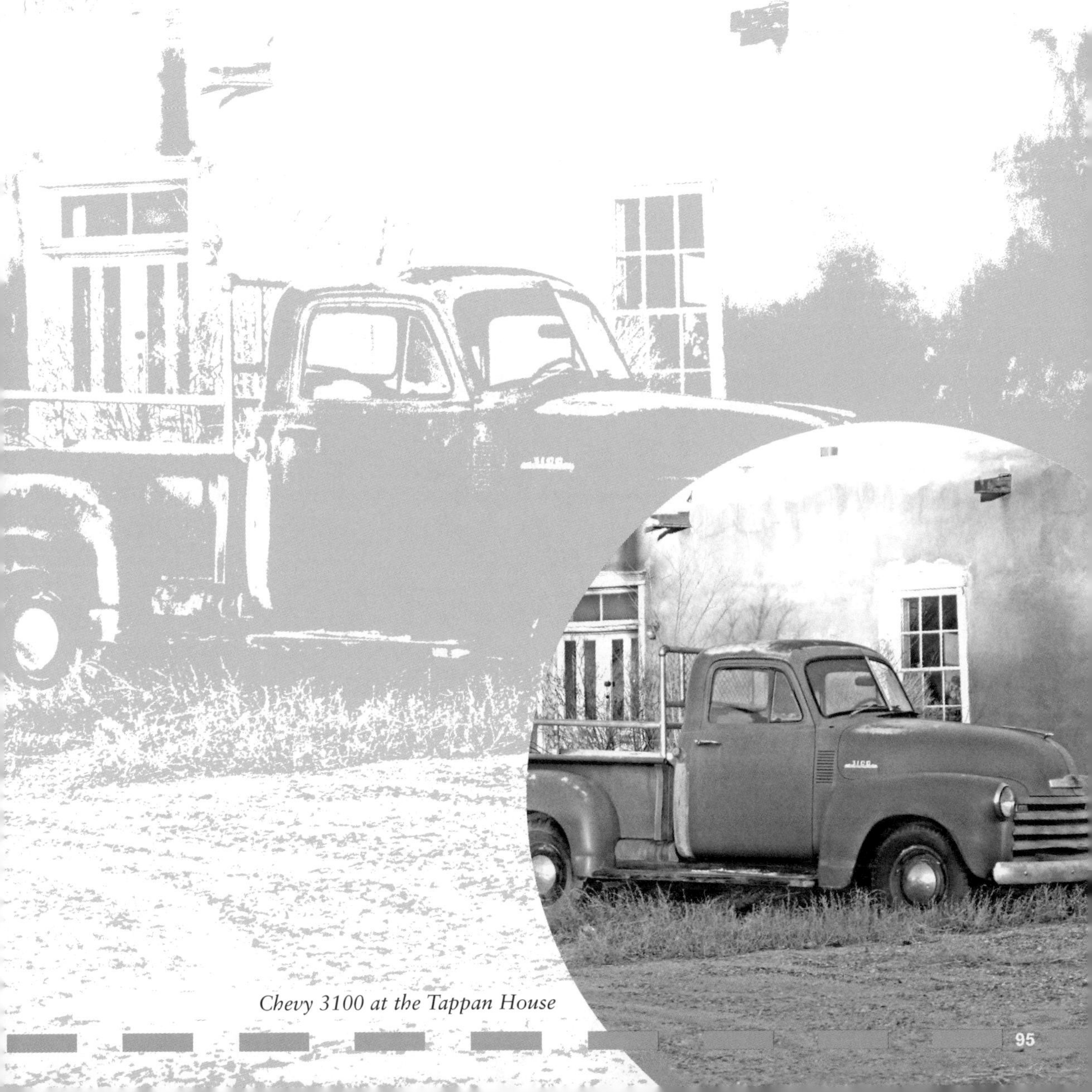

Chevy 3100 at the Tappan House

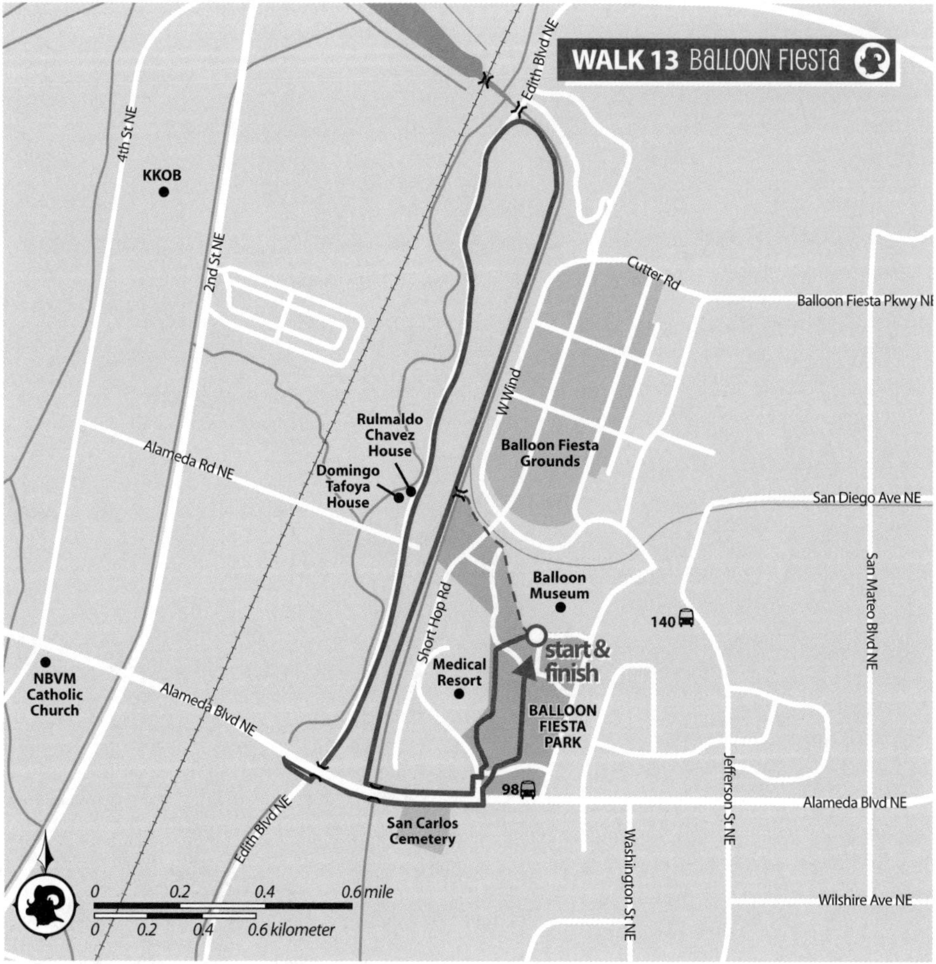
WALK 13 Balloon Fiesta
Edith Blvd NE
4th St NE
KKOB
2nd St NE
Cutter Rd
Balloon Fiesta Pkwy NE
W Wind
Rulmaldo Chavez House
Domingo Tafoya House
Alameda Rd NE
Balloon Fiesta Grounds
San Diego Ave NE
Balloon Museum
Short Hop Rd
140
start & finish
Medical Resort
San Mateo Blvd NE
NBVM Catholic Church
Alameda Blvd NE
BALLOON FIESTA PARK
Jefferson St NE
98
Alameda Blvd NE
San Carlos Cemetery
Edith Blvd NE
Washington St NE
0 0.2 0.4 0.6 mile
0 0.2 0.4 0.6 kilometer
Wilshire Ave NE

13 Balloon Fiesta: Diamonds, Dirigibles, and Other Diversions

BOUNDARIES: **Balloon Museum Dr., Alameda Blvd., Edith Blvd.**
DISTANCE: **4.25 miles; 1.75-mile shortcut**
DIFFICULTY: **Moderate (unpaved sections, narrow road shoulders); easy shortcut**
PARKING: **Free parking at the Balloon Museum**
PUBLIC TRANSIT: **Bus 98 stops on Alameda Blvd. near Balloon Museum Dr.; bus 140 stops on Jefferson St. near Balloon Museum Dr.**

What was once a barren foothill informally known as Rattlesnake Mesa is now an oasis for golf, baseball, and an international balloon fiesta. Running alongside these new fields of green is a concrete conduit that protects the city from rare but severe floods while providing a major thoroughfare for nonmotorized traffic. For the scenic route, venture beyond the end of the paved trail and loop back with a walk down an eccentric stretch of Edith Blvd. Or take the shortcut and still hit most of the highlights, the first (and best) of which is the Anderson-Abruzzo Albuquerque International Balloon Museum. Give yourself an extra hour for their multimedia exhibits on espionage, atmospheric monitoring, space exploration, and other amazing things balloons can do.

- **Start at the Balloon Museum and walk southwest toward the baseball/softball diamonds. The red-roofed building directly west of the ball fields marks the site of various healthcare facilities for the past 85 years. In 1930 the Dominican Sisters of Grand Rapids, Michigan, built the Nazareth Sanitarium to treat patients with tuberculosis. The three-story, red tile–roofed building stood at the end of a lonely dirt road high upon what was then known colloquially as Rattlesnake Mesa. In 1946, the sisters adjusted their mission, and the sanitarium became Nazareth Psychiatric Hospital. Like the insane asylum in the previous walk, Nazareth gained notoriety for its harsh conditions and practices. The original building was likely torn down in 1973, though records indicate that the sisters sold the hospital for $1 million in 1976, and Sandia Vista Hospital continued psychiatric operations there until closing in 1987. After 12 years and about as many millions of dollars in renovations, the facility reopened as the Medical Resort at Fiesta Park, a 66,000-square-foot facility offering rehabilitation services to** inpatients in an upscale setting. Now, instead of electroshock therapy and overdoses of thorazine, patients can enjoy such amenities as concierge service, spa treatments, a coffee bistro and Internet lounge, and a movie theater.

- Continue walking south past the ball parks, and turn right on Alameda. On the south side of this four-lane boulevard is San Carlos Cemetery. For those taking the shortcut, consider visiting it now to see a fascinating assortment of folk memorials. The entrance is on the west side. The most interesting graves are at the far end of the paved drive. For those in for the long haul, drop in on the way back.

  Note the blue-capped, cereal-box shaped buildings standing in the distance about half a mile past the cemetery. Those belong to General Mills. Sometimes when the wind is blowing right, you can smell freshly baked breakfast cereal. You can try to guess from the sweet aroma which sugary batch they're baking, but it always smells like cookies.

  Also note the blue-tipped towers poking up from the Nativity of the Blessed Virgin Mary Catholic Church, just under a mile west. The original church, which stood another mile west, was destroyed in the flood of 1903. The one you see today was consecrated in 1913. It's built of sandstone on a granite foundation, and local residents used wagons to haul the quarried stone from the Sandia Mountains.

- Continue west on Alameda Blvd. until you cross the bridge over the North Diversion Channel. This concrete-lined drain was dedicated with a ceremonial five-bucket dousing in 1969. As its name suggests, the NDC diverts runoff from the arroyos and channels it north into the Rio Grande, effectively providing drainage for the entire Northeast Heights and protecting the North Valley from flooding. The names of its tributary arroyos echo the canyons from which they flow: Embudo, Bear, Pino, Domingo Baca—all very familiar areas to those who enjoy hiking this side of the Sandia Mountains.

- Turn right onto the North Diversion Channel Trail (aka Paseo del Nordeste Bike Trail) and walk north along the west side of the drain. This paved, motor-free path winds 8 miles south to the University of New Mexico Psychiatric Center. Our route today covers only the remaining 0.75 mile ahead.

The escarpment on your left rises about 35 feet from Edith Blvd., giving you a commanding view over the village of Alameda, which roughly spans between Edith Blvd. and the Rio Grande. When the Alameda Land Grant was awarded in 1710, the Rio del Norte (now called the Rio Grande) defined its eastern boundary. Had you stood here then, you would see the river flowing near the base of the escarpment. Over the two centuries that followed, the river would shift its course at least three times before settling into its current course about 2 miles west.

About half a mile ahead on your left, you'll see a yard jam-packed with the stripped-down wreckage of vintage cars, mainly Chevys and Pontiacs from the 1950s–1970s. Several are (were) 1961 Impalas—a classic model for lowrider aficionados. Directly across the street are two houses on the National Register of Historic Places: The Rumaldo Chavez House is the Spanish Pueblo–style home fronting the west side of Edith; the Domingo Tafoya House is hidden somewhere in the enclave behind it. Both structures may be difficult to spot from here depending on the foliage. Both are also what remains of a mercantile plaza that was active in the 1860s. (For the nearest contemporary interpretation of a traditional mercantile, visit La Parada de Alameda at 8917 4th St. NW, farmandtablenm.com.)

● Those walking the long route today will soon get a street-level view of the historic house. For now, continue north on the dirt road ahead. (Those taking the shortcut: Turn right on the bridge just ahead and aim for the museum.) Just north of the bridge, blacktop gives way to dirt and gravel where the NDCT ends and AMAFCA Maintenance Rd. begins. On your right, the green launch fields on the Balloon Fiesta Grounds measure about a half mile long and a quarter mile wide—or roughly the size of 56 football fields. When it's not jammed with 700 balloons and thousands of spectators, the south side serves as the Albuquerque Golf Training Center. Facilities include a six-hole, par 3 practice course and a driving range. The north end of the field is often used for soccer practices and tournaments. It's also popular with electric flyers, so you might see radio-controlled airplanes buzzing around

As you approach the end of the fiesta grounds, you'll see an array of radio towers on your left. About 0.75 mile farther east is the 670-foot, 50,000-watt KKOB radio tower. Now imagine that tower with a colossal Smokey Bear head impaled upon it. That's pretty much what it looked like on the final day of the 2004 fiesta, when the Smokey

Bear balloon collided with the very top of the tower. The pilot and two young passengers had no choice but to abandon the gondola and begin a long, terrifying descent to terra firma. Spectacles like that aren't entirely rare. From 1982 to 2013 the National Transportation Board investigated 74 balloon accidents in Albuquerque. On average, less than 1 in 10 resulted in a fatality.

Close ahead, the North Diversion Channel bends northwest to cross Edith Blvd., expand into a sediment basin, and join the Rio Grande.

- Turn left on Edith. Use caution. While traffic tends to be light, the road shoulders are narrow and a couple of blind curves in the first half mile are potentially dangerous. You could opt for the ditch road along the Alameda Lateral, which starts on the west side of Edith Blvd., but its serpentine route would add an extra quarter mile to the walk, and the right-of-way gets a bit sketchy in places, particularly between Baker Ln. and Negreat Pl.

The segment of Edith in this route runs 1.5 miles. The neighborhood is a mixed bag of quirks. You may spot a garden growing in adobe ruins, or a yacht perched high upon a scrubby hilltop. There are descansos (roadside memorials), coyote fences (spruce, fir, or cedar latillas wired together to form a rustic barrier), steel windmills, and livestock. There's also an abundance of American flags and just as many PRIVATE/NO TRESPASSING signs, all of which should be properly observed. For the most part, it's a fairly quiet community, save for the occasional train—railroad tracks run about a quarter mile west of Edith—and the roosters that crow all day long.

- Cross under the bridge and turn right onto the ramp; then take a sharp right onto Alameda. San Carlos Cemetery, mentioned earlier, is a quarter mile ahead on the right. If you skipped it on the way out, now would be a more convenient opportunity to drop in.

- Turn left on Horizon Blvd. to return to the Balloon Museum.

POINTS OF INTEREST

Anderson-Abruzzo Albuquerque International Balloon Museum balloonmuseum.com, 9201 Balloon Museum Dr. NE, 505-768-6020

City of Albuquerque Golf Training Center cabq.gov/parksandrecreation, 9401 Balloon Museum Dr. NE, 505-857-8437

ROUTE SUMMARY

1. **Start at the Balloon Fiesta Museum and walk southwest past the baseball fields.**
2. **Turn right on Alameda Blvd.**
3. **Turn right on the North Diversion Channel Trail and continue straight on the dirt road. (Shortcut: Turn right on the bridge before the pavement ends and return to the museum.)**
4. **Turn left on Edith Blvd.**
5. **Cross under the bridge and turn right onto the ramp.**
6. **Turn right on Alameda Blvd.**
7. **Turn left on Horizon Blvd. to return to the Balloon Fiesta Museum.**

CONNECTING THE WALKS

Pick up Walk 12 by going 0.75 mile south on Edith to El Pueblo Rd.

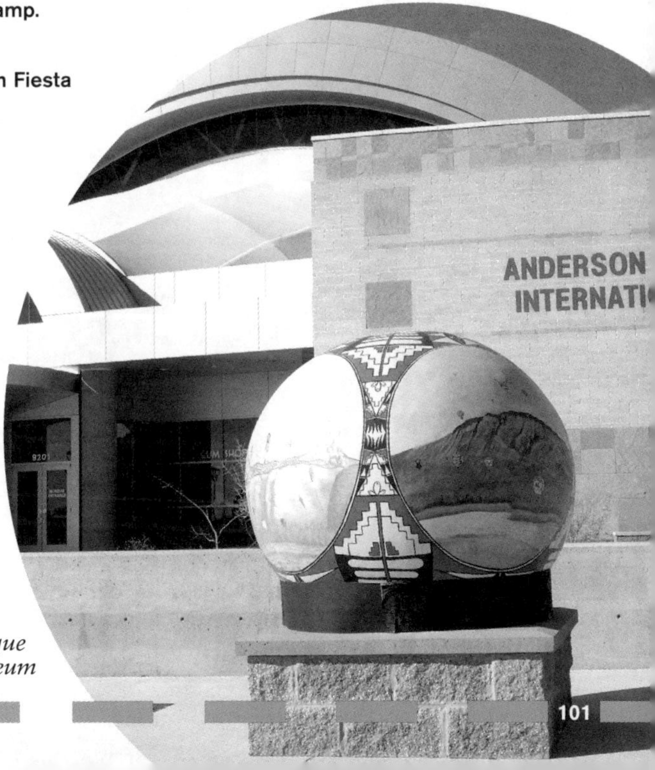

Anderson-Abruzzo Albuquerque International Balloon Museum

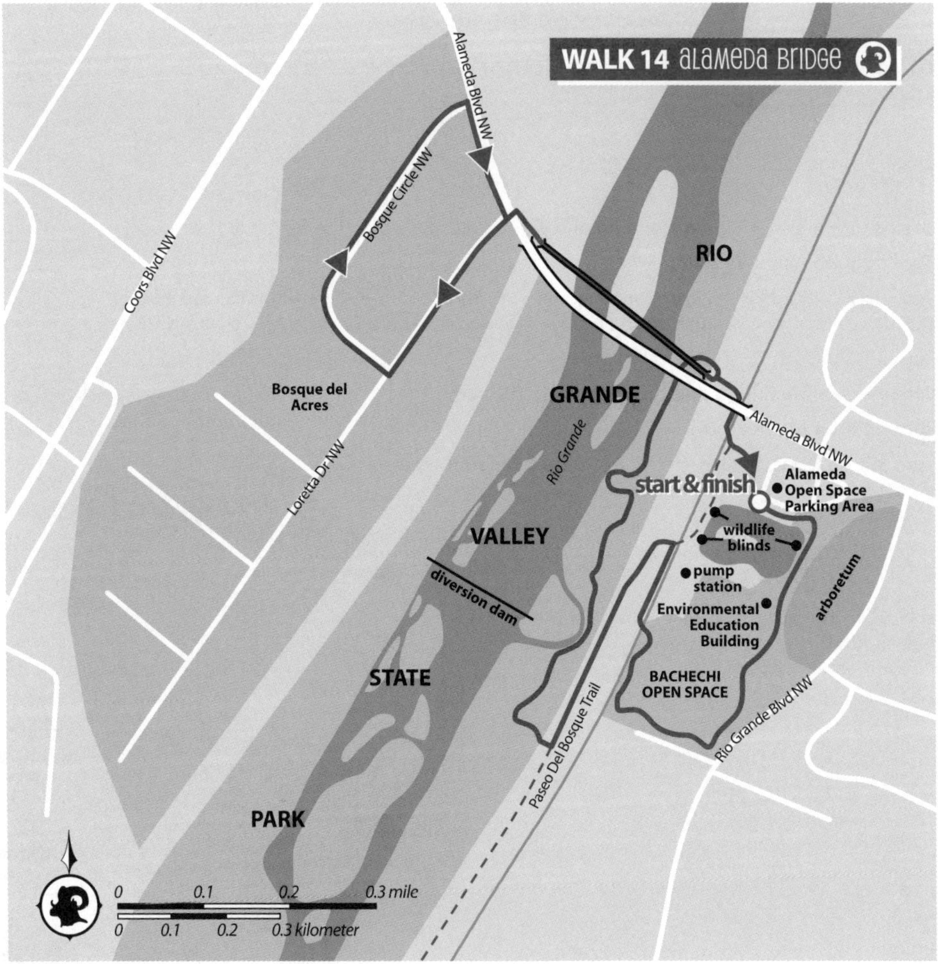
WALK 14 Alameda Bridge
Alameda Blvd NW
Bosque Circle NW
Coors Blvd NW
RIO
Bosque del Acres
GRANDE
Alameda Blvd NW
Loretta Dr NW
Rio Grande
start & finish
Alameda Open Space Parking Area
wildlife blinds
VALLEY
pump station
diversion dam
Environmental Education Building
arboretum
STATE
BACHECHI OPEN SPACE
Rio Grande Blvd NW
Paseo Del Bosque Trail
PARK
0 0.1 0.2 0.3 mile
0 0.1 0.2 0.3 kilometer

14 Alameda Bridge: Crossing the Same River Twice

BOUNDARIES: **Alameda Blvd., Rio Grande Blvd., Kitts Ln., Bosque Circle**
DISTANCE: **3 miles**
DIFFICULTY: **Moderate (dirt/sand surfaces)**
PARKING: **Parking lot closes at 9 p.m. April–October, 7 p.m. November–March**
PUBLIC TRANSIT: **Bus 98 on Alameda Blvd. at Rio Grande Blvd.**

At the northern reaches of Rio Grande Valley State Park, Alameda Open Space provides access to both the 16-mile-long Paseo del Bosque Trail and a recently established county property, Bachechi Open Space. The latter is named for Carlo and Mary O. Bachechi, who settled here in 1938 to raise a family in an agrarian environment. Less than a mile north, Bosque del Acres exists as a "living" agricultural community. This walk provides a glimpse into small family farms, both reconstructed and active, while examining elements in a complex water system that runs between them.

- **Start at Alameda Open Space and go through the gate on the south side of the parking lot.**

- **Turn left and follow the paved path east along the north side of the wetland preserve. This constructed wildlife area is part of ongoing efforts to restore the vast amounts of natural wetlands lost to development along the Rio Grande in the past 60 years. Continue to the map signboard ahead and take a moment to get oriented to Bachechi Open Space.**

- **Turn south and follow the gravel path toward the Environmental Education Building. Along the way, another path heads east and splits into an approximately quarter-mile network of trails that loop through the North Star Arboretum. Here in 1956, the McIntyre family founded the North Star Farm-Nursery to grow lumber pine and oak, in addition to plum, peach, and apple trees. They also introduced pecans. At the time, many doubted that trees originating in the Mississippi River Valley would survive in the Middle Rio Grande Valley, but they did, and New Mexico now supplies 20 percent of the nation's pecans. The nursery thrived as one of the largest in the state for more than 25 years. Many of its long-established trees remain in the arboretum. Signs**

Back Story: Crossing Two Rivers at Once

Two kinds of water flow beneath Alameda Bridge: native and imported. Native water comes from the upper reaches of the Rio Grande Basin in southern Colorado, east of the Continental Divide. Imported water starts on the west side in the Colorado River Basin and is diverted from the San Juan River, through 26 miles of tunnels beneath the Continental Divide, and into the Rio Chama in the Rio Grande Basin. Both kinds of water have been flowing through Albuquerque since 1971. At that time, the city's sole source of drinking water came from the Albuquerque Basin Aquifer, ground water beneath the city that was thought to be unlimited. But studies in the early 1990s showed that the aquifer was only half the size as originally thought and was being pumped at twice the rate that nature could replenish it. For a new source of drinking water, Albuquerque looked to the Rio Grande. However, due to the Rio Grande Compact, an archaic contract that somehow entitles Texas to most of New Mexico's water, the city lacks the right to tap native water for drinking purposes. And so in 2007 the diversion dam was installed essentially to remove only imported water and let the native water continue on its journey to Texas. The San Juan–Chama Drinking Water Project took a full decade and $400 million to implement—a fair price for water, compared to the cost of going without it.

along the way identify "habitat zones" that have been enhanced to attract Western screech owl, Woodhouse's toad, and roadrunner, among others.

Whether you stay on the direct path or detour through the arboretum, you'll eventually arrive at a boardwalk that crosses a pond and the acequia known as the Lane Lateral. This brings you to the the Bachechi Environmental Education Building (BEEB), an unimposing facility that's open only for special events and interpretive programs. Continue south to the Bachechi Family Memorial Rose Garden to see (and smell) the legacy of Mary O.'s original rose bushes.

- Continue following the walking path clockwise until you reach the Y near the south side of the pump station. Built to resemble a Spanish Mission church, the Albuquerque/Bernalillo County Water Utility Authority Raw Water Pump Station is just one stage in an elaborate process of moving water—about 80 million gallons per day—from the Rio Grande to a treatment plant about 3.5 miles southeast.

- Veer left at the Y and follow the path through the gate ahead.
- Turn right on the ditch road and go northeast to the paved Paseo del Bosque Trail. A wildlife blind stands nearby. If you opted for the arboretum detour earlier, then you probably bypassed the wildlife blinds on the east side of the wetlands. The one here is better because the Sandia Mountains provide a superior backdrop to the view.
- Go west on the footbridge to cross the Atrisco Feeder Canal, also known as the Albuquerque Riverside Drain, and follow the Paseo del Bosque Trail south. The paved trail ramps up to the top of the levee, providing a higher perspective of Bachechi Open Space. After passing its southern boundary, about a quarter mile from the bridge, keep a lookout on your right to locate a trail that descends through a gap in the flood-control fences, or jetty jacks, which resemble antitank obstacles. The U.S. Army Corps of Engineers installed more than 32,000 of these giant iron crosses throughout the Middle Rio Grande bosque to protect the levee from flood debris. Upriver damming has since rendered them obsolete, although they do prove to be useful props for postapocalyptic movies.
- Turn west to descend the steep embankment and follow the trail to a dirt road.
- Turn right on the dirt road and follow it northeast to a chain-link fence. The fence surrounds other facilities in the San Juan–Chama Drinking Water Project. An adjustable dam diverts water from the river into the diversion intake. The U-shaped canal surrounding the intake allows minnows to circumvent the dam. If it seems like a lot of effort to accommodate the little fishes, consider this: Prior to the European arrival in New Mexico, at least 28 species of fish swam in the Rio Grande. Today, only 15 of those species remain. The introduction of exotic species in the late 1800s, the loss of wetlands, and the construction of the dams mentioned earlier were exceptionally hazardous to fish populations, in particular the silvery minnow. The U.S. Fish and Wildlife Service declared it an endangered species in 1994. Since then, several silvery minnow sanctuaries have been constructed along the river. The passageway here allows them to swim upstream to better breeding grounds.
- Follow the sandy trail along the fence in a northerly direction to a maintenance road. Continue north on this dirt road to an unmarked facility. (Otherwise known as the "Re-Use Facility," it draws water from the river and pumps it to irrigation sites such as golf courses and Balloon Fiesta Park.) Take a moment to enjoy views over the river from

the walkway that encircles this structure, and then continue north on a footpath that passes beneath Alameda Bridge and its near neighbor, the old Alameda Bridge. This brings you to the Alameda Picnic Area.

A bench and plaque near the river's edge stand as an obscure memorial to Corbin Blake Hayes. On May 28, 2009, the 13-year-old Rio Rancho resident was swimming about 9 miles upstream when a current swept him away. After a five-day search involving rescue teams with helicopters, hovercraft, scuba divers, and search dogs, his body was found here. The unattributed quote on the plaque is a seemingly prophetic statement that Corbin posted on his MySpace page days before his death.

- Go southeast from the picnic area to pick up the path that hooks around and leads you up onto the old Alameda Bridge, which has been preserved for pedestrians, skaters, cyclists, and equestrians to enjoy. Views along the right railing overlook sandbar islands and restored wetlands. At the far end of the bridge, down to the right, the Upper Corrales Riverside Drain empties into the Rio Grande, while the parallel canal, Nicolls Drain, tunnels beneath Alameda Blvd. and reemerges on the south side as the Lower Corrales Riverside Drain. Continue straight on the sidewalk to the traffic light at Loretta Dr.

- Turn left and follow Loretta Dr. into the Bosque del Acres. The predominant architectural style is perhaps best summed up as "ostentatious." It's vaguely reminiscent of something from the Reagan era. A kind of J. R. Ewing vibe resonates throughout the neighborhood despite recent attempts at contemporary residential development. You'd have to explore beyond the loop and find the fake covered wagons and the big plastic cow to get the full flavor of the area, but our designated route should provide an adequate sample of the recent mansions and older split-level ranch homes that surround cultivated fields and horse pastures, all within half a mile of the megastore district at the southern fringe of Rio Rancho.

- Turn right onto Bosque Circle and follow it around to return to Alameda Blvd. Odd decorative details crop up along the way. For example, a large brick addition on one older house somewhat resembles a middle-finger gesture. Don't be offended. It seems to be directed at the newer and substantially swankier residence across the street.

- Turn right onto Alameda Blvd. and follow it back to the pedestrian bridge. Once you cross back over the river, continue straight over a footbridge that crosses back over the Atrisco Feeder Canal.

- **Turn right on Paseo del Bosque Trail and follow it back to the parking lot.**

POINTS OF INTEREST

Alameda/Rio Grande Open Space cabq.gov, 1401 Alameda Blvd. NW, 505-452-5200

Bachechi Open Space bernco.gov/bachechi-3978, 9521 Rio Grande Blvd. NW, 505-314-0398

ROUTE SUMMARY

1. Start at the gate on the south side of the Alameda Open Space parking lot.
2. Turn left and follow the paved path to the map signboard.
3. Turn right and follow the gravel path clockwise until you reach the Y near the south side of the pump station.
4. Veer left at the Y.
5. Turn right on the ditch road and go northeast to the paved Paseo del Bosque Trail.
6. Go west on the footbridge and follow the Paseo del Bosque Trail south about a quarter mile.
7. Turn right and follow the trail to a dirt road.
8. Turn right and follow the dirt road north to the Alameda Picnic Area.
9. Go southeast from the picnic area to pick up the path that hooks onto the old Alameda Bridge.
10. Cross the bridge and continue straight to the traffic light at Loretta Dr.
11. Turn left and follow Loretta Dr. to Bosque Cir.
12. Turn right onto Bosque Cir. and follow it around to return to Alameda Blvd.
13. Turn right onto Alameda Blvd. and follow it back to the pedestrian bridge.
14. Cross back over the river and continue straight over the footbridge ahead.
15. Turn right on Paseo del Bosque Trail and follow it back to the parking lot.

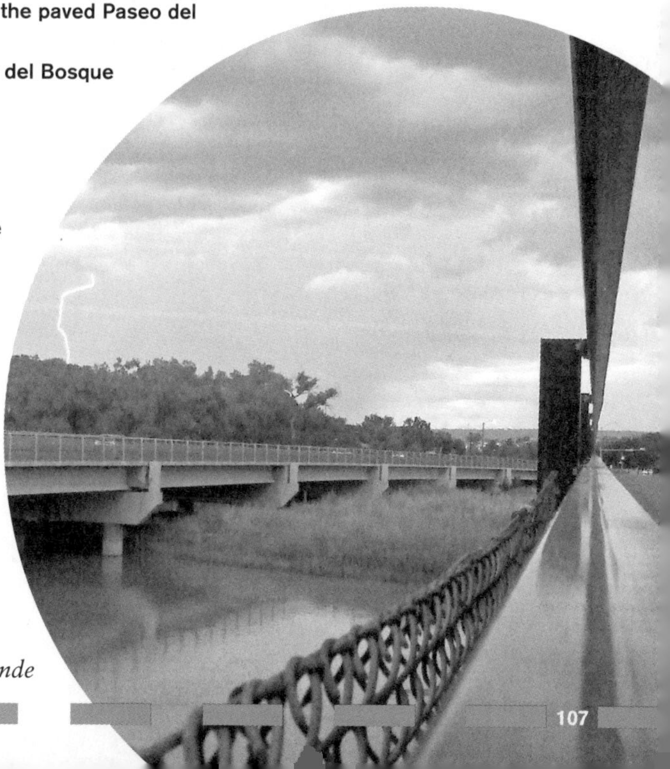

The Alameda bridges over the Rio Grande

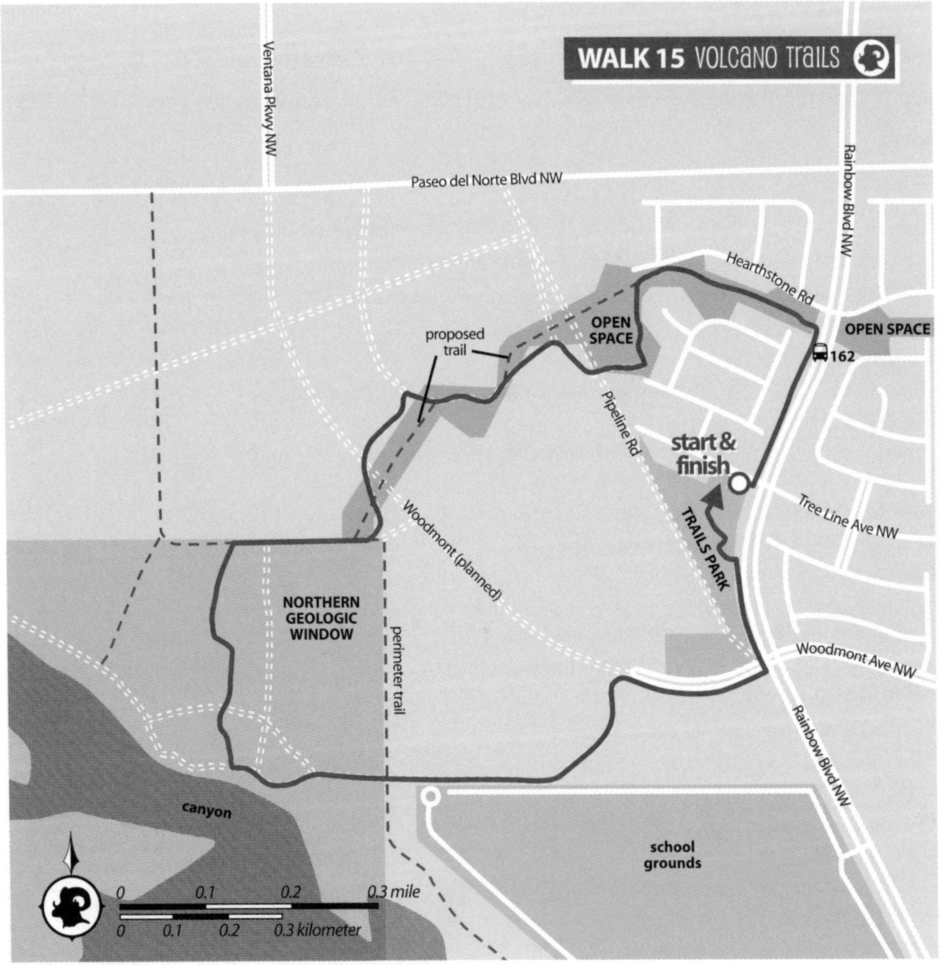
WALK 15 VOLCANO TRAILS
Ventana Pkwy NW
Paseo del Norte Blvd NW
Rainbow Blvd NW
Hearthstone Rd
OPEN SPACE
OPEN SPACE
162
proposed
trail
Pipeline Rd
start &
finish
Tree Line Ave NW
TRAILS PARK
Woodmont (planned)
NORTHERN
GEOLOGIC
WINDOW
perimeter trail
Woodmont Ave NW
Rainbow Blvd NW
canyon
school
grounds
0 0.1 0.2 0.3 mile
0 0.1 0.2 0.3 kilometer

15 Volcano Trails: Works in Progress

BOUNDARIES: **Rainbow Blvd., Tierra Antigua Elementary, Northern Geologic Window, Hearthstone Rd.**
DISTANCE: **2.25 miles**
DIFFICULTY: **Moderate (rocky, sandy terrain)**
PARKING: **Free parking at Trails Park**
PUBLIC TRANSIT: **Bus 162 on Rainbow Blvd. at Hearthstone Rd.**

The route below loops through recent residential developments and an ancient landscape within the boundaries of Petroglyph National Monument. It's the first of three walks in areas currently in the early stages of development. Describing routes like this can be exceptionally challenging because it involves both interpreting history and predicting the future; a walk description written in 2014 might not accurately reflect what visitors will find here in 2015 or later. In either case, a visit to Las Imágenes Visitor Center is highly recommended prior to setting out on this walk. There you can get the latest updates on sites throughout the monument.

- **Start at the Hailey Ratliff Trails Park parking lot on Tree Line Ave. west of Rainbow Blvd. (The 8-acre park is named for a former Tony Hillerman Middle School student who suffered a fatal collision with an SUV shortly after moving to California in 2012.) The centerpiece of this unnaturally grassy area is a sandy mound of basalt that hides the park's playground and picnic shelter. You won't find much shade later in the route, so if you packed a lunch, head for the shelter now. In mid-2014, the park was the western extent of development in Volcano Trails (now signed simply as "The Trails"), one of three sectors in the Volcano Mesa developments. A planning study in 2004 forecasted more than 100,000 additional residents at final build-out in the Volcano Mesa area and adjoining areas on the Northwest Mesa, but the invasion didn't advance as quickly as expected. Building permits peaked above 5,100 in 2004, then plummeted close to zero by 2006.**

- **Head back to Rainbow Blvd. and turn left on Rainbow Trail, a paved, protected bike lane that extends about 1.5 miles north to Irving Blvd. Follow it for just a quarter mile to the paved jogging trail at the end of the block. Everything you've seen so far in this compact development was open grassland in 2004. The blocks on the west side of Rainbow Blvd. filled in by 2005, but the east side wasn't done until 2012.**

Back Story: Pipeline Road

Imagine an arrow-straight road that begins in the heart of Albuquerque and extends on an unwavering course northwest for exactly 60 miles across some of the most spectacular landscapes on New Mexico's side of the Colorado Plateau. Historically, it begins somewhere near Central Ave. immediately west of the Rio Grande. Atrisco Dr. follows its alignment to Unser Blvd., which roughly follows it to Rainbow Blvd. In the massive sprawl of Ventana Ranch, it becomes a jogging trail, then resumes its steadfast course as a caliche road labeled as both Broadway Blvd. and Encino Rd. throughout the remainder of its journey across vacant tracts of northwest Rio Rancho. Soon after dropping over the precipitous edge of the West Mesa, it reaches the foreboding gates of a private ranch. The road becomes public again at the southwest corner of the Ojito Wilderness, but because of the gate, it's a 50-mile detour to cover the 7-mile distance between here and there. It soon blazes past the iconic volcano, Cabezon Peak. Then, near the village of Torreon, it bends slightly west. From there it makes a 40-mile beeline before US 550 picks up the alignment to Bloomington. In all, it's a 100-mile shot that skirts two national monuments and five wilderness areas. It's easy to imagine how a road like this could unite these lands for both public access and preservation. For now its primary purpose is to serve the gas industry.

- **Turn left on the jogging trail, which threads through the northernmost Volcano Trails' 41 acres dedicated to open space and parks. The jogging trail heads northwest, then soon starts to bend south. It ends at an opening in the subdivision wall.**

- **Turn right onto a dirt track and walk about 200 feet to an unmarked dirt/gravel road known as Pipeline Rd., one of the least known and most fascinating avenues in New Mexico. (See Back Story above.)**

  This is where things get a bit complicated. In 2014, plans called for an open-space corridor that connects the jogging trail to Petroglyph National Monument. Hopefully that will be developed soon and this route will be considerably easier to follow. For

now, there's little more than a tangle of dirt tracks. Our map shows the main trails as they existed in 2014, along with the proposed connecting route.

Regardless of what you find, just aim for the lone hill that peaks about 600 feet in front of you. Currently, that means crossing Pipeline Rd., veering right on a lesser road, then taking the first trail on the left. The trail ahead splits again to loop around the hill. Both branches arrive at the same dirt road on the other side. From there, you basically aim for the tallest volcano on the horizon; more specifically, toward the black scar you see just a quarter mile southwest. Head in that direction about 400 feet, or until you arrive at what will someday become Woodmont Ave. Cross the road and head south another 400 feet, and you'll arrive at an unmarked corner of Petroglyph National Monument.

This 7,532-acre park, established in 1990 and co-managed by the city of Albuquerque and the National Park Service, is best known for the estimated 25,000 rock-art images carved into basalt erupted from the approximately 200,000-year-old Albuquerque volcanic field. Ancestors of the Pueblo Indians used stone chisels and hammer stones to cut most of the petroglyphs into the basalt between 1300 and 1680 A.D. A few of the markings are much older, dating back to perhaps 2000 B.C. Spaniards and later generations of local inhabitants have produced petroglyphs, some of which are regarded as graffiti and vandalism. The monument includes about 17 miles of petroglyph-covered basalt cliffs and five volcanoes.

A corner post in a disintegrating fenceline marks the northeast corner of the monument's Northern Geologic Window (NGW). This area is characterized by blackened canyons—the scar mentioned earlier—created by the ancient lava flow. The erosion of sandhills in the area exposed these layers of volcanic rock. Hidden somewhere in the 360-acre plot are campsites dating back 3,000–4,000 years, along with a smattering of petroglyphs. The canyons were also used by Spanish shepherds in the 1800s to corral sheep.

The federal government finalized the purchase of the NGW in 2010, and plans for its use remain uncertain. Though considered sacred by Pueblo people, the land has long been—and continues to be—severely degraded by illegal dumping and off-road vehicles. In response, the national monument has considered installing sturdier fences around the NGW and limiting access to guided tours only. However, the Volcano Mesa development plan specifically requires a network of multiuse trails that provide public access to the NGW. This dilemma complicates predictions of what you'll find when you arrive here. Where you go from here may depend on the signage and fencing you encounter.

- Shortcut: Currently there's a well-defined dirt road that serves as a perimeter trail. Unfortunately, you won't see the canyon from this trail. You can take a shortcut by following it south to the first road junction. Recent signage posted here welcomes visitors into the NGW, provided they abide by a list of regulations.

- Canyon Exploratory: Follow the perimeter trail west along the north side of the NGW. Turn left on the second dirt road heading south. After a five-minute stroll through rolling sandhills, you'll arrive at the canyon rim. Along the way you'll likely scare up some rabbits. You might also find mounds of trash, most of it construction debris, which has been increasing as development creeps ever closer. Paradoxically, as the population of local residents grows, recreational use increases, along with demands to clean up and protect the monument.

  Most of the basalt that clutters the canyon walls lacks the patina of desert varnish, making it less than ideal for petroglyphs. Hence, you won't find many here. (To see bigger galleries of rock art, visit developed park sites at Boca Negra, Piedras Marcadas, and Rinconada Canyons. All are located 2–4 miles south–southeast of the Northern Geologic Window.) Explore the canyon at your leisure and watch out for rattlesnakes below the rim. When ready to continue on this route, return to the rim and follow the road east. As the canyon bends south, continue straight to the junction with the perimeter trail.

- Head east from the signed junction on the dirt road directly north of the school grounds, and follow it as it angles north to Woodmont Ave.

- Turn right on Woodmont Ave.

- Turn left on Rainbow Trail and follow it half a block north, where you'll find the east entrance to Hailey Ratliff Trails Park. Follow the walkway through the park back to the parking area.

POINTS OF INTEREST

Hailey Ratliff Trails Park cabq.gov/parksandrecreation, Tree Line Ave. and Rainbow Blvd., 505-857-8650

Las Imágenes Visitor Center nps.gov/petr, 505-899-0205, open year-round 8 a.m.–5 p.m. Serving as the Petroglyph National Monument's visitor center, Las Imágenes is located off Unser Blvd. NW at Western Trail, about a 4.5-mile drive south from Hailey Ratliff Trails Park.

ROUTE SUMMARY

1. **Start at the Hailey Ratliff Trails Park parking lot on Tree Line Ave.**
2. **Head back to Rainbow Blvd., turn left on Rainbow Trail, and go 1 block north.**
3. **Turn left on the jogging trail.**
4. **Turn right on the dirt road/open space trail and follow it southwest to the perimeter trail.**

   Shortcut: Go south on the perimeter trail to a signed junction, or

   Canyon Exploratory: Go west on the perimeter trail; then turn south on the second dirt road and follow it to the canyon rim. Go east on the rim road to the signed junction.
5. **Go east on the dirt road on the north side of the school grounds. Follow it as it angles north to Woodmont Ave.**
6. **Turn right on Woodmont Ave.**
7. **Turn left on Rainbow Trail and follow it half a block north.**
8. **Turn left into the east entrance to Hailey Ratliff Trails Park and follow the walkway back to the parking area.**

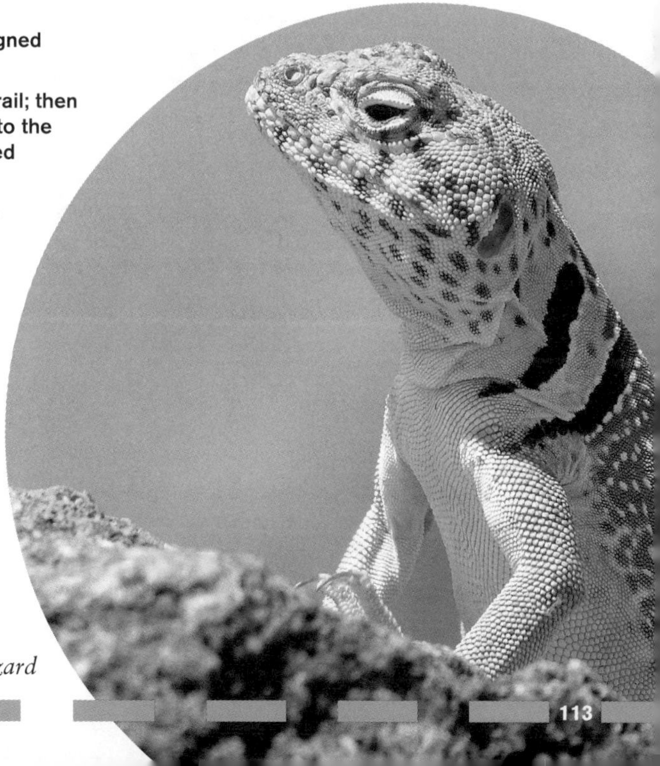

Collared lizard

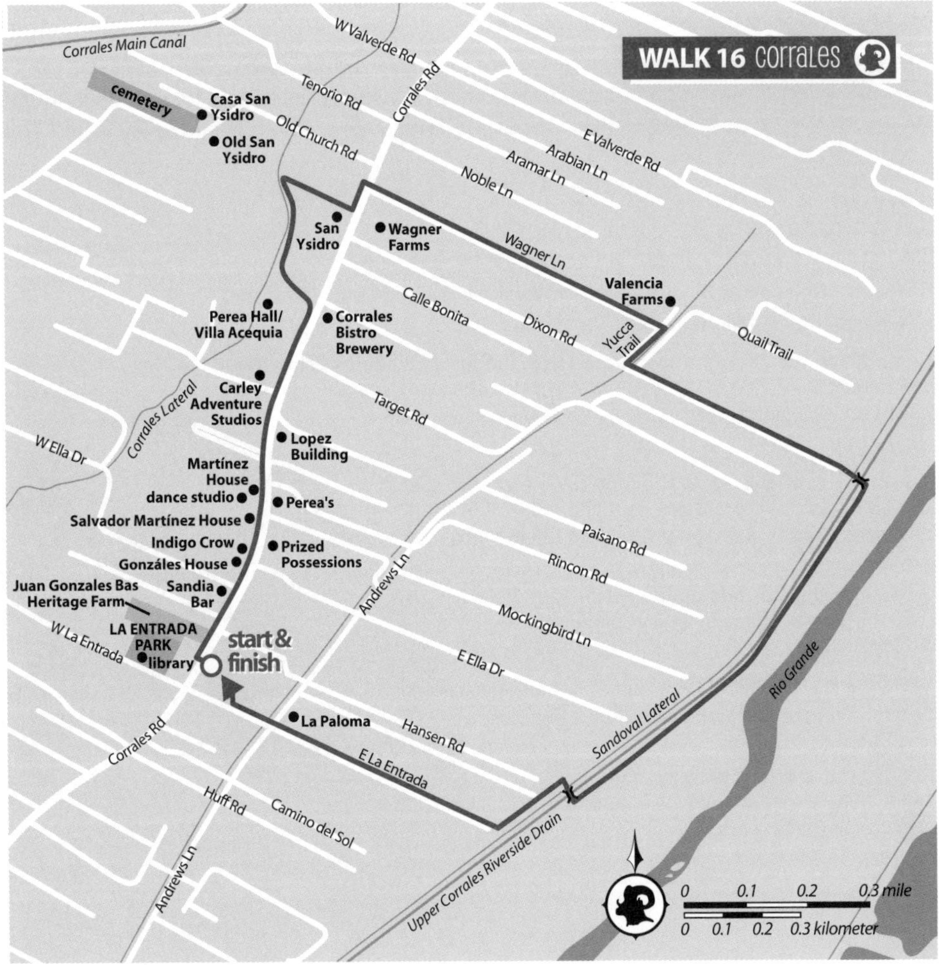
WALK 16 corrales
Corrales Main Canal
W Valverde Rd
Corrales Rd
Tenorio Rd
cemetery
Casa San Ysidro
Old San Ysidro
Old Church Rd
E Valverde Rd
Arabian Ln
Aramar Ln
Noble Ln
San Ysidro
Wagner Farms
Wagner Ln
Valencia Farms
Calle Bonita
Dixon Rd
Yucca Trail
Quail Trail
Perea Hall/ Villa Acequia
Corrales Bistro Brewery
Carley Adventure Studios
Corrales Lateral
Target Rd
W Ella Dr
Lopez Building
Martínez House
dance studio
Perea's
Salvador Martínez House
Paisano Rd
Indigo Crow
Prized Possessions
Gonzáles House
Rincon Rd
Juan Gonzales Bas Heritage Farm
Sandia Bar
Andrews Ln
Mockingbird Ln
LA ENTRADA PARK
library
W La Entrada
start & finish
E Ella Dr
La Paloma
Hansen Rd
Corrales Rd
E La Entrada
Sandoval Lateral
Rio Grande
Huff Rd
Camino del Sol
Upper Corrales Riverside Drain
Andrews Ln
0 0.1 0.2 0.3 mile
0 0.1 0.2 0.3 kilometer

16 Corrales: Horse Capital of New Mexico

BOUNDARIES: E. La Entrada Ln., the Corrales Lateral, Wagner Ln., Clear Ditch Rd.
DISTANCE: 3.25 miles
DIFFICULTY: Moderate (unpaved surfaces, narrow shoulders)
PARKING: Municipal complex at 4324 Corrales Rd.
PUBLIC TRANSIT: None

Follow the main street and back roads around the village of Corrales for a display of eclectic architecture from the past and present. Often you can identify an architectural style by the roof alone. Red tiles suggest Spanish Revival. Rounded corners are indicative of the Pueblo style. Flat roofs with stepped parapets and exposed vigas (ceiling beams) indicate Spanish-Pueblo Revival, more popularly known as Santa Fe style, which in turn developed into a craze for incorporating multiple styles into a single structure for no apparent reason. You'll find numerous examples of that on homes here. Corrales also has a long history as home to horses of all breeds, along with ample equestrian facilities, which include ditch banks, the Bosque Preserve, and the Top Form Arena. The Village of Corrales officially proclaimed itself the Horse Capital of New Mexico in 2011. You're likely to encounter a horse or two on the trails here, so be sure to review equine etiquette before setting out on this walk. (In short: Always yield to equestrians.)

- **Start at the municipal complex. You can pick up detailed information about local history, businesses, and events at the Corrales Visitor Center, if it happens to be open. If not, numerous signs out front provide useful information, though some are weathered beyond legibility. Across the street, though obscured by an office building, a shaded green with a playground and picnic table comprise La Entrada Park. The Corrales Library, built by volunteers in the 1980s, is on the west side of the park.**

- **Cross the street and go north on Corrales Road Scenic Byway. The invention of the sidewalk has not yet arrived in the rustic village, so use caution. (A good portion of municipal revenue is generated through traffic violations and towing fees, so it's in their best financial interest to preserve the inconvenience of walking.) The road gets exceptionally busy during special events—art studio tours, garden tours, wine tours, the harvest festival, and the scarecrow festival, to mention a few.**

On your left, directly north of the bank, is the Juan Gonzáles Bas Heritage Farm. In 1712 Capitan Juan Gonzáles Bas purchased the Alameda Land Grant from Francisco Montes y Vigil. He settled the land to graze cattle, horses, and sheep. He also introduced new crops such as wheat and barley and grew native produce—squash, melons, and small-cobbed corn. In 2004, villagers passed a bond for $2.5 million for obtaining conservation easements throughout the village, making Corrales the first town in New Mexico to pass bonds to preserve farmland. The Gonzáles Farm is their crowning achievement. The 6-acre property features a community garden and an ecologically sustainable farm with more than 20 Youth Conservation Corps members farming 50 varieties of crops. Some of the produce is available at the Growers' Market, which takes place by the post office Sunday mornings and Wednesday afternoons during summer and fall.

Standing on the south corner of W. Ella Dr., the Sandia Bar is a dank dive, but the beer is cheap, the folks are friendly, the pool tables are in good shape, and there's a cozy little patio out back. Ella Dr. was named for one of the daughters of Alejandro Gonzáles, "the Celery King," who owned hundreds of acres from the bluff west of Corrales to the Rio Grande. President Coolidge received a box of his celery for Christmas in 1924. The Gonzáles House, built in 1905, is now a law office at 4499 Corrales Rd.

Nearby to the north, the building that houses Indigo Crow Cafe first opened as a boardinghouse for workers on the Gonzáles farm. Reservations are recommended at the upscale cafe. Splurge on the lobster ravioli. Three doors up and standing on the east side of the road is the old Catholic Men's Society Meeting Hall. Built in 1910 the terrón building also served as a dance and wedding hall. It became a cannery during the Depression and a tractor garage during the war that followed. In the 1950s, as Corrales evolved into a budding art colony, it became an art gallery. It currently houses a jewelry and antiques store, Prized Possessions.

At 4541 Corrales Rd., the Salvador Martínez House was used as an itinerant court and headquartered the cavalry during the U.S. occupation of New Mexico in the 1840s. The house was built for Salvador Martínez, who purchased the northern half of Corrales from the Gonzáles family in the mid-18th century.

Another 50 yards north is another Martínez House, though this one is a relatively modest mud-plastered terrón home built for Cristóbal Martínez in the 1860s. Features include a symmetrical front façade, pedimented lintels over the doors and windows, and a sunken entryway. The tangentially attached building is the second of two dance halls built by the Perea family in 1946. Appropriately enough, it now serves as a dance studio.

Across the street, the "Tijuana Bar" sign on Perea's Tijuana Bar & Restaurant refers to an establishment where the Pereas honeymooned (and presumably drank) in the 1920s, when alcohol was illegal on this side of the border. One of oldest buildings in Corrales, the former home has grown considerably over the years. The addition that is now the barroom was added in 1900, the portal in the 1950s, and the walled patio in the 1980s. The Perea family has owned the building for the past century, with successive generations running the restaurant, which opened after Prohibition was repealed in New Mexico (1933).

The Lopez Building, at 4648 Corrales Rd., was built as a two-room trading post sometime between 1860 and 1898 for Jennie Weiner, who by local accounts was a Russian or German and Jewish or Arabic immigrant. In any case, with its pronounced brick coping, the building is an excellent example of Territorial-style architecture and has not changed significantly since 1927, except that the portal was added in the 1950s and the rear second story in 1988. It has a dance hall, a poker room, a pool hall, a dramatic theater, an art gallery, and a coffeehouse on its long resume. It currently offers psychotherapy services for children. A comprehensive history of the building is posted just inside the front entrance.

Grizz Carley's Adventure Studio, at 4765 Corrales Rd., seems to be the place in town for all things dealing with shooting arrows at animals and framing pictures of the results. Judging by the jeeps and Humvees

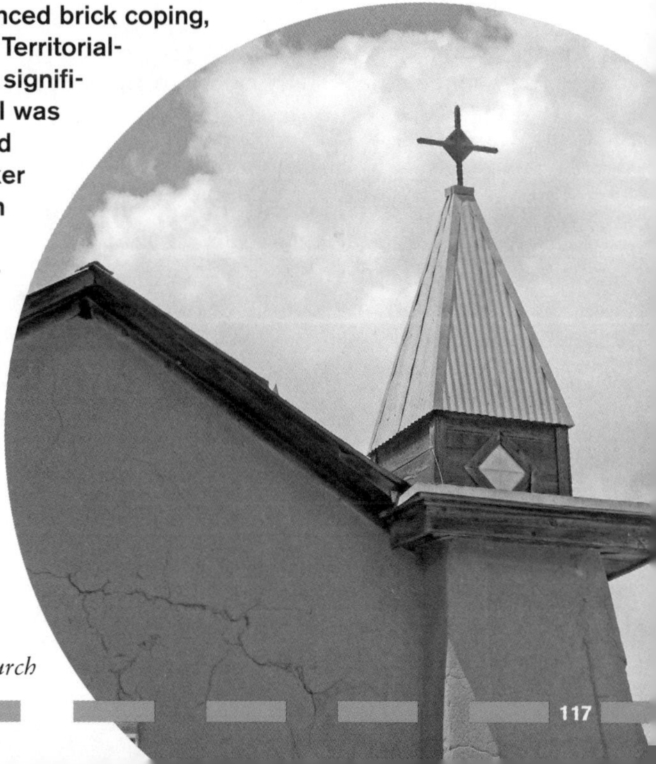

Old San Ysidro church

Back Story: L'Iglesia de San Ysidro Corrales and the Gutiérrez-Minge House

Named for the saint of the farmer and his fields, the Old San Ysidro church was built circa 1868 after a flood destroyed the first church in Corrales, L'Iglesia Jesus, Maria y Jose, which was located on the east side of Corrales Rd. Vigas and lintels from the older church were salvaged for the construction of this one. The twin towers function as buttresses to support the old adobe walls, which are nearly 3 feet thick. Every May volunteers gather to reapply mud to the walls in a weekend event known as Mudder's Day. Listed on the state and national historic registers, it's now used for village meetings, art shows, and a concert series. The historic cluster of structures located across the street began as a Greek Revival adobe rancho built for the Gutiérrez family around 1875. Historian Dr. Ward Alan Minge bought the house in 1953 and built several additions to reflect early New Mexican architectural styles. His extensive collections of New Mexico crafts, artifacts, and hand-forged farming tools are also on display here, along with Spanish Colonial furniture and handwoven rugs. The building and its collections are listed on the State Register of Cultural Properties. The complex includes a replica of a 19th-century rancho, complete with a corral, family chapel, and central plazuela. Gutiérrez-Minge House, also called Casa San Ysidro, is open to visitors during special events and for guided tours Tuesday–Friday, 9:30 a.m. and 1:30 p.m. and Saturday, 10:30 a.m., noon, and 1:30 p.m. The tour takes about an hour. Admission is $2 for children, $4 for adults. The sites are located on Old Church Rd., a mere 200 yards west of the acequia. Unfortunately, road hazards make walking it seem more like a suicide run, and the village has not yet sanctioned the path that safely connects its scenic byway to its most scenic site. For more info: 505-898-3915, **albuquerquemuseum.org/art-history/casa-san-ysidro**

parked out front, ol' Grizz is set to outfit hunting and fishing expeditions as well. His former office (the building directly northwest of the studio), is the old Abajo railroad station that once stood in Albuquerque. He also somehow managed to wrangle a few boxcars to round out the U-shaped plaza on his property.

Remember the dance hall across from Perea's? Apparently there's an Old Perea Hall, now referred to as Villa Acequia. Artist Bill Baker took over in 2005 to renovate it into his 1,000-square-foot "dream studio." One of the local art highlights in 2014 was the unveiling of its "sala grande," which showcased the work of 75 contemporary artists. Across the road is the Corrales Bistro Brewery. The food is fine, the beer is great—and if they have a band lined up, you certainly don't want to miss it.

Directly north of Old Perea Hall and across the street from the bistro is an empty lot where the historic "T-House" once stood. The T stood for "Territorial," or maybe just "Terror." Louis Imbert established a respectable vineyard here in 1883. In 1892, 10-year-old Luis Jr. accidentally shot and killed Lola Gallardo Griego as she was hanging grapes out to dry. In 1898, Louis Sr. murdered his recently divorced wife. While resisting arrest, he was killed by a one-eyed Indian named José de la Cruz. Later, in an unrelated incident, an alleged cattle thief was beaten into confession in the wine cellar, then hanged from a nearby mulberry tree.

In 1972, Monie Sanchez and former New Mexico State Police officer Bob Gilliland began renovating the homestead extensively to create the T-House bar and restaurant. Three years later, hooligan Richard Kaufman walked in brandishing a knife to settle an arm-wrestling match that Chavez had interrupted earlier in the day. Chavez disarmed Kaufman, then fired a bullet into him. Kaufman's roommate and arm-wrestling opponent, Jerry DeLorenzo, later arrived to fire a bullet into Sanchez, thus avenging Kaufman. Gilliland responded by firing 22 bullets into DeLorenzo with an M2 automatic, thus avenging Sanchez. Then noticing Kaufman was still alive, Gilliland retrieved his M1 rifle and smashed it over Kaufman's head. Moments later, Gilliland collapsed from a fatal heart attack, thus ushering vengeance to its proper conclusion. The restaurant, rechristened "Rancho de Corrales" in 1987, persisted as a decent establishment until it caught fire in February 2013. Firefighters from the station across the street, not 100 feet away, arrived hours later—perhaps too soon: An inspector later noted that the fire actually strengthened the old adobe walls, much in the way a kiln hardens clay. It was the dousing from fire hoses that destabilized the historic structure beyond repair.

- Turn left into the parking lot, giving a wide berth to this unhallowed ground, and aim northeast toward a gap in the fence at the back end of the parking lot to find a path to the Corrales Lateral. This prominent acequia, or irrigation ditch, has been channeling water to local farm fields since the early 18th century. The system has since been enhanced. Currently about 17 miles of canals and ditches course through Corrales. This walk samples a mere 200 yards, just to point it out for future reference. An extended walk from here east to, say, Mira Sol Rd. amounts to a gorgeous little hike, particularly if you return via the Clear Ditch Rd., which you'll soon see.

- Turn right on the ditch road with the least amount of mud. Ditch riders, or system administrators, use these service roads to maintain the flow of water from early May through early November. (Note the detour option in the Back Story section on page 118.)

- Turn right at the first dirt crossroad and follow it back to Corrales Rd., passing the new San Ysidro Church on your right. Wagner Farms Market and Apple Tree Cafe are straight ahead. They've been growing and harvesting crops since 1910. Make a note to pick up some fresh produce and a chile ristra before leaving town. They also operate a corn maze and pumpkin patch in September and October.

- Turn left on Corrales Rd.

- Turn right on Wagner Ln. and stroll half a mile to the end of this dirt road. Certainly by now you've noticed that Corrales smells like the City of Horses, which isn't necessarily a bad thing. Down to the left, Valencia Farms offers riding lessons, horse boarding and training, and riding camps for kids.

- Turn right on Yucca Tr. and walk along the Corrales Interior Drain.

- Turn left on Dixon Rd. This road ends with a single-lane bridge that crosses both the Sandoval Lateral and the Corrales Riverside Drain. Note the warnings about coyote activity. A shaded path follows the near side of the lateral, while the higher Clear Ditch Rd. is up on the dike on the far side of the drain. Cross the bridge for a view of the Corrales Bosque Preserve, a 662-acre ribbon of woodland between the levee and the Rio Grande. Depending on the season the air is flavored with a hint of olive, sage, or wild licorice. Spring winds bring blizzards of cottonwood fluff.

- Turn right on the dike road and go south just over half a mile. Along the way you may notice footpaths leading down the embankment on your left. These are part of an informal path system that spiderwebs between the road and the river throughout the cool deciduous woods. The paths often break up or disappear under weeds and fallen trees, but this dense floodplain habitat makes for a more interesting hike than does the linear dike road. Though rare, black bears occasionally raid nearby apple orchards and leave plenty of evidence. Detours along these trails can add a few hundred feet or a couple of miles to the hike, depending on how much you want to explore the bosque. Closer to the river, you may find tracks of porcupines, badgers, and raccoons. The dike road has the advantage of being easier to follow. Overlooking the bosque, drain, and nearby farm fields, you're more likely to spot wildlife, such as cottontails, muskrats, and any one of approximately 250 bird species—from ruby-crowned kinglets to yellow-rumped warblers. Hawks, owls, herons, and woodpeckers are also common in the area. In 2014, the Audubon Society identified the Corrales Bosque Preserve as an Important Bird Area (IBA).

- Turn right to cross a wooden bridge, and then locate the smaller bridge over the ditch ahead. Cross it and turn left. About 200 yards ahead, turn right and exit through the green gate at the end of La Entrada Ln. A block ahead, La Paloma employs adults with developmental disabilities who grow more than 28,000 plants and flowers annually, including ornamental succulents and organic wheatgrass. You can visit the greenhouse weekdays, 7:30 a.m.–3:30 p.m.

- Turn right after the solar-powered senior center to return to the municipal complex.

Points of Interest

Sandia Bar 4445 Corrales Rd., 505-897-7577

Indigo Crow Cafe indigocrowcafe.com, 4515 Corrales Rd., 505-898-7000

Prized Possessions prizedpossessionsjewelryantiques.com, 4534 Corrales Rd., 505-899-4800

Perea's Restaurant 4590 Corrales Rd., 505-898-2442

Carley Adventure Studios 4765 Corrales Rd., 505-897-4874

Corrales Bistro Brewery cbbistro.com, 4908 Corrales Rd., 505-897-1036

Wagner Farms Market wagnerfarmscorrales.com, 5000 Corrales Rd., 505-898-3903

Valencia Farms valenciafarms.com, 119 Yucca Tr., 505-899-5336

La Paloma Greenhouse arcaorganics.org, 181 E. La Entrada Ln., 505-897-2184

route summary

1. Start at the visitor center in the municipal complex.
2. Cross the street and go northeast on Corrales Road Scenic Byway.
3. Turn left after Villa Acequia and go through the gate at the far side of the parking lot.
4. Turn right on the ditch road.
5. Turn right at the first crossroad and follow it back to Corrales Rd.
6. Turn left on Corrales Rd.
7. Turn right on Wagner Ln.
8. Turn right on Yucca Tr.
9. Turn left on Dixon Rd.
10. Turn right on the Clear Ditch road and go half a mile southwest.
11. Turn right to cross two bridges.
12. Turn left and walk about 200 yards, and exit through the green gate.
13. Follow La Entrada Ln. back to the municipal complex.

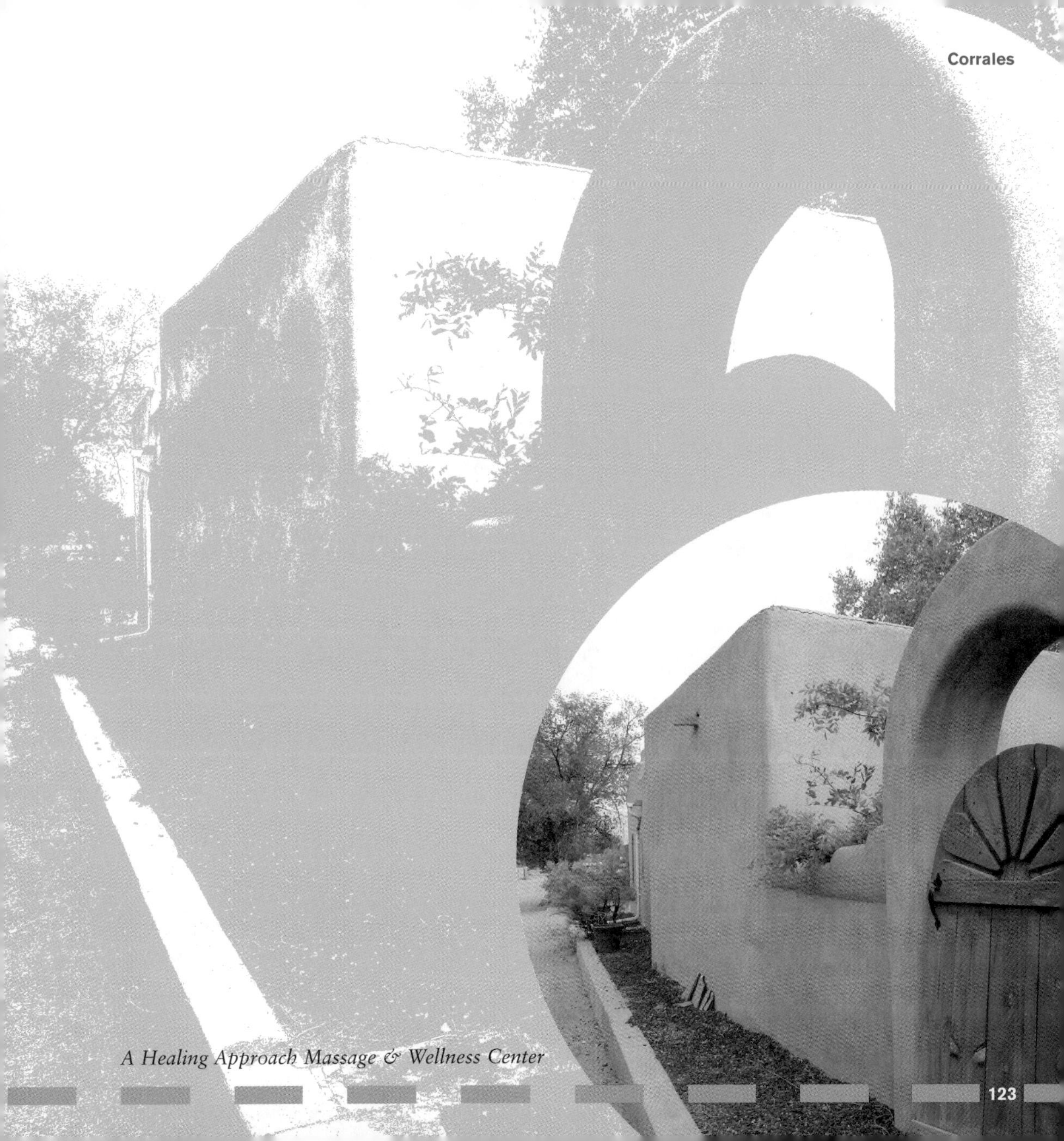

A Healing Approach Massage & Wellness Center

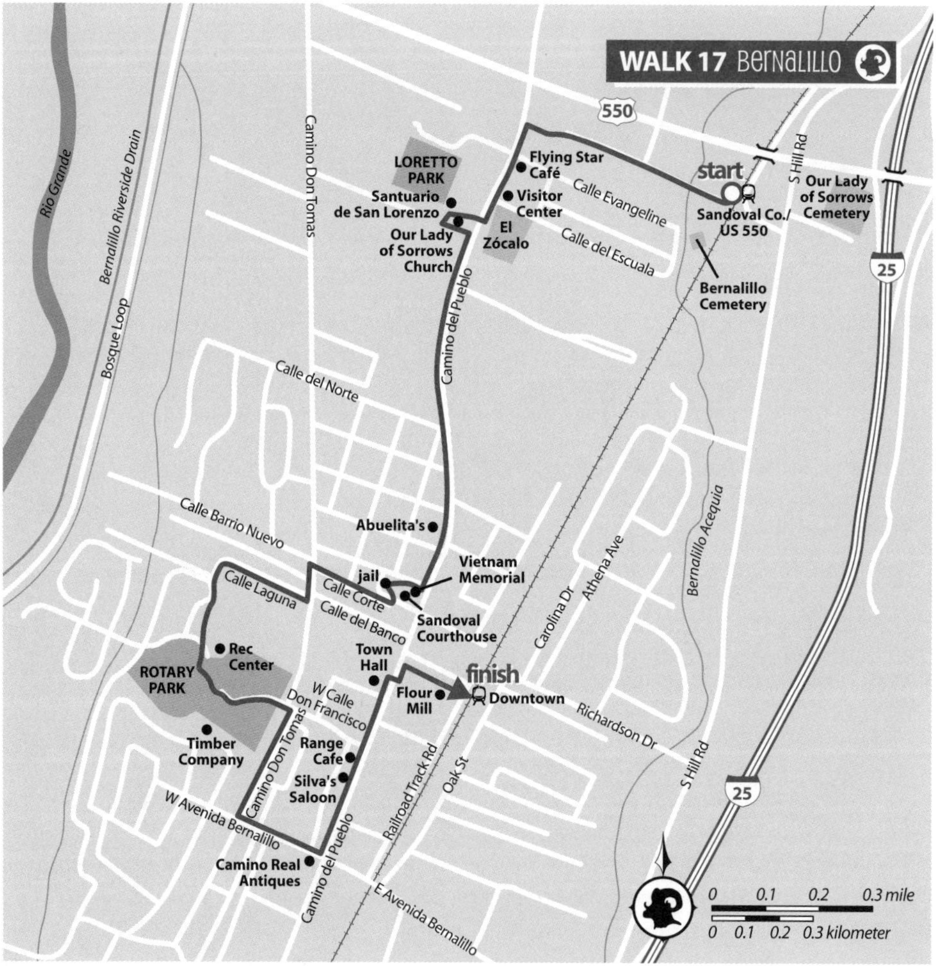
WALK 17 Bernalillo
550
25
start
Sandoval Co./ US 550
finish
Downtown
LORETTO PARK
Santuario de San Lorenzo
Our Lady of Sorrows Church
Flying Star Café
Visitor Center
El Zócalo
Calle Evangeline
Calle del Escuala
Our Lady of Sorrows Cemetery
Bernalillo Cemetery
S Hill Rd
Rio Grande
Bernalillo Riverside Drain
Bosque Loop
Camino Don Tomas
Camino del Pueblo
Calle del Norte
Calle Barrio Nuevo
Abuelita's
jail
Vietnam Memorial
Sandoval Courthouse
Calle Laguna
Calle Corte
Calle del Banco
Town Hall
Flour Mill
Rec Center
ROTARY PARK
Timber Company
W Calle Don Francisco
Range Cafe
Silva's Saloon
W Avenida Bernalillo
Camino Real Antiques
E Avenida Bernalillo
Railroad Track Rd
Oak St
Carolina Dr
Athena Ave
Bernalillo Acequia
Richardson Dr
0 0.1 0.2 0.3 mile
0 0.1 0.2 0.3 kilometer

17 Bernalillo: The City of Coronado

BOUNDARIES: Sandoval County/US 550 Rail Runner Station, Rotary Park, Avenida Bernalillo
DISTANCE: 3- and 3.5-mile options
DIFFICULTY: Easy
PARKING: Sandoval County Visitor Center, Rail Runner Stations
PUBLIC TRANSIT: Sandoval County/US 550 Rail Runner, Downtown Bernalillo Rail Runner Station

The area now known as the town of Bernalillo has been inhabited for nearly a millennium. Francisco Vásquez de Coronado made first contact with the Tiguex Pueblos here in 1540 and managed to destroy most of them by 1541. In 1598, Don Juan de Oñate began settling families on ranches and haciendas along this stretch of the Rio Grande. Mission priests established vineyards and wineries in the 1620s. In 1695, during the resettlement period following the Pueblo Revolt, Don Diego de Vargas formally established Bernalillo north of the current town site. In 1844, Bernalillo became the seat of government under the Mexican Republic. In 1857, Archbishop Lamy established the Bernalillo parish, Our Lady of Sorrows, on the north end of town. Local millionaire Jose Leandro Perea donated land to accommodate the church and convent. In his 1878 personal narrative, *The Conquest of New Mexico and California,* Philip St. George Cooke remarked: "Bernalillo is the prettiest village of the Territory. Its view, as we approached, was refreshing; green meadows, good square houses, and a church, cottonwoods, vineyards, orchards—these jealously walled in; and there were numbers of small fat horses grazing. The people seemed of superior class,— handsomer and cleaner." The AT&SF railroad found the town attractive as well and sought to establish their rail yards here. Content with living in a small town (and his power over it) Perea dissuaded them by inflating land prices from $2 to $425 per acre. The railyards went to Albuquerque instead. Still, Bernalillo profited from the rail line and the mining boom that spanned 1890–1910. A rowdy commercial district developed on the south end of town while the ecclesiastical atmosphere continued to grow on the north end. A century later, that divided pattern is still evident. However, today the bulk of Bernalillo's commercial sprawl runs along US 550, sparing the historic areas from fast-food and shopping franchises. Downtown Bernalillo is 7 miles north of Albuquerque city limits and can be accessed via I-25 or the Rail Runner.

First, a note on the route options: The directions begin at the Sandoval County/US 550 Rail Runner Station to encourage a stop at the Sandoval County Visitor Center

Back Story: Los Matachines

Las Fiestas de San Lorenzo are celebrated each August in honor of Bernalillo's patron saint. The highlight of Las Fiestas is the Los Matachines ritual, a dance-drama with roots in both Moorish culture and the earliest Spanish Colonial era. It was introduced in the New World as part of the efforts to convert indigenous peoples to Catholicism and today is one of the few dances performed by both Hispanic and Native peoples in the Southwest. In one interpretation, the elaborately costumed dancers tell the story of Montezuma, ruler of the Aztecs, and his daughter La Malinche, who influences his conversion to Christianity. El Toro, a bull representing the pre-Columbian religion and evil itself, stalks the dancers and attempts to disrupt the Montezuma's conversion. Spoiler alert: El Toro is killed in the end. The dance varies in style and meaning to those who perform it. La Malinche, for example, could be a traitor, a victim, or a heroine. In Bernalillo the ritual refers to the resettlement period that followed the Pueblo Revolt of 1680. Residents then vowed to dance in honor of San Lorenzo if he would keep them safe. The annual dance of Los Matachines has since remained an unbroken tradition.

early in the walk to the Downtown Bernalillo Rail Runner Station. The one-way route between stations is 3 miles. If not arriving by train, you can park at the visitor center and walk a round-trip route that runs 3.5 miles.

That said, welcome to the town of Bernalillo. For those interested in decrepit graveyards, Our Lady of Sorrows Cemetery and Bernalillo Cemetery are located east and south of the Sandoval County Station, respectively. Both are worth browsing if you have time to kill while waiting for a train.

- Otherwise, proceed west about a quarter mile to a road known as NM 313, Main Street, Pan American Central Highway, Old State Highway 85, Historic Route 66, El Camino Real National Scenic Byway, and the Rio Grande Pueblo Indian Trail. To avoid confusion, let's just call it Camino del Pueblo.

- Turn left on Camino del Pueblo. Flying Star Cafe is your first chance for food on this historic trail. While the cuisine at this Albuquerque-based chain is consistently good, you might want to save your appetite for local fare ahead.

  If you're in town for any of the popular events that take place in Loretto Park, the entrance is across the street. The New Mexico Wine Festival is a Labor Day weekend celebration that began in 1987 and now involves more than 20 wineries from around the state. Bernalillo was the center of New Mexico's wine industry throughout the 18th and 19th centuries. A religious order known as the La Salle Christian Brothers produced up to 10,000 gallons of wine annually. For more info on the fiesta, visit newmexicowinefestival.com.

- Continuing south on the east side of Camino del Pueblo, you'll find the aforementioned visitor center on the north corner of Calle del Escuela. On the south corner is the El Zócalo complex. Spanish for "the meeting place," El Zócalo includes a few historic structures. The Old Convent was built in 1874 and functioned alternately as a school and a cafeteria until 1966. In 2008 it was restored as a wedding and events center. To its south is the Abenicio Salazar Building. This two-story, 12,500-square-foot former Catholic high school, built in 1922, is the largest surviving example of Salazar's work. The walls are 28 inches thick and are constructed of traditional 9-by-18-inch adobe bricks. The building now houses offices and a small business–development center. Salazar was Bernalillo's master adobero from 1915 until his death in 1941. The town's historic district is also named for him. East of the convent, the Sisters of Loretto Barn was built in 1875 and renovated in 2011. The barn was part of a 34-acre farm operated by the sisters to support the school. The farm included 8,000 fruit trees, 1,000 grapevines, a brickyard, a quarry, and a devoted yard-keeper named Pablo.

- Cross to the west side of Camino del Pueblo to visit the historic mission originally dedicated in 1857 as Nuestra Señora de los Dolores. The church combines architectural features of preceding Spanish and Mexican periods with elements inspired by French-born Jean Baptiste Lamy, the first Roman Catholic bishop in New Mexico under United States rule. Native materials include 12-inch-diameter vigas, 4-foot-thick adobe walls, and an earthen floor. It served the community as the parish church for more than a century. In 1993, a new parish church was erected adjacent to the old mission. The new parish church was dedicated as Our Lady of Sorrows, while the historic church was rededicated as the Santuario de San Lorenzo. A courtyard south of the santuario contains Stations of the Cross, or Way of Sorrows.

- Go south half a mile to Abuelita's New Mexican Kitchen. Home of the "Tacopilla"—a giant sopapilla folded like a taco—Abuelita's has been dishing up hearty fare in Bernalillo for more than a quarter century. Another two blocks south, find the Bernalillo Vietnam Memorial on the north side of the Sandoval Courthouse. The original courthouse, a Victorian mansion that had belonged to the Perea family, burned in 1926, along with all records dating back to 1903. In the parking lot behind the courthouse is the old stone jailhouse. A weathered sign indicates that it was built in 1896 by Agenicio [sic] Salazar Sr. and repaired in 1976.

- Exit the parking lot on the south side and turn right on Calle Corte. This narrow street becomes a footpath that squeezes down an alley to Camino Don Tomas between Calle del Banco and Calle Barrio Nuevo.

- Turn left on Camino Don Tomas.

- Turn right on Calle Laguna. Follow the road past the housing service projects and around the bend, then continue straight onto Rotary Park Rd. Bernalillo Recreation Center is ahead on the left. Facilities in the vicinity include a swimming pool, five baseball fields, soccer fields, a picnic shelter, and a playground. On the south side of Rotary Park are a water tower and silo left over from the New Mexico Timber Co., a sawmill operation that began in 1924 as White Pine Lumber. In its early years, lumberjacks logged with two-man saws and hauled the timber 40 miles by horse-drawn wagon from the top of Stable Mesa in the Jemez Mountains to a mill pond located where the park is today. The red locomotive in the park is the engine that eventually replaced the horses. The Santa Fe Northwestern Railroad line ran from Porter Landing, through the Gilman tunnels, down the Jemez River, and crossed the Rio Grande north of Coronado State Monument. (To fully appreciate the arduous journey, take the hike at Stable Mesa described in *60 Hikes Within 60 Miles: Albuquerque.*) At the peak of operations, 500 men worked the forest, trains, and mill. White Pine Lumber shut down in March 1931, but the mill reopened four months later as New Mexico Lumber and Timber. The branch line railroad was abandoned in 1940, the tracks were scrapped for the war effort, and trucks of 180-ton capacity replaced the train until the mill closed in 1951.

- Continue on Rotary Park Road past the murals on the east side of the park.
- Turn right on Calle San Lorenzo. Many houses on this street date back to the mill era.
- Turn left on Avenida Bernalillo and return to Camino del Pueblo. There on the southwest corner, Camino Real Antiques occupies the former Azteca Ballroom and Casa Blanca Bar, a hopping establishment in the 1940s. During World War II, Albuquerque's military bases deemed it too rowdy and set the entire town of Bernalillo off-limits to GIs. In the late 1960s, police officer Clemente Salazar, son of Abenicio, attempted to quell a fight in the Casa Blanca parking lot. He was shot to death with his own gun.
- Turn left on Camino del Pueblo. Ahead on the left is Silva's Saloon. The bar and pool hall are packed with antiques, memorabilia, and fascinating weirdness. Professional bootlegger Felix Silva Sr. officially opened the establishment in 1933, one day after Prohibition ended. He always wore an apron and kept nine loaded guns stashed throughout the building until suffering a fatal stroke on the job in 1995.

  Nearby to the north, the building that houses The Range Cafe previously served as a warehouse, Greyhound bus stop, mercantile building, and drugstore with a soda fountain. This family restaurant still boasts its original tin ceiling, two gift shops, its own cookbook, and extraordinary food. The huevos rancheros are a local favorite, though certainly Matt's Ultimate Hoosier ranks in the top four of the world's best pork-based sandwiches. Tucked in the back of the restaurant is a full bar called Lizard Rodeo Lounge.
- Continue north to Town Hall, cross the street, and locate the footpath between the car wash and the First Baptist Church. Follow it to the Downtown Bernalillo Rail Runner Station. West of the station are the ruins of the molino known as L. B. Putney Flour Mill. Built in 1915 by Abenicio Salazar, the molino milled flour, sugar, salt, and coffee until the Putney family declared bankruptcy in 1939. The building burned in the 1950s and again in the 1960s. The three-story, 9-by-18-inch adobe-brick walls remain standing. The Bernalillo Youth Conservation Corps had partially restored the building before losing their funding in 2014.

POINTS OF INTEREST

Flying Star Cafe flyingstarcafe.com, 200 S. Camino del Pueblo, 505-404-2100

Sandoval County Visitor Center sandovalcounty.org, 264 S. Camino del Pueblo, 505-867-TOUR or 800-252-0191

Our Lady of Sorrows olosbernalillonm.org, 301 S. Camino del Pueblo, 505-867-5252

Abuelita's New Mexican Kitchen abuelitasnmkitchen.com, 621 S. Camino del Pueblo, 505-867-9988

Bernalillo Recreation Center townofbernalillo.org/depts/recreation, 370 Rotary Park Rd., 505-771-2078

Camino Real Antiques 1100 S. Camino del Pueblo, 505-867-7448

Silva's Saloon 955 S. Camino del Pueblo, 505-867-9976

The Range Cafe rangecafe.com, 925 Camino del Pueblo, 505-867-1700

ROUTE SUMMARY

1. **Start at Sandoval County/US 550 Rail Runner Station and go west to Camino del Pueblo.**
2. **Turn left on Camino del Pueblo.**
3. **Turn right at the Sandoval Courthouse and cross the parking lot.**
4. **Turn right on Calle Corte.**
5. **Turn left on Camino Don Tomas.**
6. **Turn right on Calle Laguna.**
7. **Bear left on Rotary Park Rd.**
8. **Turn right on Calle San Lorenzo.**
9. **Turn left on Avenida Bernalillo.**
10. **Turn left on Camino del Pueblo and go north to Town Hall.**
11. **Turn right on the footpath north of the crosswalks and follow it to the Downtown Bernalillo Rail Runner Station.**

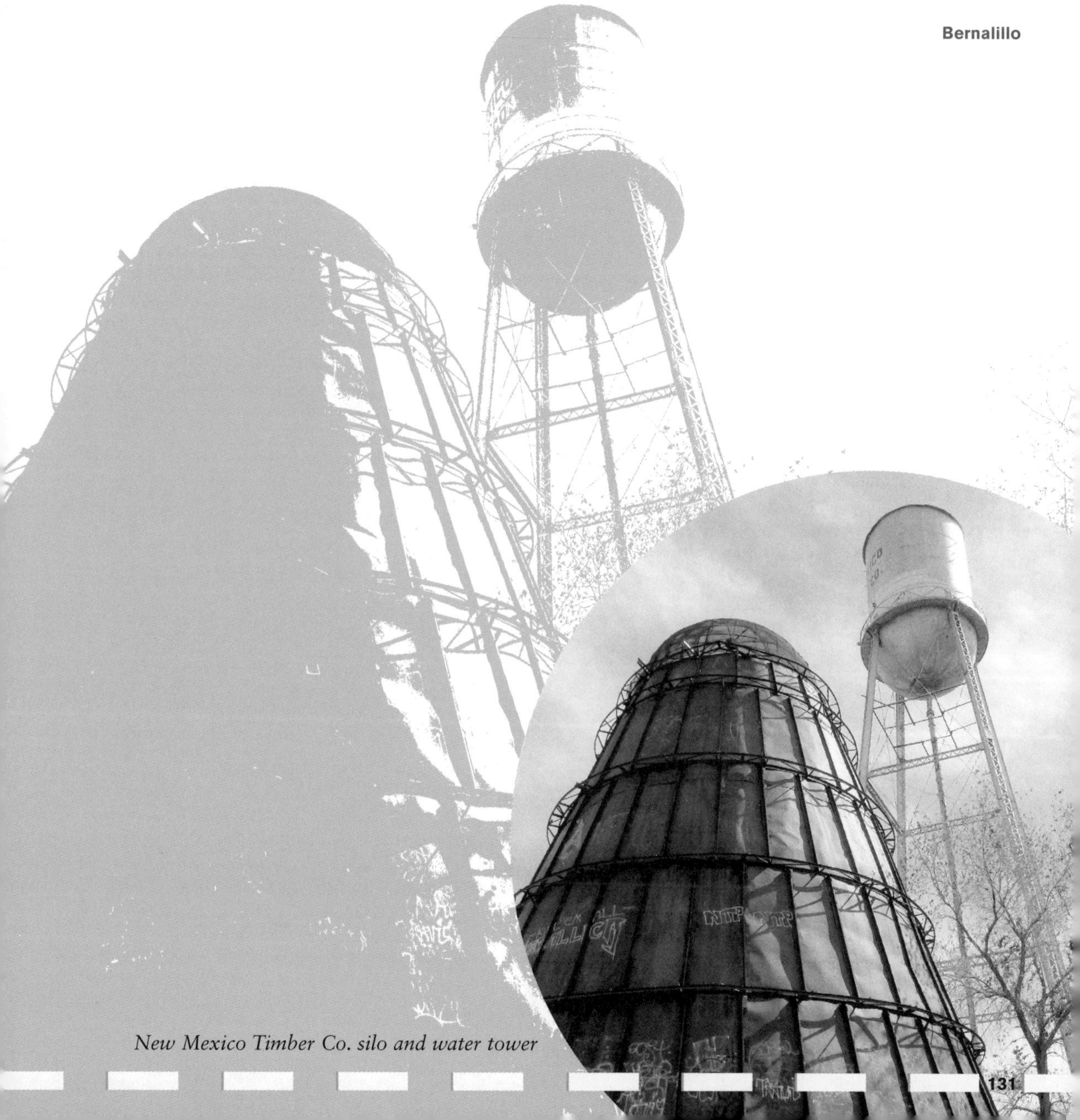

New Mexico Timber Co. silo and water tower

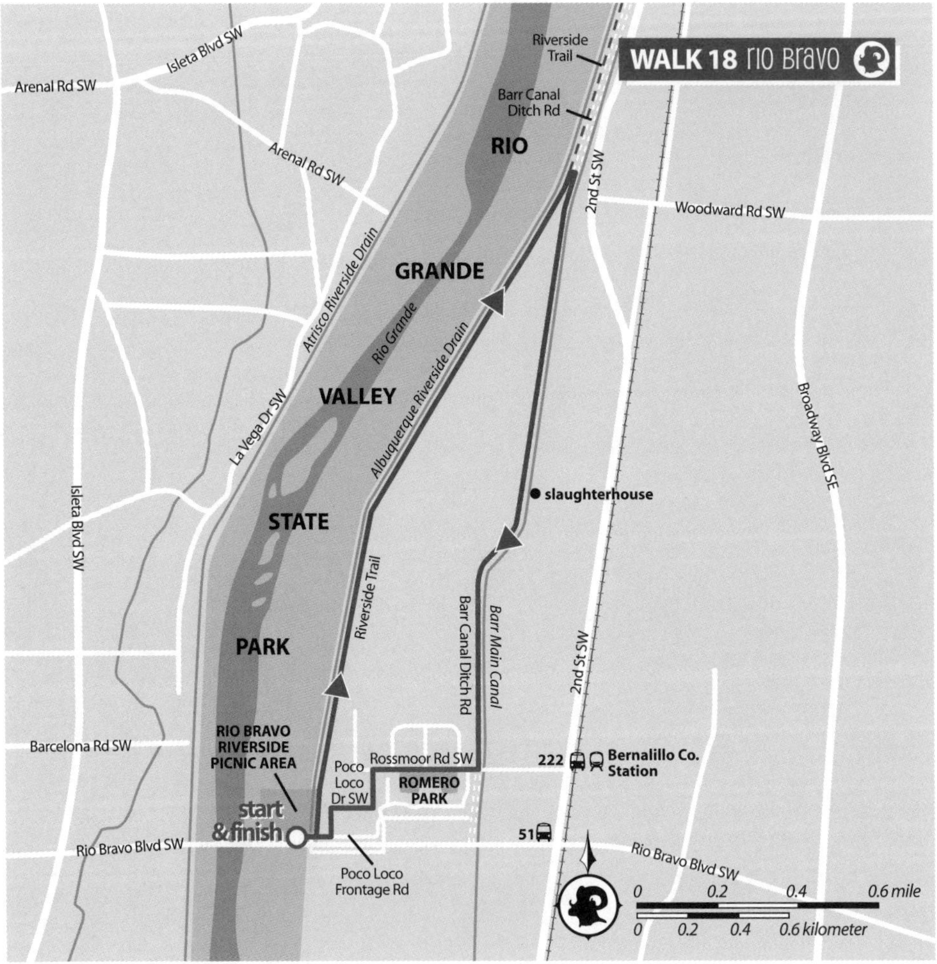
WALK 18 rio bravo
Riverside Trail
Barr Canal Ditch Rd
Isleta Blvd SW
Arenal Rd SW
Arenal Rd SW
RIO
2nd St SW
Woodward Rd SW
GRANDE
Atrisco Riverside Drain
Rio Grande
Albuquerque Riverside Drain
VALLEY
La Vega Dr SW
Broadway Blvd SE
slaughterhouse
Isleta Blvd SW
STATE
Riverside Trail
Barr Canal Ditch Rd
Barr Main Canal
PARK
2nd St SW
Barcelona Rd SW
RIO BRAVO RIVERSIDE PICNIC AREA
Poco Loco Dr SW
Rossmoor Rd SW
ROMERO PARK
222
Bernalillo Co. Station
start &finish
51
Rio Bravo Blvd SW
Rio Bravo Blvd SW
Poco Loco Frontage Rd
0 0.2 0.4 0.6 mile
0 0.2 0.4 0.6 kilometer

18 Rio Bravo: Still a Little Crazy

BOUNDARIES: **Rio Bravo Blvd., Rio Bravo Riverside Picnic Area, 2nd St.**
DISTANCE: **4 miles**
DIFFICULTY: **Moderate (unpaved sections)**
PARKING: **Parking lot closes at 9 p.m. April–October, 7 p.m. November–March**
PUBLIC TRANSIT: **ABQ Ride 51 westbound stops on Rio Bravo Blvd. west of 2nd St. Rail Runner stops on 2nd St. north of Rio Bravo Blvd.**

Wedged between the natural splendor of the Rio Grande Valley State Park and the industrial gloom of 2nd St. are more than 126 acres of agricultural land poised for residential development. If the description so far sounds less than enticing, then take a moment to assess your options at the Rio Bravo Riverside Picnic Area parking lot: To the west, a fully accessible nature trail leads to picnic sites and continues in a quarter-mile loop that visits the edge of the Rio Grande. To the north, wood fences mark a trail that winds beneath a canopy of majestic cottonwoods. Informal paths split from the main trail and weave deeper into the bosque. To the south, numerous paths squeak beneath the Rio Bravo bridge, allowing further exploration of these wooded banks. And to the east is Poco Loco Frontage Road, the beginning (and end) of a search for remnants of a vanishing past.

- **Start by walking east from the gravel parking lot, the way you came in. Just beyond the gate, a dirt road runs north along the west bank of the Albuquerque Riverside Drain. Perched over this narrow canal is a fully accessible fishing pier—a popular spot to angle for rainbow trout.**

- **Cross the drain and turn north on Paseo del Bosque, a paved multiuse trail on the east side of the Albuquerque Riverside Drain. Two nearby signs identify it as "Riverside Trail" and, to compound confusion, "Bridge Blvd. to 2nd St." (To clarify, this section runs from Rio Bravo Blvd. to Bridge Blvd.) Yet another sign welcomes you to Dr. John A. Aragón Bosque Park. The namesake doctor was a pioneer of multicultural education at the University of New Mexico and served as president of New Mexico Highlands University from 1975 to 1985.**

Back Story: Camp Albuquerque

More than 425,000 German POWs were shipped to the United States during World War II. Many stayed in camps in El Paso, Lordsburg, and Roswell. Some were destined to be housed in Civilian Conservation Corps buildings in Rio Grande Park, north of what is now the Rio Grande Zoo, but Albuquerque citizens vehemently opposed the idea. So in 1943 Camp Albuquerque received a shipment of Mussolini's men instead, and nobody complained. Then one day in July 1944, it was all gone. The Italians were transferred to undisclosed locations. The barracks came down, only to reappear on an 8-acre plot down by the slaughterhouse on the south edge of town. The first to arrive at the Schwartzman iteration of Camp Albuquerque were German soldiers captured in North Africa and trucked up from Camp Roswell. Demands for both food and farm labor had already escalated to critical limits, so the Germans worked farms in a 40-mile span from Corrales to Los Lunas, receiving 80 cents per day for their labor. June Mann was 10 years old when they came to work her father's farm on Rio Grande Blvd. "They did everything," she recalled decades later. They drove tractors and picked strawberries. The celery they grew and harvested was shipped to the White House. One Nazi grafted Bing cherries onto sour pie cherries, the result being larger and sweeter pie cherries. Up to 171 soldiers crowded the Schwartzman facility. Only three attempted to escape, one successfully. The camp passed inspection by the International Red Cross shortly before the prisoners were released in March 1946. Major renovations soon transformed Camp Albuquerque into the Schwartzman Apartments. This real estate venture lasted about 20 years before the buildings were uprooted once again and relocated to Los Lunas. Concrete foundations are the only trace of history that remains on the weedy 8-acre lot.

- **As you continue north-northeast, dense vegetation obscures views of the canal flowing in the opposite direction alongside the trail. The elms and cottonwoods here aren't as massive as those closer to the river, but in places their limbs arch overhead while their roots rumple the asphalt underfoot. (Watch your step.) The sturdy, 850-foot fence on your right ends to reveal empty lots where three 400-foot radio towers stand in a row to transmit 5,000 watts of sports jabber, courtesy of KNML.**

("The Sports Animal" is 610 on your AM dial.) Directly north of these scrubby lots are cultivated fields—the western extent of what remained of the Schwartzman properties as of 2014. In 1883 Josef Schwartzman left Austria at the age of 14, established a meat market on Central Ave. in 1889, and acquired 200 acres in the South Valley in the early 1900s. By the 1930s the Schwartzman family had amassed more than 1,000 acres to grow crops and raise cattle—up to 10,000 head jammed their feedlots. The cows are gone now and the main crops in recent years are alfalfa and chile. A network of irrigation ditches attracts waterfowl. In fall and winter, the harvested fields are a popular refueling stop for sandhill cranes. In November you might hear the sound of their rattling kar-r-roo calls and catch the scent of green chile wafting from a distant roaster. Enjoy the moment while you can. The fields are prime for a master-planned community, according to the new property managers. For now, the northern-most field ends in a point, and a dirt road merges on your right.

- Take a hairpin turn onto the dirt road and walk south through the pedestrian access in the gate ahead. A nearby acequia gate here crosses the Barr Canal. Three ditch roads run alongside this waterway. The low road is in better shape, while the upper roads afford better views. Best to stay on the low road for now. Portable latrines crowd the storage lot on the east side of the Barr Canal. An additional warning for those with bikes and dogs: goat heads (*Tribulus terrestris*) tend to grow thicker on the high roads and are capable of damaging tires and bare paws. The roads continue south another half mile with cultivated fields on both sides. A farmhouse and silo stand at the south end of the fields on your left. Closer to the canal, the ruins of a slaughterhouse lurk behind a cluster of trees. The Schwartzman Packing Plant started in the early 1900s to supply Schwartzman's meat market. In 1966 an equipment malfunction caused an explosion that damaged the plant, but it remained in operation, processing up to 25 million pounds of meat per year before shutting down in 1981. Now its cinder block walls serve as canvases for graffiti artists whose talents have improved dramatically in recent years.

- Continuing south you're likely to catch a whiff of petrol wafting from an asphalt-recycling operation. Mounds of crushed roads stand among mountains of wrecked vehicles on both sides of the canal. Environmental records are disturbing in the industrial area along 2nd St., yet minnows and crayfish seem to thrive in the adjacent irrigation system. They're easiest to spot when the water runs low. Irrigation season normally runs from March 1 through the end of October. Shells scattered along the canal belong to the Asian clam (*Corbicula fluminea*), an invasive species introduced to the Rio Grande in 1966. The ditch road continues south, squeezing between shanties on the east side of the Poco Loco neighborhood and an abandoned paint-supply warehouse on Rossmoor Rd.

- Turn right at Rossmoor Rd, the first paved cross street. Ambassador Edward L. Romero Park lies ahead on the left. Equipped with a basketball court, picnic area, and climbing wall, this award-winning park acts as a buffer zone between the new developments of Westbrook Commons and an established hamlet known as "Poco Loco" (a little bit crazy). Edward L. Romero served as ambassador to Spain during the Clinton administration, and the park named in his honor represents a diplomatic effort to neutralize tension between the two communities it serves.

- Turn left on Poco Loco Dr. and follow it as it zigzags back to the parking area at the end of Poco Loco Frontage Rd.

Points of Interest

Rio Bravo Riverside Picnic Area cabq.gov/parksandrecreation, Poco Loco Frontage Rd. SE, 505-452-5200

Ambassador Edward L. Romero Park bernco.gov/parks, 310 Rossmoor Rd. SE, 505-314-0400

Route Summary

1. Start at the Rio Bravo Riverside Picnic Area parking lot. Walk east on Poco Loco Frontage Rd.
2. Turn north on the Riverside Trail.
3. Turn south onto the Barr Canal ditch road.
4. Turn west on Rossmoor Rd.
5. Turn south on Poco Loco Dr.
6. Turn west on Poco Loco Dr.
7. Turn south on Poco Loco Dr.
8. Turn west on Poco Loco Frontage Rd.

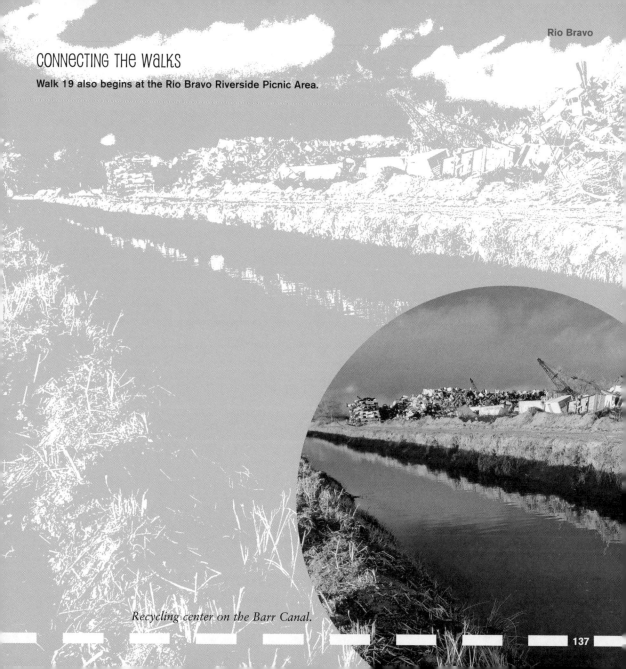

CONNECTING THE WALKS

Walk 19 also begins at the Rio Bravo Riverside Picnic Area.

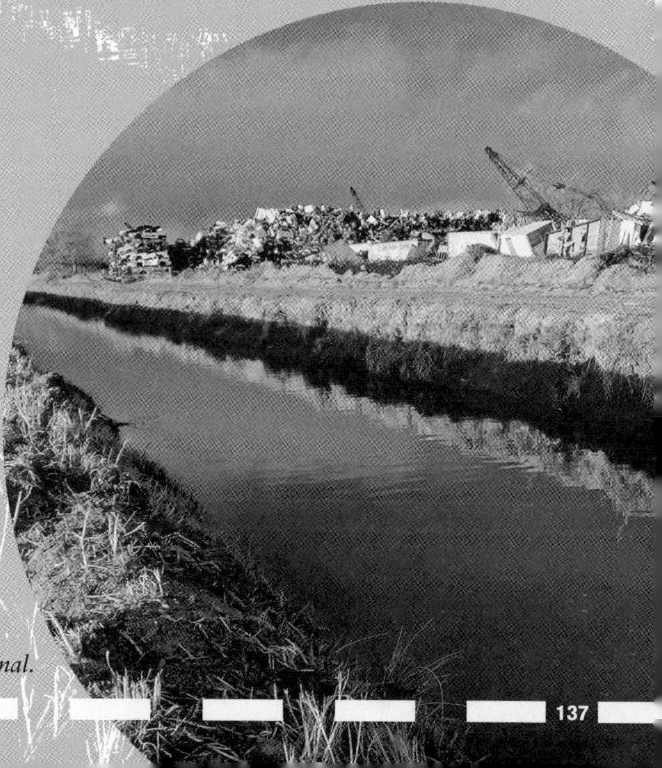

Recycling center on the Barr Canal.

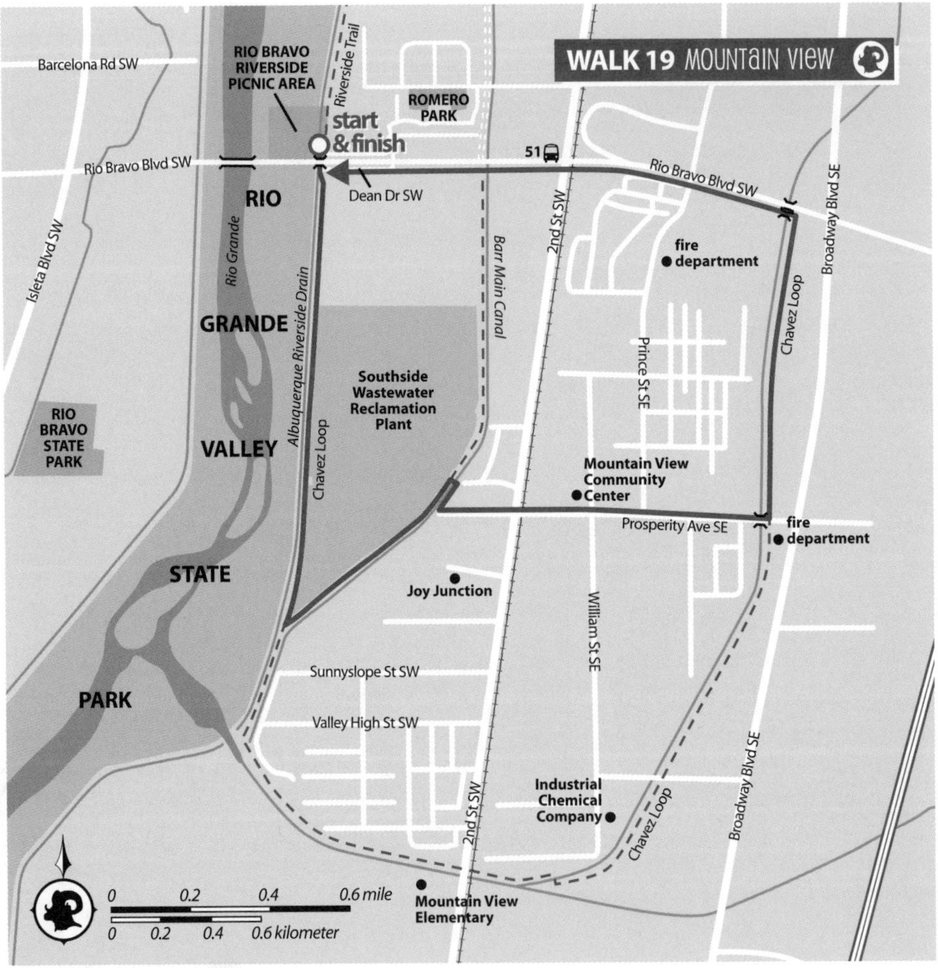
WALK 19 MOUNTAIN VIEW
Barcelona Rd SW
RIO BRAVO RIVERSIDE PICNIC AREA
Riverside Trail
ROMERO PARK
start & finish
51
Rio Bravo Blvd SW
Rio Bravo Blvd SW
Dean Dr SW
RIO
Rio Grande
GRANDE
VALLEY
STATE
PARK
Isleta Blvd SW
Albuquerque Riverside Drain
Chavez Loop
Barr Main Canal
2nd St SW
fire department
Broadway Blvd SE
Chavez Loop
Prince St SE
Southside Wastewater Reclamation Plant
RIO BRAVO STATE PARK
Mountain View Community Center
Prosperity Ave SE
fire department
Joy Junction
William St SE
Sunnyslope St SW
Valley High St SW
Industrial Chemical Company
Chavez Loop
Broadway Blvd SE
2nd St SW
Mountain View Elementary
0 0.2 0.4 0.6 mile
0 0.2 0.4 0.6 kilometer

19 MOUNTAIN VIEW: CHAVEZ LOOP

BOUNDARIES: **Rio Bravo Riverside Picnic Area, Tijeras Arroyo, Broadway Blvd.**
DISTANCE: **3-, 4.5-, and 5.5-mile options**
DIFFICULTY: **Moderate (unpaved sections on shortcuts)**
PARKING: **Parking lot closes at 9 p.m. April–October, 7 p.m. November–March**
PUBLIC TRANSIT: **Bus 51 on Rio Bravo Blvd. at 2nd St. Rail Runner on 2nd St. north of Rio Bravo Blvd.**

Chavez Loop is a 5.5-mile extension on the south end of the 14-mile Paseo del Bosque Trail. (Technically, they overlap, but for the sake of simplicity, we'll discuss them separately for now.) Paseo del Bosque flanks the Rio Grande Valley State Park from Alameda Blvd. to Rio Bravo Blvd. Pedestrians, equestrians, skaters, bicyclists, wheelchairs, baby strollers, dog walkers, and bird-watchers share this motor-free multiuse thoroughfare. You might also spot a deer, coyote, or roadrunner. Bridges at cross streets keep the entire length of it uninterrupted by traffic. Attractions along the way include the Rio Grande Nature Center, the BioPark (Aquarium, Botanic Garden, and Zoo), Tingley Beach, and the National Hispanic Cultural Center. By contrast, Chavez Loop doesn't stick to the bosque. Features along its route include a sewer treatment plant, industrial sectors, and salvage lots. However, it's not without its merits. For one, it never gets crowded. And while its "attractions" might not be attractive in the conventional sense, a walk here leads to a deeper understanding of the city.

- **Start at the fishing pier at the Rio Bravo Riverside Picnic Area, between the Rio Grande and the Albuquerque Riverside Drain. The small but fully accessible pier is a popular spot to catch rainbow trout and discarded shopping carts. The previous walk describes other nearby amenities. Walk directly south to pick up Paseo del Bosque and cross beneath Rio Bravo Blvd. (Rio Bravo was the name given by the Spanish to the Rio Grande north of El Paso.) The trail then briefly jogs east on Dean Dr. to cross the drain before turning south again to overlap Chavez Loop. (If you'd prefer more nature and less industry, follow the dirt road on the west side of the drain.) From there the paved trail squeezes between the tree-lined drain and a small industrial compound, the razor wire–crowned walls of which soon end at the edge of a lightly wooded tract.**

- Just under half a mile into the walk, you arrive at the junction of the Albuquerque Riverside Drain and the San José Drain. (If you're on the dirt road and want to take the shortcut, switch over to Paseo del Bosque here.) Cross the arched bridge over the San José Drain.

  Walk 14 describes Albuquerque's innovative strategy for diverting water from the Rio Grande, the nation's fifth largest watershed, for use in the city's water system. What's even more brilliant are the processes at work for releasing it back to the river after it's run its course through the city. The massive facility ahead on the left is the Southside Wastewater Reclamation Plant (SWRP), which cleans approximately 55 million gallons of wastewater every day. Isleta Pueblo, located about 10 miles downstream, uses water from the Rio Grande for ceremonial purposes, so cleaned-water quality requirements are stringent. The task of reclaiming water from sewage takes a complex system of clarification tanks, aeration basins, digesters, and generators. And those are just the parts you can see from behind the fence. (For a full behind-the-scenes virtual tour, click the Education link at abcwua.org. Tours can also be scheduled for student groups, grades 4–12.) A fortified pair of discharge pipes on the west side of the trail muffle gushing water as it's expelled into the Rio Grande, unseen below about 100 yards on your right. The volume of water entering the river here ranks the SWRP as the Rio Grande's fifth largest tributary.

- Continue south past a field of solar panels to the point where the Barr Canal comes in from your left. This is where to decide whether to take the shortcut or the full loop. Allow wind conditions to influence your decision. The odor emitted from the SWRP is reminiscent of swamp gas, or an estuary at low tide. It's not an unbearable stench, though it's not entirely pleasant to be caught downwind in a mild breeze.

  5.5-mile loop: Continue straight another quarter mile or so to the next bridge. The berm ahead is an embankment for the Tijeras Channel. Chavez Loop turns southeast and ramps up to the edge of the concrete-lined channel. It's the last leg in an otherwise natural drainage. Tijeras ("scissors") Arroyo, Bernalillo County's largest, is a conduit for runoff from the mountains 15 miles east. Fossils found in its higher reaches include ancient species of land tortoise, camel, llama, and mammoth. With the South Diversion Channel as a tributary, the Tijeras Channel streams runoff from parts of Central Ave., Yale Blvd., and the Albuquerque International Sunport, combined with effluent from Kirtland Air Force Base and Sandia National Laboratories. It all enters the Rio Grande here, just half a mile downstream from SWRP's discharge. Contaminants from the base and the labs occasionally seem to negate SWRP efforts. Close ahead, Mountain View Elementary School, home of the Mountain Lions, stands on the channel's south bank.

From here the trail dips into the channel to pass beneath 2nd St. and the railroad tracks. Cross the next bridge and follow the paved path as it splits away from the Tijeras Channel and bends northeast to follow the South Diversion Channel. On your left is a stock warehouse for Industrial Chemical Corporation, distributors of leaded premium racing fuel, aircraft deicing fluid, chloroform, and hundreds of other beneficial chemical products. On your right is Crane Service Inc., where you might spot Grove's flagship all-terrain crane, the GMK7550. This seven-axle beast has a 550-ton capacity and a standard 230-foot twin-lock boom that can be extended to 430 feet with attachments. Ahead on the right, the red six-story tower is part of a training facility for the Bernalillo County Fire Department. Cross Prosperity Ave. The 4.5-mile route rejoins the main loop here.

4.5-mile loop: From the Y junction of the paved trail and the Barr Canal, hook left on the dirt road and walk northeast. Ahead on your right, look for a 50,000-square-foot brick schoolhouse and gymnasium. The facility began with Congregational Church sponsorship as the Rio Grande Industrial School in 1911. A 1920 issue of the Prescott Journal-Miner reported that the institution "has been doing good for the Spanish speaking population of New Mexico." Archbishop Reverend R. A. Gerkin purchased the property in 1937 to establish a Catholic school for boys. Brothers of Our Lady of Lourdes arrived from Oostakker, Belgium, to run the school, which was equipped with carpentry shops, a printing plant, and a dairy. Our Lady of Lourdes Chapel, a Pueblo-style structure, was later built directly south of the school. Athletic records from other schools in the district remark that Lourdes Catholic School closed in 1944 and reopened in 1962. Attendance records indicate that enrollment declined after the opening of St. Pius in 1958. In either case, Lourdes finally shut down in 1966 and soon became the Drug Addicts Recovery Enterprises Treatment Center. Joy Junction, Albuquerque's largest emergency homeless shelter, has managed the property since 1983 and purchased it from the New Mexico Girls' Ranch in 1998. The chapel has since been partially restored, but the schoolhouse is on the verge of collapse.

Its extensive deterioration caught the eye of filmmaker Wally Pfister, and in 2013 he brought actors Johnny Depp and Morgan Freeman here to film scenes for the sci-fi thriller *Transcendence.* Some residents from the homeless shelter were hired onto the film crew. Absent from all historic registers, the schoolhouse will likely be demolished soon.

- Continue northeast to the next bridge. For the 3-mile loop, continue following the Barr Canal north to Rio Bravo Blvd., where you'll turn left to return to the Rio Bravo Riverside Picnic Area.

- Otherwise, turn right, cross the bridge, turn right again, and follow the dirt road down to the concrete barricade at Bowers Rd.

- Turn left on Bowers Rd. and walk to its end, where you'll find the Joy Junction Thrift Store. Once you cross 2nd St. and the railroad tracks, you're on Prosperity Ave. Look up the tracks to see the downtown skyline 5 miles north. Walk past the brickyard and the Mountain View Community Center, where you can score a free lunch if you get there on time. A couple of auto salvage lots and small ranches also flank the road. Cross the South Diversion Channel to rejoin Chavez Loop.

- Turn left on Chavez Loop, indicated with bollards and a sign prohibiting motor vehicles. Salvage lots flank the next half mile. The South Valley is home to at least a dozen car and truck salvage lots with a combined inventory of roughly 20,000 discarded vehicles. The lots have thinned out noticeably in recent years, likely in response to increasing prices of certain metals.

  Ahead at the corner of Rio Bravo Blvd. is a memorial kiosk offering shaded benches and a brass bas relief titled *Spinning* by sculptor J. D. Adcox. The memorialized rider, Christopher Jerome Chavez, was killed in a hit-and-run on June 30, 1999, while bicycling to work westbound on Rio Bravo Blvd. He was a 14-year veteran of the Albuquerque Fire Department.

- Turn west on Rio Bravo Blvd. and stay in the protected lane for the next mile to return to the Rio Bravo Riverside Picnic Area.

Points of Interest

Rio Bravo Riverside Picnic Area cabq.gov/parksandrecreation, Poco Loco Frontage Rd. SE, 505-452-5200

Albuquerque Wastewater Utility abcwua.org, 4201 2nd St. SW, 505-768-2500

Joy Junction Thrift Store joyjunction.org, 107 Bowers Rd. SW, 505-873-8372

Mountain View Community Center bernco.gov, 201 Prosperity Ave. SE, 505-314-0297

Route Summary

Start at the fishing pier at the Rio Bravo Riverside Picnic Area and walk south.

5.5-mile loop: Continue straight and follow Chavez Loop back to the Rio Bravo Riverside Picnic Area.

4.5-mile loop: From the Y junction of the paved trail and the Barr Canal, hook left on the dirt road and walk northeast. Continue north to the next bridge. Cross the bridge, turn right again, and follow the dirt road down to the concrete barricade at Bowers Rd.

- Turn left on Bowers Rd., which becomes Prosperity Ave. Continue straight to cross the South Diversion Channel.
- Turn left on Chavez Loop and follow it back to the Rio Bravo Riverside Picnic Area.

3-mile loop: From the Y junction of the paved trail and the Barr Canal, continue north to Rio Bravo Blvd.

- Turn left to return to the Rio Bravo Riverside Picnic Area.

Connecting the Walks

Walk 18 also starts at the Rio Bravo Riverside Picnic Area.

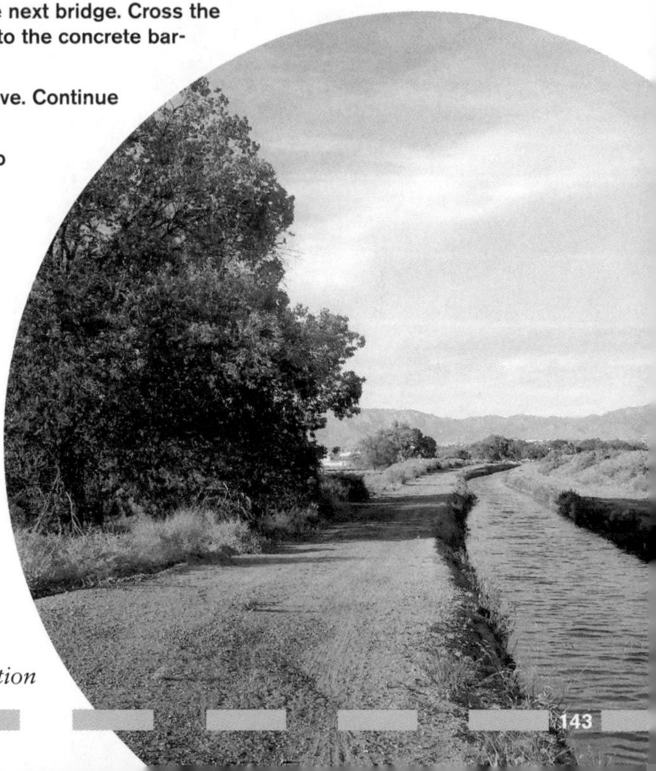

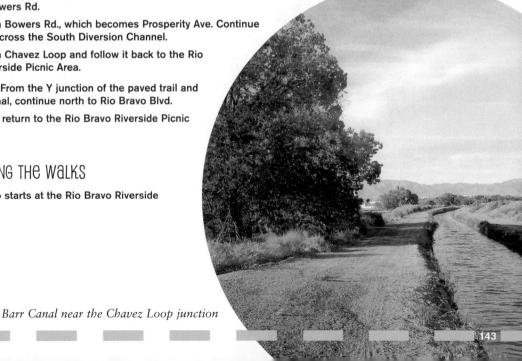

Barr Canal near the Chavez Loop junction

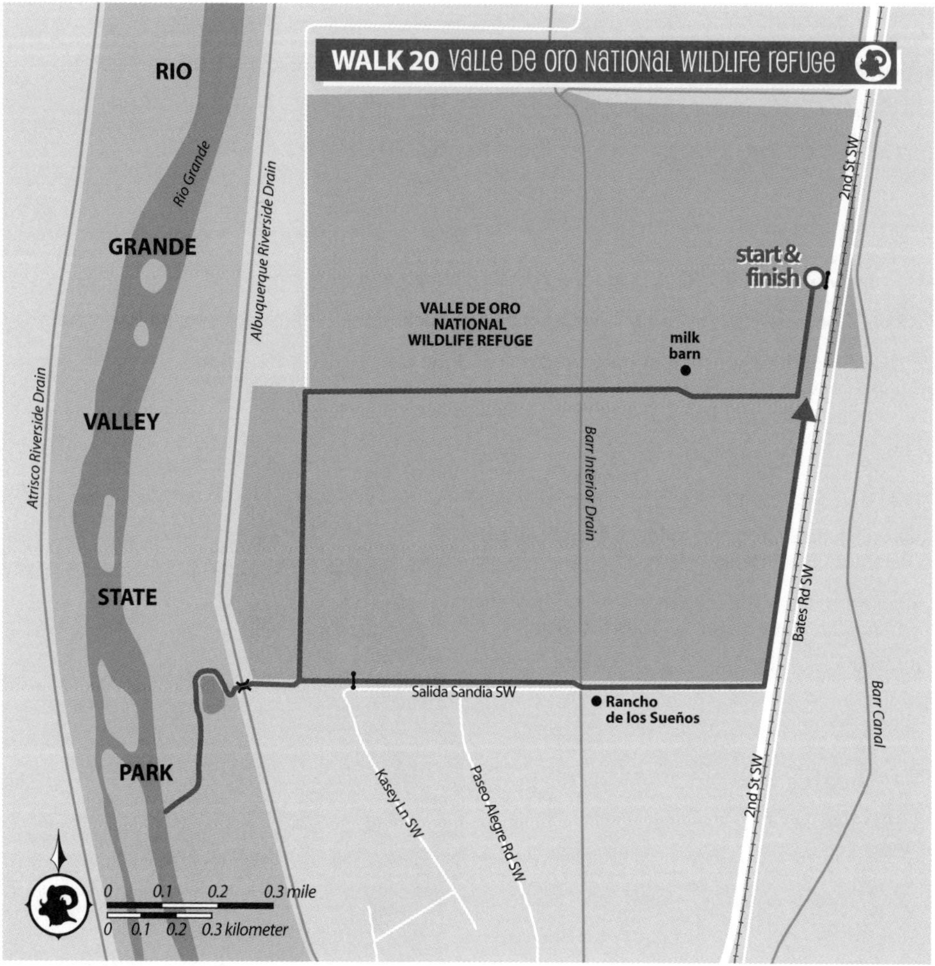
WALK 20 Valle de Oro National Wildlife Refuge
RIO
GRANDE
VALLEY
STATE
PARK
Rio Grande
Atrisco Riverside Drain
Albuquerque Riverside Drain
VALLE DE ORO
NATIONAL
WILDLIFE REFUGE
Barr Interior Drain
milk
barn
start &
finish
2nd St SW
Bates Rd SW
Barr Canal
Salida Sandia SW
Rancho
de los Sueños
Kasey Ln SW
Paseo Alegre Rd SW
2nd St SW
0 0.1 0.2 0.3 mile
0 0.1 0.2 0.3 kilometer

20 Valle de Oro National Wildlife Refuge

BOUNDARIES: **2nd St., Salida Sandia, the Rio Grande, Lagunitas Ln.**
DISTANCE: **4 miles on current roads and trails**
DIFFICULTY: **Moderate (unpaved surfaces)**
PARKING: **Free parking near Valle de Oro NWR entrance on 2nd St.**
PUBLIC TRANSIT: **None (yet)**

Valle de Oro, the Southwest's first urban wildlife refuge, is billed as an oasis for both wildlife and people. Located 5 miles south of downtown Albuquerque and within a 30-minute drive for half the state's population, the former dairy farm formally received approval for refuge status from the U.S. Department of the Interior in 2012. Since then the managing agency, the U.S. Fish and Wildlife Service, has been scrambling to finalize the purchase of the 570-acre property—along with its substantial water rights. Projects are also underway to develop the land for recreation while restoring the environment for the benefit of wildlife.

As is often the case, a harmonious balance between preservation and public access poses significant challenges. The slow rate of progress here might be attributed to the number of collaborating agencies. Bernalillo County, the Trust for Public Land, Friends of Valle de Oro, the U.S. Bureau of Reclamation, and the Albuquerque Metropolitan Arroyo Flood Control Authority are among the entities eager to contribute their respective visions to the refuge's mission. Add to that any attempts to address individual desires in a diverse local community and it becomes clear that delays don't necessarily arise from inabilities to get things done but from the process of finding agreement on what should be done. That said, once the final plans are approved, changes to the refuge will likely be quick and dramatic. Hence, a walk description written in the summer of 2014 might not accurately reflect what visitors will find here in, say, the winter of 2015.

At present one of the most striking features is the expanse of the land and its emptiness. Not much obstructs the view over the refuge. On its diagonal length—from its northeast corner on 2nd St. to the bridge over the Albuquerque Riverside Drain—elevation drops a mere 15 feet over the span of a mile. Some might describe it as bland, almost Midwestern. At this time it might be easy to say there's nothing here and walk away. That will change. And in the meantime, the refuge has been hosting a growing flurry of public activity. Events include monthly

BACK STORY: VALLEY GOLD TO VALLE DE ORO

The refuge project frequently changed names before its final christening. "Middle Rio Grande" and "Price's Dairy" were on the table before the final christening with the Spanish translation of "Valley Gold." The story goes back to 1906, when El Paso widow Mary Price bought a cow. Her older boys delivered milk from that one cow to 11 customers. The dairy doubled production within its first month. Now they had two cows. They didn't stop there. The family farm grew into a conglomeration that supplied dairy products to distributors throughout west Texas and southern New Mexico. In 1932 Price's Producers acquired Matthew's Dairy on Rio Grande Blvd. and renamed it Valley Gold Dairies. (One of the investors was New Mexico native Conrad Hilton. The Prices returned the favor when Hilton's fledgling hotel empire began to crumble during the Depression.) In response to milk shortages following World War II, Valley Gold purchased a dairy on the site of what is now the wildlife refuge. Price's Valley Gold Dairies Inc. eventually expanded to 1,600 cows and developed into one of New Mexico's top 100 private companies with $10–$20 million in annual revenues and 85 employees. Mary's grandson Dudley Price closed the dairy in 1998. His farmland in Bernalillo, big enough to require its own airport, became the city's largest residential development.

open house tours, sunset walks, bird-watching, kite flying, archery training, art challenges, field trips, gardening workshops, and Youth Conservation Corps projects. Or if you'd prefer to tour the site on your own, contact the Valle de Oro NWR. (See page 149 for contact info.)

Though site plans have yet to be finalized, a few recurring details hint at the shape of things to come. The map here is based on what currently exists, while the route description below required some speculation. With that in mind . . .

- **Start in the parking area off 2nd St. Ideally, you'll find a visitor center nearby, and maybe some gardens. With the eastern section being slightly higher in elevation and farther from the river, you might expect an upland habitat cultivated here with desert shrubs and grasses.**

- As you walk west, you might come across a trail that indicates an original alignment of El Camino Real de Tierra Adentro. The Spanish Colonial "royal road of the interior," used by settlers, missionaries, soldiers, and traders for almost 300 years, once traversed this site north–south, passing directly in front of the milk barn (if that's still standing). Running parallel to El Camino is the Barr Interior Drain, which takes irrigation water from the Albuquerque Riverside Drain and carries it to the Williams Lateral, both of which you'll cross later. Senior water rights attached to the property were valued at $18.6 million but reduced enough to account for less than half the property's overall $18.5 million price tag. Without them, neither crops nor restoration would be possible, and then the whole place would succumb to suburban sprawl. (At least that's what happened to Price's dairy farm in Bernalillo.)

- Continue west across the Barr Drain and into the western section of the refuge. Plans for this area tentatively call for ridges and swales that allow for oxbow ponds and cattail marshes, which in turn will help support a dense riparian habitat of cottonwood, willow, buffalo berry, and native olive. You may find ponds, wetlands, and a saltgrass meadow. The main idea is to expand the bosque into the refuge.

- Follow whatever path or road leads to the southwest corner of the refuge. There you should find access to Salida Sandia.

- Turn right and cross the parallel ditches ahead. Hopefully you'll find Paseo del Bosque. The paved, 16-mile recreation trail currently extends south to the Tijeras Channel, which is about 3 miles north of the bridge. West of the trail is the riverside forest known as the bosque, or what's left of it. Recent restoration projects have substantially deforested the banks and carved out shallow basins. It was a shocking sight at first, but runoff that would otherwise flood nearby residential areas now flows into the hollows to foster newly planted cottonwoods and willows. Within a decade we should see a densely wooded wetland habitat that better represents the natural state of the bosque, however you define it. Humans have been altering this riparian environment for more than a millennium. Conditions varied under the Pueblo periods, the Spanish Colonial era, and (most drastically) in the post-WWII age, when the U.S. Army Corps of Engineers set out to solve the city's flooding problem once and for all.

A 20-mile ribbon of bosque is formally designated as the Rio Grande Valley State Park, totaling 4,300 acres spanning from Sandia Pueblo south to Isleta Pueblo. Perhaps you've grown familiar with the multifaceted woodland during previous walks in Alameda, Corrales, Los Poblanos, and elsewhere. You can decide for yourself what looks natural, but as you wander these 90 acres of it, don't be too quick to judge. It just needs more time. (Also note that this portion of the RGVSP is managed by the State Land Office, which has its own peculiar set of rules, so be sure to observe any posted signage for access and regulations.)

I've walked the refuge grounds and perimeter roads three times in as many years, each visit in a different season. The built environment changed little over time. It would've been easy to say there was nothing and leave it at that. Instead I walked and waited for the land to reveal something a little different. Snowy mountains loomed behind a brilliant red barn. Tumbleweeds the size of sumo wrestlers cartwheeled down ditch roads. Kestrels came to perch on every fencepost I passed. Or maybe it was the same bird just following along. Either way, it was one of many memorable experiences.

● Return to the parking area via the perimeter trail, or Salida Sandia and 2nd St., if necessary. Attractive farms and estates face the south side of the refuge. None seem too keen on strangers dropping in, so observe the No Trespassing signs. Rancho de los Sueños, however, does welcome visitors by appointment. The 30-acre horse breeding and training facility has produced such champions as Pikko del Cerro, winner of the 2009 Dressage at Devon Stallion Championship, and Pikturesk, the 2007 U.S. Dressage Foundation Horse of the Year.

Concluding this walk, Refuge Manager Jennifer Owen-White notes: "Whenever I take people to the refuge I ask them to stop for a moment, look out over the farm fields and imagine what this place will look like in five years, in ten years. Imagine diverse habitats with lots of wildlife, wetlands, forest, gardens, families enjoying the outdoors, and school kids learning about conservation. Imagine what this land will become and what it will mean to both people and wildlife, a true refuge for all."

POINTS OF INTEREST

Valle de Oro National Wildlife Refuge fws.gov/refuge/valle_de_oro or facebook.com/valledeoronationalwildliferefuge, 7851 2nd St. SW, 505-933-2708

Rio Grande Valley State Park Albuquerque Open Space cabq.gov, 505-897-8831

NM State Land Office nmstatelands.org, 505-272-7525

Horses Unlimited (Rancho de los Sueños) horsesunlimited.us, 850 Salida Sandia SW, 505-873-9043

ROUTE SUMMARY

1. **Start at the entrance on 2nd St.**
2. **Walk to the southwest corner of the refuge.**
3. **Turn right on Salida Sandia and cross the bridge.**
4. **Wander the bosque at your leisure.**
5. **Return via the perimeter trail or Salida Sandia and 2nd St.**

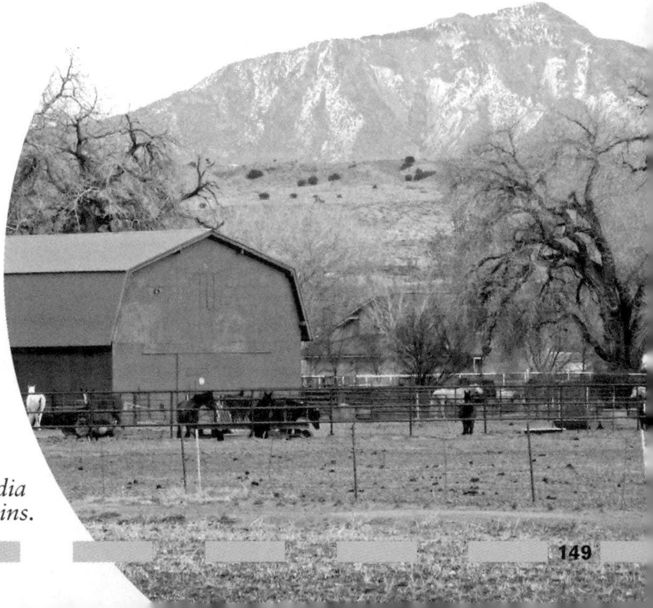

Red barn at the end of Salida Sandia fronts the Manzano Mountains.

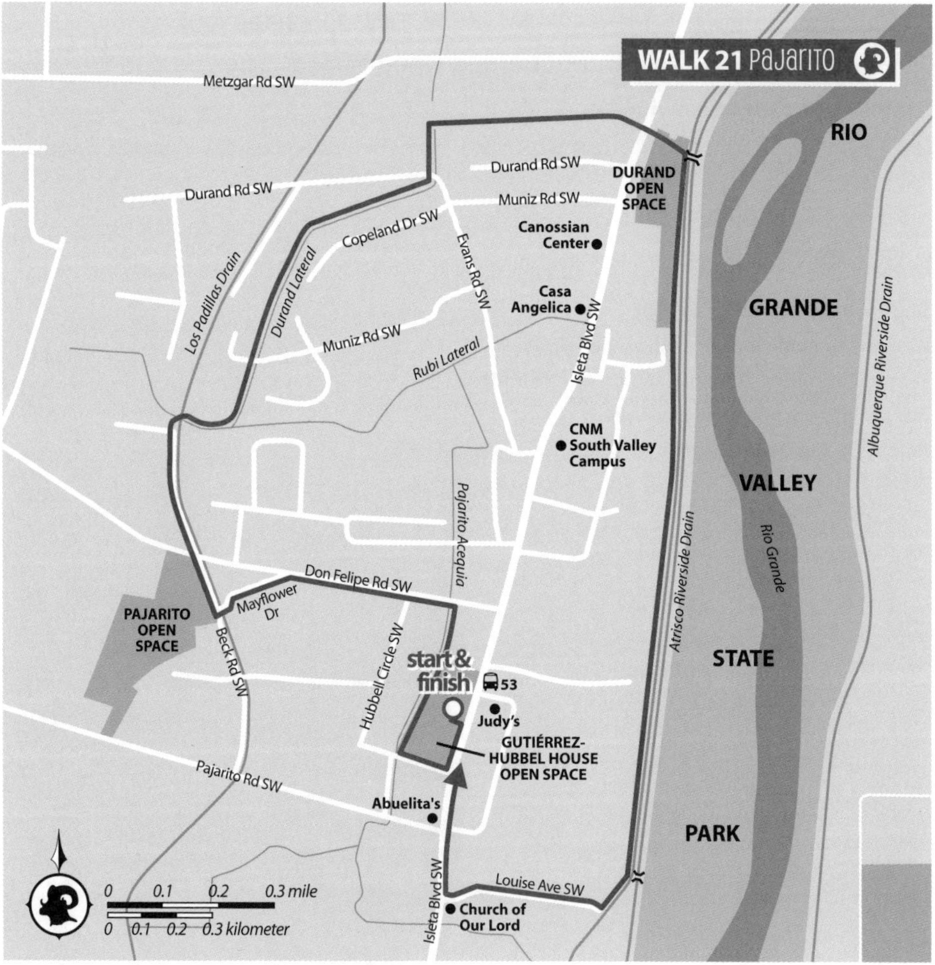
WALK 21 Pajarito
Metzgar Rd SW
Durand Rd SW
Durand Rd SW
Muniz Rd SW
DURAND OPEN SPACE
RIO
Canossian Center
Copeland Dr SW
Evans Rd SW
Casa Angelica
Los Padillas Drain
Durand Lateral
Muniz Rd SW
Rubi Lateral
Isleta Blvd SW
GRANDE
Albuquerque Riverside Drain
CNM South Valley Campus
VALLEY
Pajarito Acequia
Rio Grande
Don Felipe Rd SW
Mayflower Dr
PAJARITO OPEN SPACE
Beck Rd SW
Hubbell Circle SW
start & finish
53
Judy's
GUTIÉRREZ-HUBBEL HOUSE OPEN SPACE
Atrisco Riverside Drain
STATE
Pajarito Rd SW
Abuelita's
PARK
0 0.1 0.2 0.3 mile
0 0.1 0.2 0.3 kilometer
Isleta Blvd SW
Louise Ave SW
Church of Our Lord

21 Pajarito: Rx Trail Trifecta

BOUNDARIES: **Beck Rd., Los Padillas Spillway Diversion, Los Padillas Feeder, Louise Ave.**
DISTANCE: **3.5- and 4.5-mile options**
DIFFICULTY: **Moderate (mostly unpaved)**
PARKING: **Free parking sunrise–sunset at all Open Space parks**
PUBLIC TRANSIT: **Bus 53 on Isleta Blvd. at Don Felipe Rd.**

Pajarito grew from a series of estancias, or farming communities, settled along the west bank of the Rio Grande in the 17th century. Spain granted the sitio, or tract, of San Ysidro de Pajarito to Josefa Baca in the 1730s. Baca's 1746 will deeded the land to her children, who in turn sold it to Clemente Gutiérrez by 1785, sometime after his marriage to Josefa's granddaughter. Following the U.S. war with Mexico in 1848, the Treaty of Hidalgo assured that grants made under Mexican or Spanish control would be upheld by the U.S. government. However, of the 272 land grant claims from New Mexico, the U.S. Court of Private Land Claims confirmed only 69. Pajarito was one of the lucky ones. Thus the 47,000-acre property remained in the sole possession of the Gutiérrez family. Their holdings spanned from the Rio Puerco east to the Rio Grande, south to Los Padillas and north to Atrisco. Today the village of Pajarito sits just south of Albuquerque city limits. Recent developments by Bernalillo County Open Space Division include three parks, each offering a "Prescription Trail." Prescription Trails is a program designed to promote healthy lifestyles for families. (For more info, visit **prescriptiontrails.org.**) Walk this route to visit the three Rx Trail sites and find out what makes each unique.

- **Start at the Gutiérrez-Hubbell House, built for Juliana Gutiérrez and her husband James "Santiago" Hubbell in the 1860s. The union of these powerful families boosted their collective holdings to 165,000 acres. However, it would be sold off piece by piece over the years, and the house would become a trading post, stagecoach stop, and post office. By the time the county stepped in to protect the house in 2000, the property was down to a mere 10 acres. After a decade of restoration efforts on the 5,700-square-foot adobe house, the handsome property is a slice of life on the farm during New Mexico's territorial period. Features on-site include a cultural center, wildlife habitats, farming workshops, trails, a museum, and a gift shop. The house is open for tours Tuesday, Thursday, and Saturday, 10 a.m.–2 p.m. It's also a venue for special events, lectures, and festivals.**

Back Story: The Vanishing Mayordomo

Acequias were established on the Atrisco Land Grant in 1692, on the Pajarito Land Grant in 1746, and in Lagunitas in 1826. Combined they irrigated about 30,000 acres throughout the South Valley. That's about half the acreage farmed in the Middle Rio Grande Conservancy District (MRGCD), which stretches from Sandoval to Socorro counties. Farms in this region consume nearly six times as much water as the cities. The elaborate system of canals, ditches, laterals, and drains is driven almost entirely by the force of gravity; hence, fields at higher elevation are the first to receive water. Farmers are allowed a certain number of inches of water per year per acre. Once the upper fields receive their allotted amount, their gates are closed and the water flows down to the next fields. Checks are devices that resemble gates but are used to slow water flows, thereby raising the level to the point that it backs up through a tap box or overflows a turnout. In locations where checks are not effective, siphons carry water underground and out to nearby fields. In traditional acequia systems, the mayordomo, or ditch boss, is responsible for managing these devices in a precise order. One mistimed gate could ruin a field with too much or too little water. It's all part of a strict rotation and scheduling plan laid out by the MRGCD, which monitors 1,200 miles of ditches and drains. In 2008 the MRGCD implemented a computer modeling program called the Decision Support System (DSS) to help ditch bosses and farmers determine when, how often, and for how long they should irrigate. The DSS uses satellite monitoring, moisture sensors, and other high-tech devices to optimize delivery. It's credited with conserving a considerable amount of water, but as technology develops, tasks of the mayordomo are becoming increasingly automated.

- **Locate the trailhead on the east side of the house and follow it clockwise around the property. It wraps around agricultural fields and up the Pajarito Acequia. Ancient cottonwoods shade this historic ditch.**

- **Turn left on the first paved street, Don Felipe Rd. There aren't any sidewalks, but the shoulders are wide on this quiet street, and the horses are friendly. Just watch out for tractors and oversized farm vehicles that occasionally rumble by.**

- At the Y ahead, veer left onto Mayflower Dr., which squeezes between modest farms and a grand estate. It crosses the Los Padillas Drain and ends at Beck Rd. Across the road is the parking area for the 20-acre Pajarito Open Space. Though pajarito is Spanish for "little bird," here you're likely to spot feathered fliers of all sizes, from hummingbirds in summer to bald eagles in winter. Wood ducks, sandhill cranes, egrets, warblers, bluebirds, roadrunners, and flycatchers also make frequent appearances. The park was part of the Beck dairy farm before the county acquired it in 1999. Its Rx Trail circles fields of alfalfa, grown and harvested for dairy cattle feed, along with a variety of grasses for wildlife forage. Numerous interpretive signs along the way describe the history and ecology of the South Valley.

- Go north on Beck Rd. It crosses Don Felipe Rd. and runs alongside Los Padillas Drain before ending at the Durand Lateral. Note the innovative construction of this intersection of waterways: The drain flows beneath the lateral. Near to the west is a small farm with llamas and emus.

- Cross the Durand Lateral and turn right. It soon arrives at the Rubi Lateral, a gorgeously shaded ditch that would be a pleasure to walk along were it not for razor-wire fencing that obstructs it.

- Turn left to continue following the Durand Lateral. It passes near backyards and becomes increasingly shaded before reaching the first paved street, Durand Rd. Cross the road and continue north on the ditch road. The lateral soon arrives at a wide ribbon of fields known as Los Padillas Spillway Diversion, which was established in 2011. The power lines in the spillway diversion went up in the 1980s.

- Turn right and follow the gravel path on the south side of this wide, shallow channel. The path leads to a structure that formerly housed an automotive repair shop, a used car dealership, and a gas station. The first paved road it crosses is Isleta Blvd., which follows an original alignment of the Camino Real, the oldest European road in the continental U.S. At 1,500 miles, it's also the longest historical route in the Western hemisphere. Though the Camino Real normally followed the east bank of the Rio Grande, a ford near the founding site of Barelas (Walk 3) led to a branch on the west bank. This vital route of commerce contributed to the prosperity of Pajarito's estancias.

Shortcut: The Gutiérrez-Hubbell House is just a mile south, and a right turn here would shave a mile off your walk while leading you past a few notable sites. Canossian Spirituality Center was established by the Canossian Daughters of Charity in 1996. The serene retreat features meditation gardens, a library, and a chapel. Casa Angelica, just south of the center, is a home for "children with pervasive needs." Directed by the Canossian Daughters of Charity since 1967, the 15-acre facility provides therapies, direct care, and a family environment for individuals with severe disabilities. Warning: Traffic on Isleta Blvd. can get busy, due in part to the Central New Mexico (CNM) Community College South Valley Campus, located about half a mile south. Again, sidewalks are absent, but road shoulders are wide enough for safe walking.

- To stick with the 4.5-mile route, cross the boulevard to enter the 10-acre Durand Open Space. The asymmetrical Quonset hut north of the park is a remnant of Westernair, a local aviation company founded in the 1950s by Dick Durand Jr. Born at home in Pajarito in 1926, Durand grew up to become a celebrated aviator. The park itself was a grassy landing strip known as Pea Patch. The aforementioned power lines brought an end to aviation here, and the runway reverted to an alfalfa field. A cockpit-shaped sign east of the parking area explains more about Durand and his remarkable achievements in aviation.

- Turn right on the Rx Trail on the east side of the park and follow it to the south end of the former airstrip. A gate in the corner provides access to a ditch road on the west bank of the Los Padillas Feeder. The first intersecting road is a mile south. You won't find access to Isleta Blvd. on this stretch. It's a pleasant stroll between bosque and farmland. Look out for longhorn cattle.

- Turn right on Louise Ave. and follow this short residential street to a modest worship hall identified as Church of Our Lord, or COOL for short.

- Turn right on Isleta Blvd. Ahead on the left, Abuelita's rivals the restaurant of the same name in Bernalillo (Walk 17). It's well worth stopping in for a chile relleno and cerveza after a long walk. Just need to cool off? Try the ice-cream counter tucked in the back corner of Judy's Trading Post. Take time to wander the labyrinth of unusual wares in this local consignment shop—especially on hot summer days. Unlike the Gutiérrez-Hubbell House directly across the street, this place is air-conditioned.

Points of Interest

Gutiérrez-Hubbell House gutierrezhubbellhouse.org, 6029 Isleta Blvd. SW, 505-244-0507

Pajarito Open Space bernco.gov, 6000 Beck Rd. SW, 505-314-0400

Durand Open Space bernco.gov, 4750 Isleta Blvd. SW, 505-314-0400

Canossian Spirituality Center canossianspiritualitycenter.org, 5625 Isleta Blvd. SW, 505-452-9402

Abuelita's New Mexican Kitchen 6083 Isleta Blvd. SW, 505-877-5700

Judy's Trading Post and Auction www.judystradingpost.com, 6016 Isleta Blvd. SW, 505-877-6000

Route Summary

1. Start at the Gutiérrez-Hubbell House.
2. Follow the Rx Trail clockwise.
3. Turn left on Don Felipe Rd.
4. Bear left onto Mayflower Dr.
5. Turn right on Beck Rd.
6. Turn right on the Durand Lateral.
7. Turn left at the next ditch junction.
8. Turn right at the Los Padillas Spillway Diversion.
9. Follow the Durand Rx Trail south to the gateway.
10. Continue south on the Los Padillas Feeder ditch road.
11. Turn right on Louise Ave.
12. Turn right on Isleta Blvd. to return to the Gutiérrez-Hubbell House.

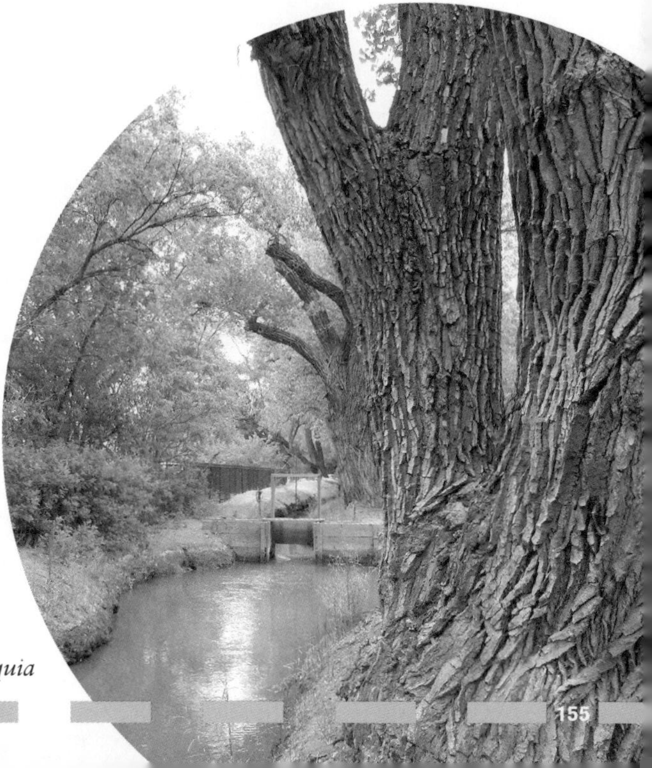

Pajarito Acequia

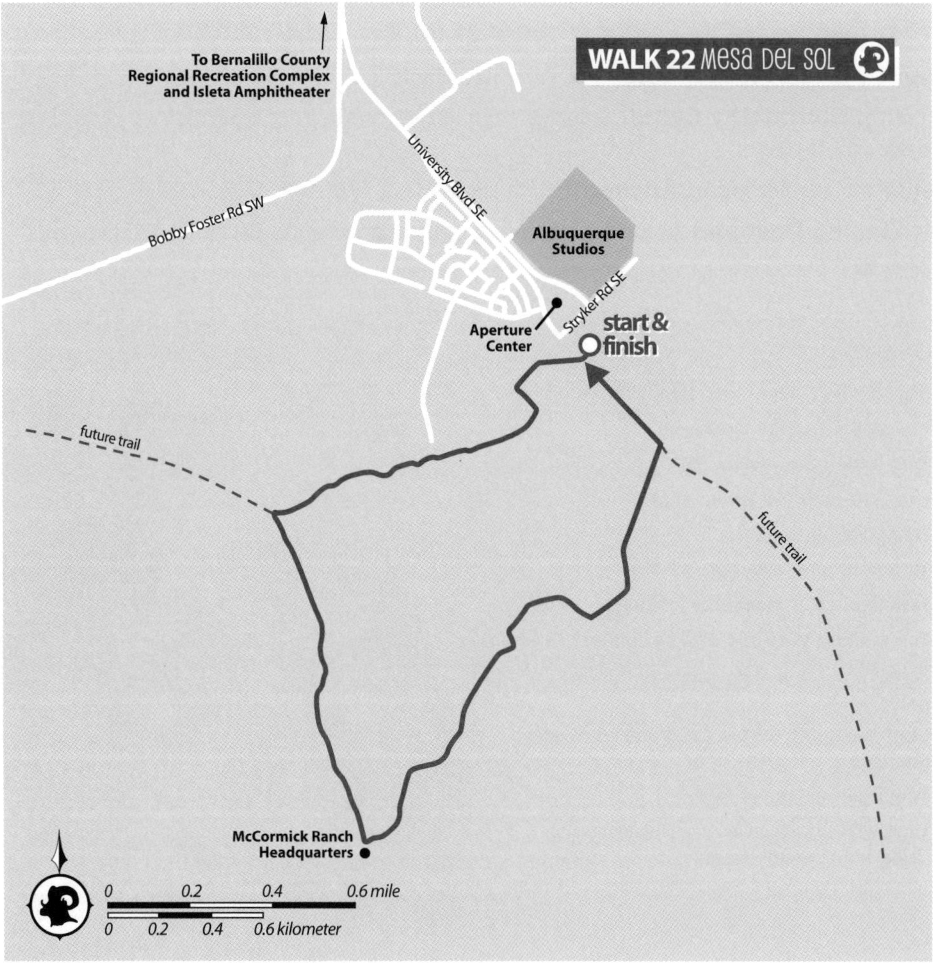

WALK 22 Mesa del Sol
To Bernalillo County Regional Recreation Complex and Isleta Amphitheater
University Blvd SE
Bobby Foster Rd SW
Albuquerque Studios
Stryker Rd SE
Aperture Center
start & finish
future trail
future trail
McCormick Ranch Headquarters
0 0.2 0.4 0.6 mile
0 0.2 0.4 0.6 kilometer

22 Mesa del Sol: Future Perspectives

BOUNDARIES: **University Blvd., Perspectives Trail**
DISTANCE: **3.1 miles (5K)**
DIFFICULTY: **Moderate (unpaved trail)**
PARKING: **Free at University Blvd. and Stryker Rd.**
PUBLIC TRANSIT: **MDS shuttle from George Pearl Hall on UNM Main Campus**

Located on the southern outskirts of town, Mesa del Sol is a large-scale mixed-use master planned community. At 12,900 acres—nearly the size of the borough of Manhattan—it occupies about 12 percent of the city of Albuquerque. Much of the land is held in state trust primarily for the University of New Mexico. In May 2001, the State Land Office named Forest City as the master developer. Everything about their plan looked good on paper. The community would be the largest and most ambitious New Urbanist development in the Southwest. Homes, parks, shops, schools, and offices would be built within walking distance of each other. And instead of cookie-cutter homes thrown down in assembly-line fashion, 37,000 signature houses would be constructed in eight distinct villages over a 50-year period.

But in 2006, just as construction workers were breaking ground, the U.S. housing bubble began to burst. To complicate matters further, reports emerged of a so-called Radioactive and Mixed Waste Management Facility (RMWMF) just over a mile east of Mesa del Sol property. It's essentially a hole in the ground where Sandia National Laboratories dumped 1.5 million cubic feet of chemical and nuclear waste—and then covered it up with 3 feet of dirt. News of the toxic mess would've sent normal investors running for the nearest exit. (It's likely what prompted Forest City to sell off their interests and retreat to their headquarters in the relatively pristine city of Cleveland, Ohio.) But Mesa del Sol is a public-private partnership built with city, state, and federal funds. And though the RMWMF debacle still remains unresolved, development on the mesa continues.

Attractions on the mesa include the **Bernalillo County Regional Recreation Complex,** a 640-acre facility with 44 sports fields and the **Isleta Amphitheater.** Formerly known as the Mesa del Sol Amphitheater, the Journal Pavilion, and the Hard Rock Pavilion, the outdoor music venue has a capacity of 15,000 and hosts events like Tim McGraw's Sundown Heaven Town

Back Story: Mark 17 Impact Site

On May 27, 1957, a B-36 bomber approached Kirtland Air Force Base with a crew of 20 airmen and a Mark 17 hydrogen bomb. With a design yield of 20 megatons of TNT, it was potentially 1,000 times more destructive than the atomic bombs dropped on Japan. At an altitude of 1,700 feet, and for reasons still unclear, the bomb dropped from its sling and tore through the closed bomb bay doors. The sudden loss of the 42,000-pound payload sent the plane skyrocketing as the H-bomb nosedived into grazing land. Though the plutonium pit had been removed as a safety precaution for "broken arrow" events such as this, the bomb was loaded with 300 pounds of high explosives and various uranium/plutonium components. The resulting explosion blasted a 25-foot crater in the mesa top and scattered shrapnel nearly a mile. At least one cow was killed by flying debris. Despite immediate and repeated cleanup efforts, souvenir hunters with metal detectors and Geiger counters continue to find radioactive fragments in the northeast corner of Mesa del Sol. In 1996, the Center for Land Use Interpretation placed a small monument on the Mark 17 Impact Site. It has since been removed, and currently nothing remains on-site to acknowledge the historic incident.

Tour, Wiz Khalifa's Under the Influence Tour, and Mötley Crüe's Final Tour. (Let's hope they mean it this time.)

Albuquerque Studios, a 28-acre site with eight state-of-the art sound stages, opened in 2007 as the largest media production facility in the Southwest and has since hosted such productions as *The Avengers, Terminator Salvation, The Book of Eli, Hieroglyph,* and all six seasons of *Breaking Bad.* Across the street, construction of the Phase One Residential area began in 2011 and neared completion in 2014 with 213 homes.

Between the studio and the neighborhood, and marking the southern terminus of the University Blvd. extension, is the curved glass façade of **Aperture Center,** an 80,000-square-foot structure completed in 2008. World-renowned architect (and New Mexico native) Antoine Predock designed this award-winning, LEED-certified building to accommodate restaurants and retail stores on the first floor and office space on the upper floors. So far, no retailers have moved in, and **Rose's Table Café** is the only food option. Fortunately, it's a good one, specializing in flavors from the proprietor's hometown of Merida. For breakfast, get the huevos motuleños, the Yucatán version of huevos rancheros. For lunch, try the soft tacos made with cochinita pibil, pork slow-roasted Mayan style. For dinner, well, the nearest dinner option is about an 8-mile drive. (See Walk 28.)

Also housed in the Aperture Center is the academic arm of UNM's **Interdisciplinary Film and Digital Media** program. (See Walk 25 for the research arm, ARTS Lab.) The program is designed to advance technology in numerous fields, including gaming, engineering, marketing, journalism, and fine arts. Check their schedule for exhibitions, film fests, and other events.

For now, most of Mesa del Sol remains a vacant, arid plain, but another feature developers have long envisioned is a 30-mile natural-surface trail system for runners, walkers, bicyclists, and outdoor enthusiasts. By mid-2014, the Perspective Trail was the only trail completed, and it's popular for both 5K races and slow, contemplative walks. Of course there's a chance you'll find it rumbling with construction projects in the immediate vicinity. Or you might find it as I did on a midsummer walk in 2014—under a commotion of Western kingbirds, agitated at my presence, apparently, because there wasn't another human soul anywhere to be seen.

- **Start at the south corner of the parking lot behind the Aperture Center. A trailhead sign there maps out the route, and trail markers can guide you through the rest of it. Head west and follow the route counterclockwise. The first mile skirts around the proposed school site and along the south side of a residential area yet to be built. A junction near the end of the first mile is the site of the proposed Central Park trailhead, according to the development plan. Eventually, two trails should split from here, one aiming northwest toward Mount Taylor, the other southwest toward Sierra Ladrones.**

- **Turn left and continue another 0.75 mile on Perspective Trail to the remnants of old corrals. The trail map identifies the site as Historic McCormick Ranch Headquarters. The ranch began in the early 1900s and grew to nearly 20,000 acres by 1941, roughly spanning east–west from present-day I-25 to the Manzano foothills, and north–south from Tijeras Arroyo to Isleta Pueblo.**

  At the onset of World War II the National Defense Research Committee recruited UNM physics professor Jack Workman, along with researchers from Columbia University,

Johns Hopkins, Princeton, and the University of Michigan, to develop top-secret weapons. Workman acquired A. W. McCormick's land lease along with 10,000 acres of adjacent property to create the New Mexico Proving Ground (NMPG). Projects here included the development of armor-piercing projectiles and proximity fuzes. The latter was instrumental in stopping the Nazi V-1 rocket attacks on Britain. During tests conducted at the NMPG from 1941 to 1952, researchers fired a total of 15,923 rounds of ordnance and rockets. The mess they left behind is the subject of an astonishing 500-page South Kirtland Operations Area (SKOPA) report, released in 2006.

The eastern part of the NMPG eventually became the site of Mesa del Sol, while the larger western portion would become SKOPA. By then it had expanded deep into the neighboring Sandia Ranger District of Cibola National Forest. That massive tract of public land still remains strictly off-limits to the public, and maintained signage on the trails there warns of an "unmarked unexploded ordnance area."

- Turn left and follow the trail 1.25 miles northeast. A trail planned for the junction here should someday lead to La Semilla, a 2,880-acre nature reserve and environmental education center that doesn't yet exist. The mile-wide strip of recreational land shares a 4.5-mile boundary with the military installation. La Semilla ("the seed") also serves as a buffer zone between the Mesa del Sol community and explosive activities to the immediate east. Although it isn't mentioned in the La Semilla Master Plan, the Mark 17 Impact Site is located on the northern end of the property. (See Back Story on page 158.)

- Turn left and follow the trail a quarter mile northwest to return to the parking area.

POINTS OF INTEREST

Bernalillo County Regional Recreation Complex bernco.gov, 5601 University Blvd. SE, 505-314-0400

Isleta Amphitheater isletaamphitheater.net, 505-452-5100

Albuquerque Studios abqstudios.com, 5650 University Blvd. SE, 505-227-2000

Aperture Center 5700 University Blvd. SE

Rose's Table Café rosestablecafe.com; 5700 University Blvd. SE, Suite 130; 505-433-5772

Interdisciplinary Film and Digital Media Program ifdm.unm.edu, 505-277-2286

Mesa del Sol mesadelsolnm.com, 505-452–2600

route summary

1. Start at the south corner of the parking lot behind the Aperture Center.
2. Follow Perspective Trail counterclockwise.

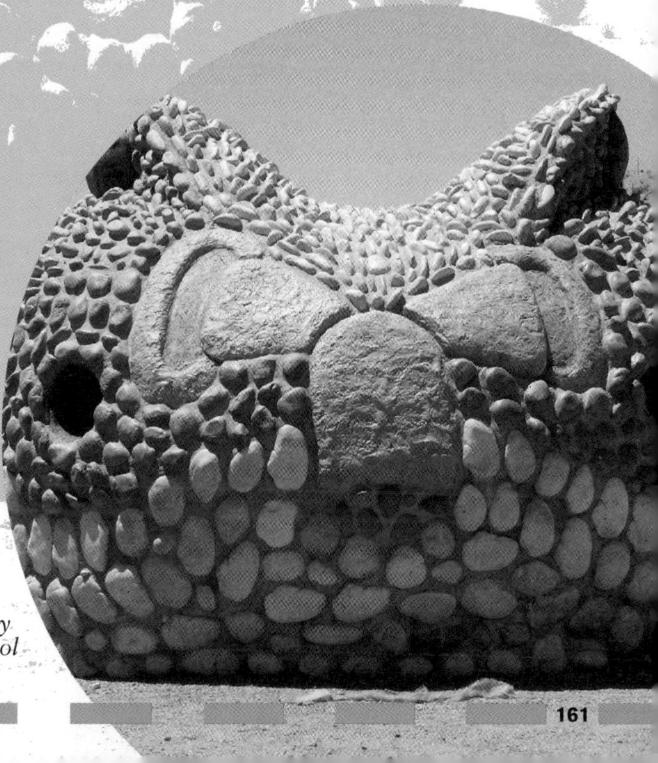

A 450-foot rattlesnake sculpture on the University Blvd. median, about 3 miles north of Mesa del Sol

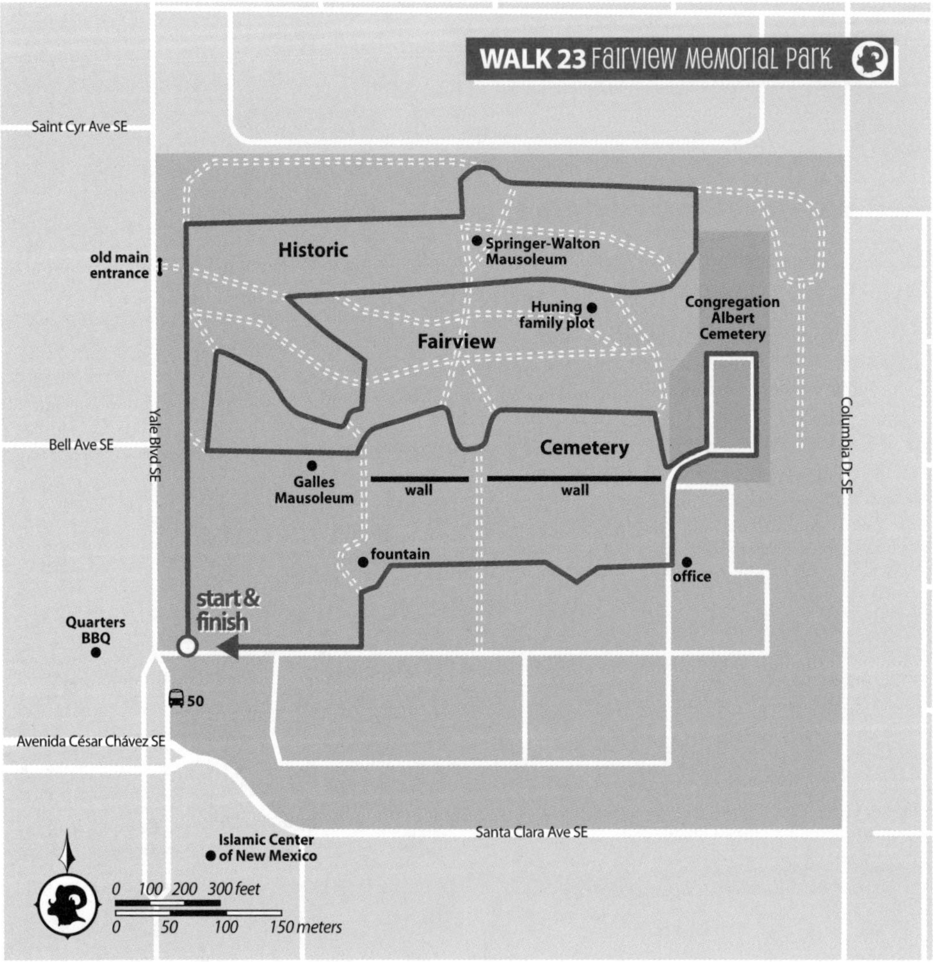
WALK 23 Fairview Memorial Park
Saint Cyr Ave SE
old main entrance
Historic
Springer-Walton Mausoleum
Huning family plot
Congregation Albert Cemetery
Fairview
Bell Ave SE
Yale Blvd SE
Cemetery
Columbia Dr SE
Galles Mausoleum
wall
wall
fountain
office
start & finish
Quarters BBQ
50
Avenida César Chávez SE
Islamic Center of New Mexico
Santa Clara Ave SE
0 100 200 300 feet
0 50 100 150 meters

23 Fairview Memorial Park: Gone But Not Forgotten

BOUNDARIES: **Yale Blvd., Garfield Ave., Columbia Dr., Santa Clara Ave.**
DISTANCE: **1.5 miles**
DIFFICULTY: **Moderate (unpaved roads and paths)**
PARKING: **Free parking within the cemetery**
PUBLIC TRANSIT: **Bus 50 on Yale Blvd. at Avenida César Chávez**

People have been living—and dying—in the Albuquerque area for 12,000 years, so it's difficult to pinpoint exactly when the custom of burying corpses began around here. The oldest local Anasazi burial sites date back to A.D. 500–900. Spanish camposantos in town date to the early 1700s. The first graveyard to serve modern Albuquerque was Fairview Cemetery, now Fairview Memorial Park, established in 1881 2 miles east of the new town center. Essentially, it was a landfill in a sandhill, a simple place where people went to deposit their departed friends and relatives. In 1892, an editorial in the Albuquerque Morning Journal lamented the "present excuse for a cemetery." Written by Elias Sleeper Stover, then serving as the first president of the University of New Mexico, the letter called for the formation of an association to designate and manage a "proper cemetery worthy of the growth and promise of Albuquerque." The town's new business elite—Franz Huning, William Hazeldine, and Sleeper himself—soon answered the call by forming the Albuquerque Cemetery Association and transforming Fairview into a symbol of urban prosperity. It has since expanded to 36 acres with an overall body count exceeding 30,000.

Note: For liability reasons, No Trespassing signs are posted throughout the park. For one, the park attracts more than its fair share of vagrants and vandals. Also, exploring old cemeteries is inherently risky. Do not lean on headstones or railings. Avoid walking on grave sites, as it may cause the casket to collapse and expose you to a potentially infectious corpse. Avoid any rodents (ground squirrels, mainly) you may encounter. Keep any kids close at hand. Dogs are not permitted in the memorial park. You can also check with the park office for a quick overview of cemetery etiquette and precautions.

Back Story: The White Plague

By the latter part of the 19th century, 150,000 Americans were dying annually from tuberculosis, otherwise known as consumption, phthisis, scrofula, and the White Plague. For every death, an estimated 10–20 others were suffering the early stages of the agonizing disease. The best treatment at the time was clean, dry, high-altitude air. The arrival of the railroad in Albuquerque was perfectly timed to profit from the grisly epidemic. Pamphlets distributed throughout eastern cities promised "sunshine and health in Albuquerque" but also warned, "DON'T come to Albuquerque for health if you are broke." Sanatoriums sprang up throughout the state. Railroad Ave., now Central, was known as San Row, and one out of every three people in the state was a "lunger." Throughout the health-seeking movement, nearly 25 percent of patients died in treatment, while 50 percent of those released succumbed within 5 years of discharge. New Mexico's lucrative TB industry ground to a halt in 1944 with the discovery of the antibiotic streptomycin. However, drug-resistant strains of the disease emerged in the 1980s, and currently an estimated 500,000 new cases of multidrug-resistant tuberculosis occur annually worldwide.

- **Start at the entry gate, located in the southwest corner of the park. This side is the original Fairview Memorial Park, created by Strong-Thorne Mortuary in 1935 to the immediate south of the 1881 cemetery. These 19 acres are characterized by robust trees, tidy grounds, green turf, grid patterns, straight roads and paths, and headstones that remain largely intact. Depending on wind conditions, the smoker at Quarters BBQ across the street may torment you with the delicious scent of brisket and ribs. A breeze from the east, however, might smell of something overcooked. That would be coming from the crematory.**

- **Go north on the nearest road, a narrow corridor lined with trees. This pleasant 100-yard stretch leads you directly to the barren chaos of the historic cemetery. Funds for perpetual care end here in the historic section, and everything that characterizes the south side is largely absent from the north side. The treeline straggles to an end with a few surviving elms. Invasive species such as salt cedar and Russian olive have taken hold in small patches. And like so many other neglected landscapes in town,** ground cover is a carpet of goat heads. Stick to the roads to avoid picking up and carrying their thorny seeds into groomed areas of the park.

Susan Schwartz, historian for Fairview Cemetery, devotes time to organizing cleanups and leading tours of this section. For a positive perspective, she suggests introducing it this way: "Historic Fairview Cemetery takes one back in time when Albuquerque was still in its infancy. As you walk through more than a century of burials, a sense of community starts to form in your mind. As your walk continues, you see thousands of names on headstones, bringing to mind streets, buildings, and businesses with these same names. It makes you curious and holds you captive wanting to know more about the individuals buried here. It is not just a cemetery, it is the final resting place for countless founders and the infamous people in this Land of Enchantment."

- Continue north on the dusty road. The old main entrance is ahead on the left. The gates were constructed in 1925 by artist/contractor Angelo DeTullio. His obituary, published the same year, credits him as "the first man to introduce motion pictures into Albuquerque" for the newsreels he screened in 1898.

- Take the first right north of the old gates. Many of the cemetery's earliest individual graves are in the grid on your left. Ahead on the right, members of the Benevolent and Protective Order of Elks are laid out in a distinctive half-moon formation. Burials in this section date from 1921 to 1985. To the immediate east is the Springer-Walton mausoleum, a simplified Classical Revival structure with a tiered roof that's now vegetated with prickly pear cactus. The west-facing doorway is securely bolted with rebar to prevent trespassing, escape, or both.

- Turn left, followed by a quick right at the T-junction. A historical map indicates this section, 17E, is subdivided between "colored" and "Indian." Most of the markers have gone missing, and in an unfortunate twist, a Confederate soldier somehow ended up in the colored section. Shards of glass and chinaware, some of it predating World War I, are inexplicably scattered throughout the Indian section. Continue east along the south side of 17D, the "stillborn" section.

- Turn right on the next road, and bear left at the Y ahead. The Huning family plot is on the left. Franz, buried in the middle, developed the Highland neighborhood explored in Walk 2. By now you may have noticed subtle curves in the roads. Some are based on the original layout, which mimicked Victorian designs popularized in bigger cities decades earlier. Others are unintended changes to the cemetery's circulation patterns, with "cut-off" roads plowed through sections. The hook through the colored section destroyed individual grave sites, while the curved approach to the Huning plot destroyed entire family plots.

- Follow the winding roads back to the southwest corner of the old cemetery, taking time to note the various designs in curbing, wrought iron, and headstones. Also note causes of death where indicated for a perspective on how efficiently tuberculosis populated these hallowed grounds. (See Back Story on page 164.)

- As you approach the point where you entered the old cemetery, turn left on the road heading east alongside section 14. With white mulberry, elm, spruce, and juniper shading the graves, this section hints at the original landscaping intent. It also contains the Galles Mausoleum. H. L. Galles founded Galles Motor Company in 1908 and sold the first 11 cars in the New Mexico Territory. The company remains as the oldest and largest family automotive business in the state.

- The road bends northeast to pass between two Masonic sections, with graves dating 1898–1922 on the left (section 6) and 1916–1987 on the right (section 11A). Directly east of 11A is the bigger of the cemetery's two Woodmen of the World sections. Resembling amputated trees and stacked logs, the WOW monuments are the most unusual and elaborate in the cemetery. Classic symbols of the fraternal organization include the ax, mallet, wedge, and Latin inscription Dum Tacet Clamet (though silent, he speaks).

- Continue winding your way east to the brick entrance of the Congregation Albert Cemetery. Established in 1882 by the B'nai B'rith Lodge No. 336 and acquired in 1902 by the Congregation Albert, the Reform Jewish Temple in Albuquerque, this secluded section is a tranquil, green oasis. An old wrought iron entry arch set on rock posts (now blocked off) indicates where the original entry was located. Walk the paved loop and exit the way you came in.

- Turn left to exit the old cemetery and go south to the parking lot. On the left is a hollow tile and white stucco building designed in the California Mission style by Brittelle and Ginner and constructed in 1934 by Kilbourne L. House. It originally functioned as

New Mexico's first crematorium. After a fire in 1982, the building was internally redesigned to hold offices, a family consulting room, and the columbarium for cremains. The cremator was relocated to a building just east of its original site.

- Turn right and walk west from the parking lot to the fountain, where you'll find Clyde and Carrie Tingley. In 1910 the couple was bound for Arizona when Carrie suffered a tuberculosis attack. They disembarked the train in Albuquerque and decided to stay. Though his grammar often betrayed his lack of formal education, Clyde's unique way with words made him a popular politician. He was a progressive leader who, quite simply, got things done, bringing paved streets, public parks, hospitals, and numerous other projects to the city. As governor of New Mexico, he mastered the art of obtaining and allocating New Deal funds to shepherd his impoverished state through the Depression. (Those closest to the Tingleys credited Carrie for 90 percent of Clyde's success.) In the end, however, his greed for power would grow to overshadow his 40-year political career, and he is remembered today as much for his bullying and corruption as his unparalleled achievements.

- Turn left at the fountain and return to the entry road. A right turn will take you back to the gate. If you wish to explore more of the park, a current map labels sections along the south wall from west to east accordingly: Cremation, Greek, Fellowship of the Desert, Baby Land, and the Islamic Center of New Mexico. (Either many Muslims ended up in Baby Land or the current map is slightly out of order.) The domed mosque at the Islamic Center can be seen beyond the cemetery walls. Visitors are welcome for tours by appointment. You'll also find veterans memorials near the southeast corner of the park.

POINTS OF INTEREST

Fairview Memorial Park facebook.com/historicfairviewcemetery, 700 Yale Blvd. SE, 505-262-1454

Quarters BBQ thequartersbbq.com, 801 Yale Blvd. SE, 505-843-6949

Islamic Center of New Mexico icnm-abq.org, 1100 Yale Blvd. SE, 505-256-1450

route summary

1. Start inside the entry gate and walk north.
2. Take the first right north of the old gates.
3. Turn left at the Springer Mausoleum, followed by a quick right at the junction, and follow the road around east about 100 yards.
4. Turn right toward the brick wall; then go left at the Y ahead.
5. Follow the winding roads back to the southwest corner of the old cemetery.
6. Near the point where you entered the old cemetery, turn left on the road heading east.
7. Wind east to the brick entrance of the Congregation Albert Cemetery.
8. Walk the paved loop and exit the way you came in.
9. Turn left to exit the old cemetery and go south to the parking lot.
10. Turn right in the parking lot and walk west to the fountain.
11. Proceed southwest to return to the entry gate.

connecting the walks

Walk 24 visits Isotopes Park on Avenida César Chávez less than a half mile west of Fairview Memorial Park.

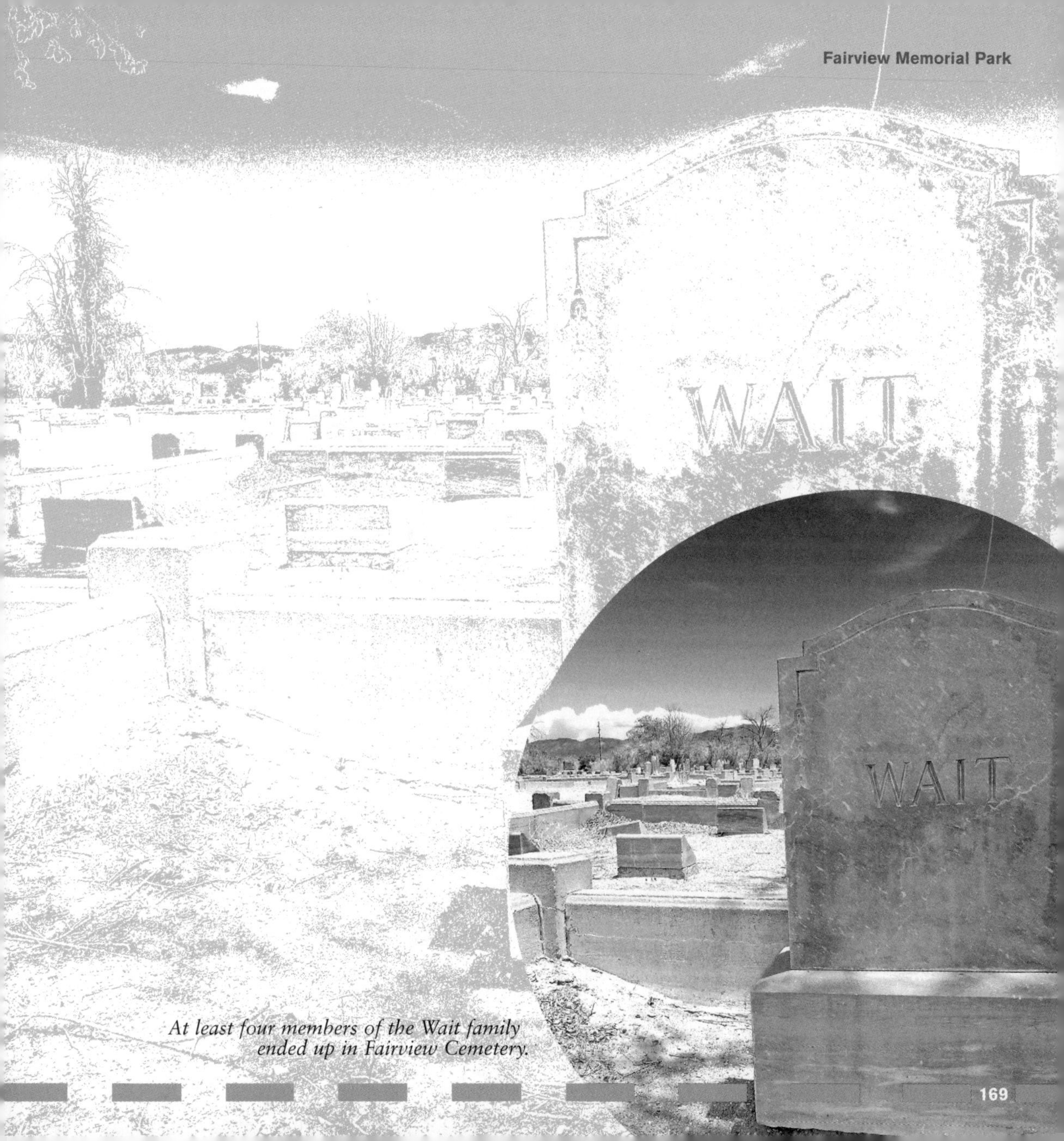

At least four members of the Wait family ended up in Fairview Cemetery.

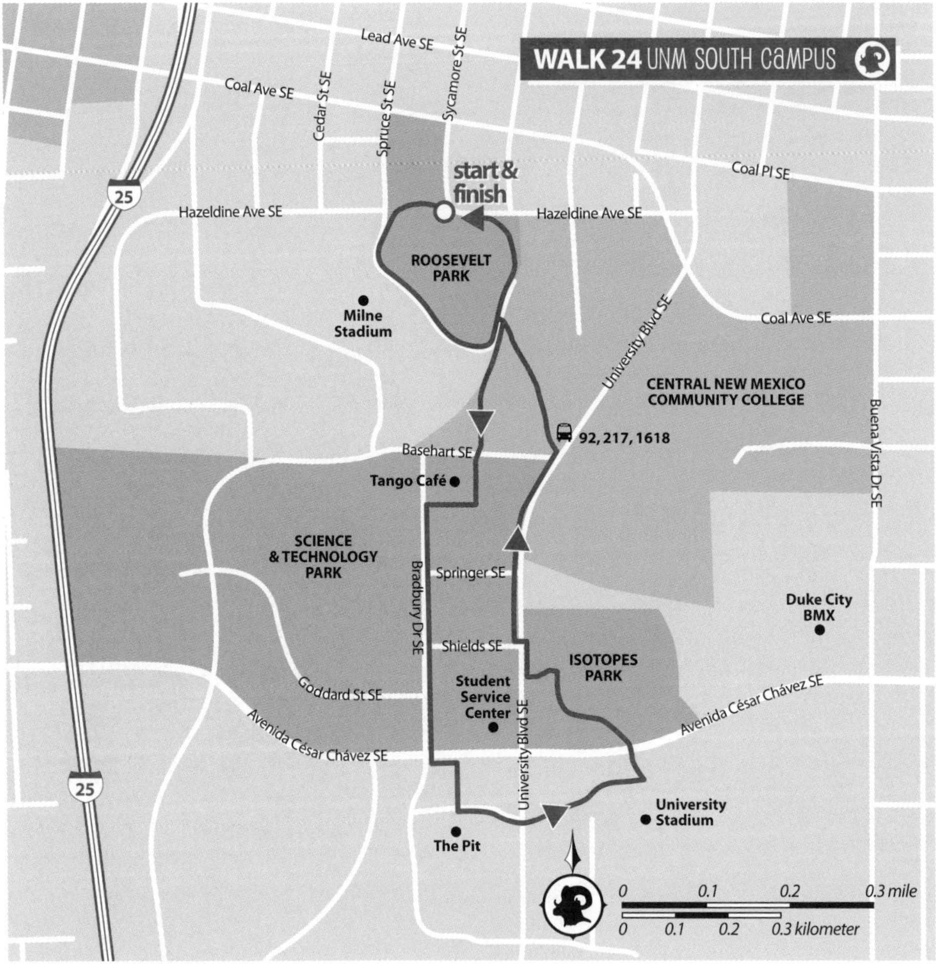
WALK 24 UNM SOUTH CAMPUS
Lead Ave SE
Coal Ave SE
Cedar St SE
Spruce St SE
Sycamore St SE
Coal Pl SE
start & finish
25
Hazeldine Ave SE
Hazeldine Ave SE
ROOSEVELT PARK
Milne Stadium
Coal Ave SE
University Blvd SE
CENTRAL NEW MEXICO COMMUNITY COLLEGE
Buena Vista Dr SE
92, 217, 1618
Basehart SE
Tango Café
SCIENCE & TECHNOLOGY PARK
Bradbury Dr SE
Springer SE
Duke City BMX
Shields SE
ISOTOPES PARK
Student Service Center
Goddard St SE
University Blvd SE
Avenida César Chávez SE
Avenida César Chávez SE
25
University Stadium
The Pit
0
0.1
0.2
0.3 mile
0
0.1
0.2
0.3 kilometer

24 UNM SOUTH CAMPUS: JOCKS AND NERDS

BOUNDARIES: **Coal Ave., Bradbury Dr., Avenida César Chávez, Buena Vista Dr.**
DISTANCE: **2 miles**
DIFFICULTY: **Easy**
PARKING: **Free parking at Sycamore St. and Hazeldine Ave.**
PUBLIC TRANSIT: **Buses 92, 217, and 1618 on University Blvd. at Basehart Rd.; UNM shuttle system (free)**

While the University of New Mexico south campus is a center of intellectual and athletic achievement, it lacks the consistent aesthetic and identity of the older central campus. The district is divided into disconnected parts. There are $250 million worth of athletic facilities and a comparable amount invested in cutting-edge laboratories. There are also massive tracts of undeveloped land and even greater acreage devoted to parking lots that largely sit vacant except during athletic events. Both UNM and city planners recognize the faults and potential for the area, and their goals seem to be in sync, at least in terms of developing public spaces and amenities that connect people and consistently populate the area. On an average workday, about 5,000 employees occupy the south campus. During events, the population can increase tenfold. Depending on your preferences between jocks and nerds, you can make the most of this walk by timing it to attend or avoid the games. Or as a compromise, check with the sports venues for smaller events and activities, such as training camps and scrimmage matches, that will allow you access to the grand interiors of these modern coliseums without the hassle of frenzied fanatics. And to make the most of your intellect, check with the Science & Technology Park for enlightening seminars that are free and open to the public.

- **Start at Roosevelt Park, a 15-acre city park designed by a local landscape architect and built with federal Civil Works Administration funding in the midst of the Great Depression. It was originally named Terrace Park, but Mayor Clyde Tingley had it changed to honor his close friend and benefactor, President Franklin Roosevelt. The project employed 275 CWA laborers to plant more than 2,250 trees and bushes, including umbrella catalpas and Siberian elms. The abutment along the south side of the park was built with stone recovered from the demolition of a county jail across town. The land's transformation from a sandy arroyo to a verdant oasis took little more than a year, and the landscape has changed little since—except perhaps for the**

$2.8 million renovation it received in 2007. The shaded hollow now contains a disc golf course, a playground, and a 0.65-mile perimeter path.

- Follow the path around to the west side of the park. This ridge overlooks both the park and Milne Stadium to the immediate west. The view of the football field from here is as good as anywhere in the stands. Built in 1939, the stadium hosts Albuquerque Public School football, track and field, and community events. Continue on the trail to the east side of the park, where the wall is just high enough to deter the feeble and infirm from hopping over it. But keep going and eventually you should find an open gate.

- Exit through the gate and turn right into a parking lot on the campus of Central New Mexico Community College. Serving 30,000 students across seven campuses, CNM boasts the largest higher-education enrollment in the state. The main campus is the 60 acres extending east and southeast from Roosevelt Park.

- Walk south toward the building with the giant soccer ball on the roof. Actually, that's a data-receiving antenna at the Center for Rapid Environmental Assessment and Terrain Evaluation (CREATE). It receives MODIS data from NASA's Aqua and Terra satellites, and data from NOAA's HRPT satellites. These data sets can be used in Decision Support Systems in hydrology, meteorology, ecology, and climatology, as well as decision models for rapid-response situations such as terrorist attacks and major environmental disasters. In other words: don't call it a giant soccer ball.

  The CREATE Receiving Station is on the north side of the UNM Science & Technology Park. Established in 1965, the STP currently consists of 662,662 square feet of research and development, laboratory, office, and mixed-use space, about half of which is currently developed. CREATE's neighbor to the west is the Manufacturing Training and Technology Center. It houses the auditorium where public seminars are held, but one of its most impressive facilities is Tango Café (open Monday–Friday, 7 a.m.–3 p.m.). The daily specials are always good, and unless you plan to hit the concession stands at a ball game later on, this is your only dining option on the route.

- Turn right at the circle in the plaza and walk about 100 yards west.

- Turn left on Bradbury Dr. The homely building ahead on the right houses the Albuquerque Institute for Mathematics and Science. In 2014, U.S. News & World Report ranked it as the best high school in New Mexico and the 17th best charter school in the nation.

Across the street is the Advanced Materials Lab, which hosts collaborative researchers from UNM, Sandia National Laboratories, and "qualified" U.S. companies. You probably don't want to know what really goes on in there. Ahead on the left is the Center for High Technology Materials, an interdisciplinary research organization involving faculty and students from the departments of electrical and computer engineering, physics and astronomy, and chemical and nuclear engineering. The building at the corner of University Blvd. and Avenida César Chávez is the Student Support & Services Center, where you can obtain maps and additional information about features and attractions in the area.

- Cross Avenida César Chávez, named for the American labor leader, civil rights activist, and recipient of the U.S. Medal of Freedom. Straight ahead is The Pit, home to UNM Lobos basketball since 1966. The name comes from its unique construction. The 338-by-300-foot roof was built first, and then 55,000 cubic yards of earth were excavated beneath it to form the bowl of the arena. There are no supporting pillars in the seating area of the arena to obstruct views of the court, which is set 37 feet beneath street level. Initial cost was a mere $1.4 million, though $60 million worth of improvements in 2010 raised its profile while reducing its seating capacity.

The most memorable sports moment from this arena didn't involve the Lobos, but rather the Wolfpack. North Carolina State's upset over Houston in the 1983 NCAA Final Four championship set coach Jimmy Valvano running around the court in search of someone to hug. His heartwarming display of elation would become more famous than the buzzer-beating dunk that won the game.

The Pit is also famous for noise and has often been rated as one of the loudest basketball venues in the nation, thanks to rabid Lobos fans and subterranean acoustics. Also, the Rolling Stones played here in 1972. Stevie Wonder was an opening act. Tickets were $5.50. David Bowie, Elvis Presley, and James Brown have also rocked this arena.

- Walk east to University Stadium. Like Roosevelt Park, it was built in a natural arroyo. The Lobos played their first game here on September 17, 1960, defeating the National University of Mexico by a score of 77-6. The largest turnout on record stands at 44,760 for the game against New Mexico State in 2005—back when the stadium was built to hold 38,634 fans. Unless you catch a game or special event here, you won't find a way inside, though the field is partially visible from the gates on the north side.

- Cross back to the north side of Avenida César Chávez. Here you have the option of a quarter-mile detour to Duke City BMX, the largest covered BMX facility in the country. Best to call or check their online schedule before venturing up that way; otherwise all you might see are mounds of dirt under a big roof. There's supposed to be a $17 million velodrome nearby, but, well, remember that Simpsons episode where Springfield bought a self-destructing monorail? Um, that's pretty much what happened with Albuquerque's velodrome. And remember the episode where the Springfield Isotopes moved to Albuquerque? Well, welcome to Isotopes Park.

  The original ballpark that stood on this site was Albuquerque Sports Stadium, built in 1969 for the Albuquerque Dukes. The first batter to stand at the plate was Willie Mays. In 2000, the Dukes moved to Portland, where they became the Beavers, and Albuquerque was left without a pro team for the first time in 41 years. Eager to attract a new team, city voters approved a $25 million renovation of the stadium. In 2003, the Calgary Cannons arrived in the Duke City, where they became the Isotopes. Though "the Lab" (as the stadium is known) seats little more than 13,000 spectators, the 'Topes have been known to draw standing-room-only crowds exceeding 15,000. Like many other Triple-A ballparks, the Lab is a place to experience major league fanfare on an intimate level. If you can't coordinate your walk with a game, you can get a peek at the field from the gates. Or consider scheduling an exhaustive tour of the stadium—well in advance.

- Go northwest across the parking lot to University Blvd. and turn right. The small, bunkerlike building on the right is the Crystal Growth Facility. They do things like grow laser material directly onto silicon chips so that someday we might enjoy ultrafast light-driven computers. Ahead on the left, the institutional-green building houses the Regional Computer Forensics Laboratory, self-billed as "a one-stop, full service forensics laboratory" for digging up digital evidence in criminal investigations. Unfortunately, you have to prove yourself as a legitimate member of a law enforcement agency before they'll go sleuthing through any cell phones or hard drives you bring them.

- Continue straight to the northwest corner of Basehart Rd., and cut diagonally across the CNM parking lot to return to Roosevelt Park.

POINTS OF INTEREST

Roosevelt Park cabq.gov/parksandrecreation, 525 Sycamore St. SE, 505-857-8650

Central New Mexico Community College cnm.edu, 525 Buena Vista Dr. SE, 505-224-3000

Manufacturing Training and Technology Center 800 Bradbury Dr. SE

Public Lecture Series stc.unm.edu, 505-272-7310

Tango Café tangocafeabq.com, 505-224-2980

Student Support & Services Center unm.edu, 1155 University Blvd. SE, 505-277-8503

The Pit golobos.com, 1414 Bradbury Dr. SE, 505-925-5608

University Stadium unmtickets.com, 1111 Avenida César Chávez SE, 505-664-8661

Isotopes Park abqisotopes.com, 1601 Avenida César Chávez SE, 505-924-2255

Duke City BMX dukecitybmx.org, 1011 Buena Vista Dr. SE, 505-890-1269

route summary

1. Start at Roosevelt Park and walk to the west side.
2. Follow the perimeter trail to the gate on the east side.
3. Exit through the gate and turn right.
4. Walk south to the Science & Technology Park.
5. Turn right at the plaza and go to Bradbury Dr.
6. Turn left and walk south to The Pit.
7. Turn left and go to the north side of University Stadium.
8. Go north to Isotopes Park.
9. Go northwest to University Blvd. and turn right.
10. Go north to Basehart Rd.
11. Walk northwest across the parking lot to return to Roosevelt Park.

connecting the walks

Walk 23 begins near the northeast corner of Avenida César Chávez and Yale Blvd., less than half a mile east of Isotopes Park.

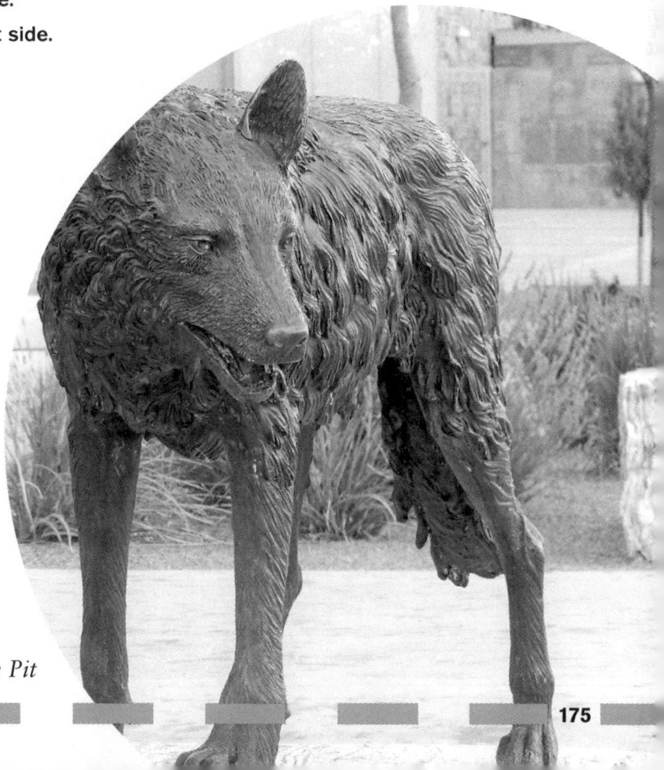

Lobo sculpture at the Pit

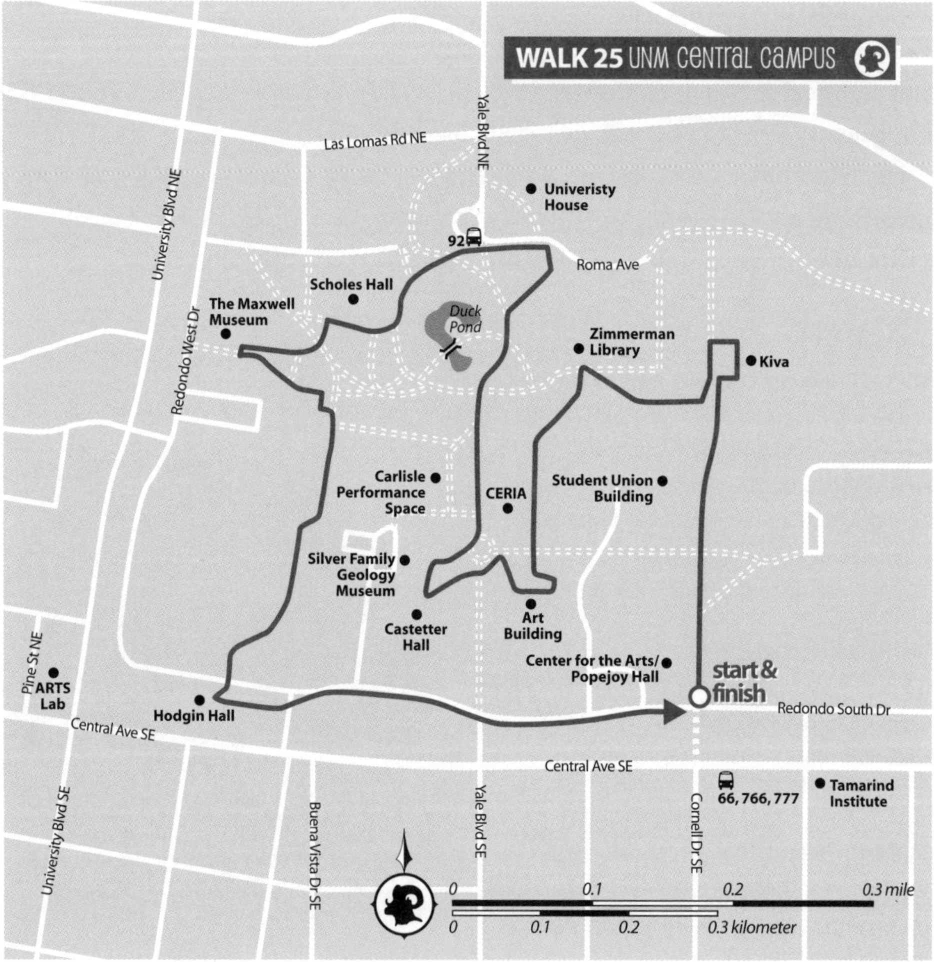
WALK 25 UNM Central Campus
Las Lomas Rd NE
Yale Blvd NE
University Blvd NE
Univeristy House
92
Roma Ave
Scholes Hall
The Maxwell Museum
Redondo West Dr
Duck Pond
Zimmerman Library
Kiva
Carlisle Performance Space
CERIA
Student Union Building
Silver Family Geology Museum
Castetter Hall
Art Building
Center for the Arts/ Popejoy Hall
start & finish
Pine St NE
ARTS Lab
Hodgin Hall
Central Ave SE
Redondo South Dr
Central Ave SE
66, 766, 777
Tamarind Institute
University Blvd SE
Buena Vista Dr SE
Yale Blvd SE
Cornell Dr SE
0
0.1
0.2
0.3 mile
0
0.1
0.2
0.3 kilometer

25 UNM Central Campus: Back to School

BOUNDARIES: **Central Ave., Las Lomas Rd., University Blvd., Stanford Dr.**
DISTANCE: **1.75 miles, plus interiors**
DIFFICULTY: **Easy**
PARKING: **Cornell Visitor Parking Structure on Stanford Dr. and Redondo Dr.; free parking on Ash St.**
PUBLIC TRANSIT: **Bus 66 on Central Ave. at Cornell Dr.; bus 92 on Yale Blvd. at Las Lomas Rd.; UNM shuttle system (free)**

Created by an act of the Territorial Legislature in 1889, the University of New Mexico has since evolved into a showcase of regional Southwest architecture. At least 30 structures on campus are the design of John Gaw Meem. Some call it Pueblo Revival overkill. Frank Lloyd Wright's critique of the campus publicly condemned Meem for using concrete and steel to imitate ancient indigenous designs. Meem shrugged it off, and the campus retains his spirit of simplicity and elegance. But there's more than architecture to contemplate here. This short route visits numerous art galleries, performance spaces, science exhibits, designed landscapes, and more. To make the most of this walk, time it with events posted at **unmevents.unm.edu.** For more info on UNM parking and the free shuttle system, visit **pats.unm.edu.**

- **Start on the west side of the Cornell Visitor Parking Structure and walk north to *Fiesta Dancers* by Chicano sculptor Luis Jiménez. Like so many of his other works, the garish sculpture has generated considerable controversy since the unveiling in 1996. Jiménez often used elements of kitsch and commercialism to comment on widespread misperceptions of Hispanic culture.**

  On your left is the main entrance of the UNM Center for the Arts, which houses five major arts facilities: With seating for more than 2,000 patrons, Popejoy Hall is the largest venue of its kind in the state. Its signature series brings a world-class spectrum of live theater, ballet, modern dance, jazz, classical, and international music performances. Keller Hall, the recital home of the department of music, seats about 300 and hosts about 170 instrumental performances each year. Facilities include an orchestra pit, recording studios, and a 1967 Holtkamp organ. With 2,741 pipes, it's the largest organ in the state. The UNM Art Museum claims to hold the largest collection

of fine art in the state—nearly 30,000 objects in more than a dozen specialized collections ranging from Old Master Painting to Art Since 1950. Rodey Theatre is a 400-seat convertible proscenium/thrust theater designed by George Izenour. Performances showcase student and faculty theatrical productions. Theatre X is a 100-seat convertible space dedicated to experimental performances.

- Continue north past the Student Union Building on your left. The SUB houses eight eateries, a convenience store, a barbershop and salon, a game lounge/pool hall, a computer lab, an arts and crafts center, a grand ballroom, and a movie theater. On your right is Mesa Vista Hall, another one of Meem's Pueblo Revivals. Built in 1950 with decorative yet inaccessible balconies, it resembles something from a B-Western movie set.

- Continue straight and go downstairs to a sunken courtyard. The Campus Arboretum tour brochure indicates that English ivy, India hawthorn, Chinese photinia, and golden rain trees are somewhere in this stand of honey locust. The domed structure on the right is the Kiva Lecture Hall, built in 1968. To its north and built the same year is Masely Hall, named for the founder of the art-education program in 1947. In room 105 you'll find the Masley Art Gallery, which exhibits works by art-education students and faculty and by art teachers and students from the local community.

- Go back up the stairs and turn right. Smith Plaza, ahead, is the site of UNM's first football field. On the north side of the plaza is Zimmerman Library, named for former UNM President James Fulton Zimmerman (1927–1944). Originally built in 1938 as a Public Works Administration project, the library has since been expanded three times to house a collection that now exceeds one million books. Beam carvings throughout the massive ceilings were crafted by Taos, Navajo, and San Juan Pueblo artists. The tour brochure from the Institute for Environmental Education instructs visitors to "lie on the floor and look at the herringbone patterns in latillas between the vigas." So do that now, if nobody is looking. Then visit the Herzstein Latin American Gallery on the second floor.

- Exit the library the way you came in and head toward the west side of the humanities buildings on the south side of the plaza. Walk south and up the stairs to get on the overpass. Continue straight to the art building. At the end of the walkway, the doors on the left open to the John Sommers Gallery. The gallery has two rooms totaling 1,000 square feet. Its rotating program showcases student artwork.

- Exit the art building on the ground level and walk west toward the fountain (Tribute to Mother Earth, by Youn Ja Johnson, 1994). On your right, the CERIA building contains the Museum of Southwestern Biology, which houses collections of plants and animals from the American Southwest and Central and South America. Though primarily a research museum, tours of the facility can be scheduled by appointment. Southwest of the fountain is Castetter Hall, the main building for most biology courses and labs. The Potter wing on the west side has a two-story public Greenhouse Conservatory. To its north is Northrop Hall, home of the Silver Family Geology Museum. Established in the 1930s by Stuart Northrop, the modest display is but a small sample of the 20,000 specimens from the geological collections of the department of earth and planetary sciences.

- Return to the fountain and walk north past the Carlisle Performance Space. Built in 1928 as UNM's first gymnasium, it still retains its original maple floor, which now functions as the stage in a 144-seat dance theater. UNM is the only school in the nation that offers an MFA in flamenco. Posters from the last three decades of its Flamenco Festival are on display inside.

- Continue north to The Center of the Universe, a concrete portal (with sodium vapor lights) that transports you to an alternate dimension known as the Duck Pond. This busy little water feature is especially popular among kids and wedding photographers. However, accommodating waterfowl was not part of the original plan. Shortly after the pond was installed in 1976, people mysteriously began showing up with ducks and leaving without them.

- Follow the path on the right side of the pond. Castetter Cactus Garden is on your right at the former main entrance to Zimmerman Library.

- Bear right at the Y ahead, and go to Roma Ave. On the north side of the street is University House. Built in 1930, this 7,000-square-foot Pueblo Revival home stands on a beautifully landscaped 1-acre lot. President Zimmerman and his family were the first residents. It was listed on the National Register of Historic Places in 1987.

- Turn left on Roma to rejoin the loop around the pond; then turn right after the next building ahead to enter Ash Mall. This pastoral, modernist landscape is characterized by undulating hills covered with seemingly randomly placed trees. The building on the north side of the mall is Scholes Hall, built in 1936 to resemble the Mission church at Acoma Pueblo. It was the first UNM building by Meem to be added to the National Register. The mural on first floor corridor is Union of the Americas by Jesús Guerrero Galván, UNM's artist in residence in 1943.

On the west side of the mall is the Alumni Chapel. This Meem building, built in the Franciscan style, is dedicated to alumni who have died in various wars. Carillon bells chime on the hour and play the UNM fight song at 8 a.m.; "O, Fair New Mexico" at noon; and the alma mater at 5 p.m. Behind the chapel is the Maxwell Museum, founded as the Museum of Anthropology of the University of New Mexico in 1932–which makes it the first public museum in Albuquerque. It holds more than 10 million items in multiple collections. Exhibits and programs relate to cultures around the world, with an emphasis on the cultural heritage of the Southwest. A 46-foot totem pole from British Columbia towers over the courtyard on the east side. The main entrance is on the south side.

- Walk east from the Maxwell Museum and turn right (south) after passing Bandelier Hall. Continue south past the Centennial Engineering Center and Logan Hall. On the west side of Logan is a plaza with a small restaurant, outdoor seating, and a motley collection of abstract sculptures. Cross the plaza and continue south across Redondo Dr. to Hodgin Hall.

Detour 1: Cut southwest through the grove to the corner of Central and University. Across the street to the west is the Arts, Research, Technology, and Science Laboratory, or ARTS Lab. Immersive installations, dome mapping, and other innovative events occur on an irregular schedule in this modest facility, which is described on its website as its "Digital Media Garage."

- Hodgin Hall, UNM's first administration/classroom building, was originally designed in the Richardsonian Romanesque style. Shortly after construction in 1892 the building appeared to be on the verge of collapse due to poorly designed roof trusses. Obsessed with the Spanish Pueblo–Revival style, University President William G. Tight ordered the building to be remodeled accordingly. The overhaul, completed in 1908, included removing the hipped roof and fourth story, with the remaining levels set back in tiers to resemble a terraced pueblo. Its redbrick exterior was stuccoed, the arched windows squared, the corners of the building rounded, and a viga-topped portal added to the east entrance. The new look set the standard for campus buildings to follow. A 10-page brochure from the UNM Alumni Association (unmalumni.com) provides a detailed tour of Hodgin Hall. The aforementioned Institute for Environmental Education tour brochure instructs visitors to "find a partner and make a Roman arch with your bodies," which presents an interesting challenge for those touring alone.

- Go about half a mile east on Redondo to return to the start. Alternately, you could walk along Central to catch a whiff of the many restaurants facing campus. Most cater to student tastes and budgets. Either way you'll pass Yale Park, where stands *Cultural Crossroads of the Americas,* a 1996 sculpture by Bob Haozous. The billboard-sized work made a bolder statement before UNM officials insisted on removing the razor wire that crowned it.

Detour 2: Continue east another block to Stanford Dr.; then go south to Central to visit the Tamarind Institute, UNM's renowned center for fine art lithography. The gallery, hallways, and store are packed with works by master artisan-printers from around the world.

Albuquerque aficionado Rudolfo Carrillo recaps the route with nostalgia: "I first walked UNM's main campus more than 30 years ago and countless times since. As a student stagehand at Popejoy Hall, and later the manager of Keller Hall, I was fascinated by the spacious architecture of UNM's Center for the Arts. Hearing and seeing the Holtkamp organ in Keller Hall still evokes a sense of wonder in me. Wandering north along Mesa Vista Hall when the mall is verdant evokes memories of Professor Berthold's office festooned with a giant papier-mâché phallus and a Palestinian flag. The campus is dynamic, constantly changing, and compelling for the architecture, history, and culture that makes it one of our city's real treasures." Carrillo is the founder of Infinity Report, an award-winning experimental writing site: infinityreport.blogspot.com.

Points of Interest

UNM Center for the Arts finearts.unm.edu, 203 Cornell Dr. NE, 505-277-3824

Popejoy Hall popejoypresents.com, 505-277-8010

Keller Hall music.unm.edu, 505-277-4569

Rodey Theatre theatre.unm.edu, 505-277-4332

Theatre X theatre.unm.edu, 505-277-4332

UNM Art Museum unmartmuseum.org, 505-277-4001

Student Union Building sub.unm.edu, 505-277-2331

Masley Art Gallery, Masley Hall unm.edu/~arted, 505-277-4112

Herzstein Latin American Gallery, Zimmerman Library library.unm.edu, 505-925-9554

John Sommers Gallery, Art Building finearts.unm.edu, 505-277-5861

Museum of Southwestern Biology, CERIA Building msb.unm.edu, 505-277-1360

Silver Family Geology Museum, Northrop Hall epswww.unm.edu, 505-277-4204

Carlisle Performance Space, Elizabeth Waters Center for Dance theatre.unm.edu, 505-277-4332

Maxwell Museum, Anthropology Building maxwellmuseum.unm.edu, 505-277-4405

UNM Arts Lab artslab.unm.edu, 1601 Central Ave. NE, 505-277-2253

Tamarind Institute tamarind.unm.edu, 2500 Central Ave. SE, 505-277-3901

route summary

1. Start at Popejoy Hall.
2. Walk north to Kiva Auditorium.
3. Walk west to Zimmerman Library.
4. Walk south to the art building.
5. Go west to Northrop Hall.
6. Walk north past the Duck Pond to University House.
7. Go to the west side of the Duck Pond.
8. Turn right and go to the anthropology building.
9. Turn around and go east past Bandelier Hall.
10. Turn right and go south to Hodgin Hall.
11. Go east on Redondo Dr. to return to the start.

CONNECTING THE WALKS

Connect with Walk 26 by continuing five blocks east of the Tamarind Institute on Central.

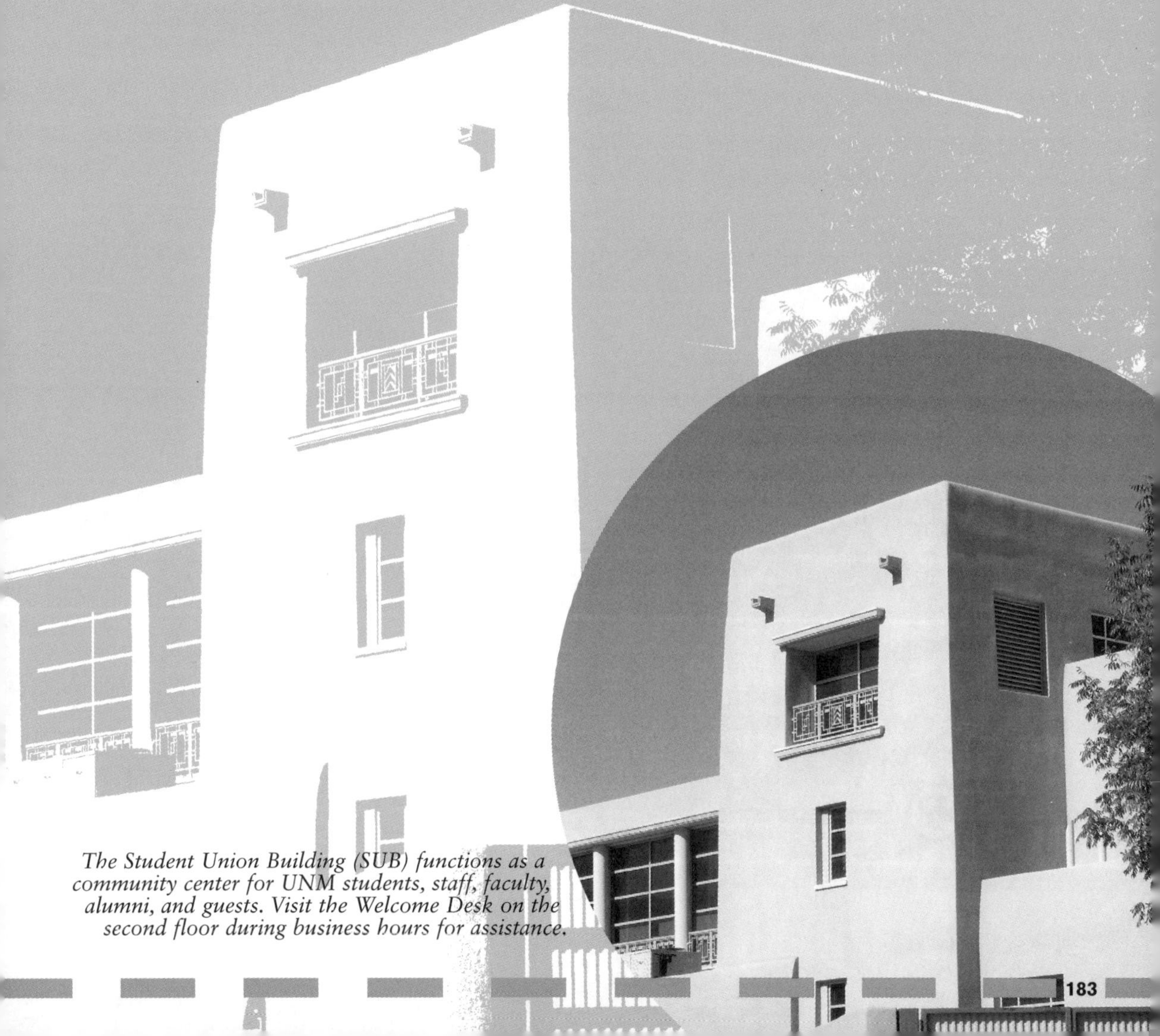

The Student Union Building (SUB) functions as a community center for UNM students, staff, faculty, alumni, and guests. Visit the Welcome Desk on the second floor during business hours for assistance.

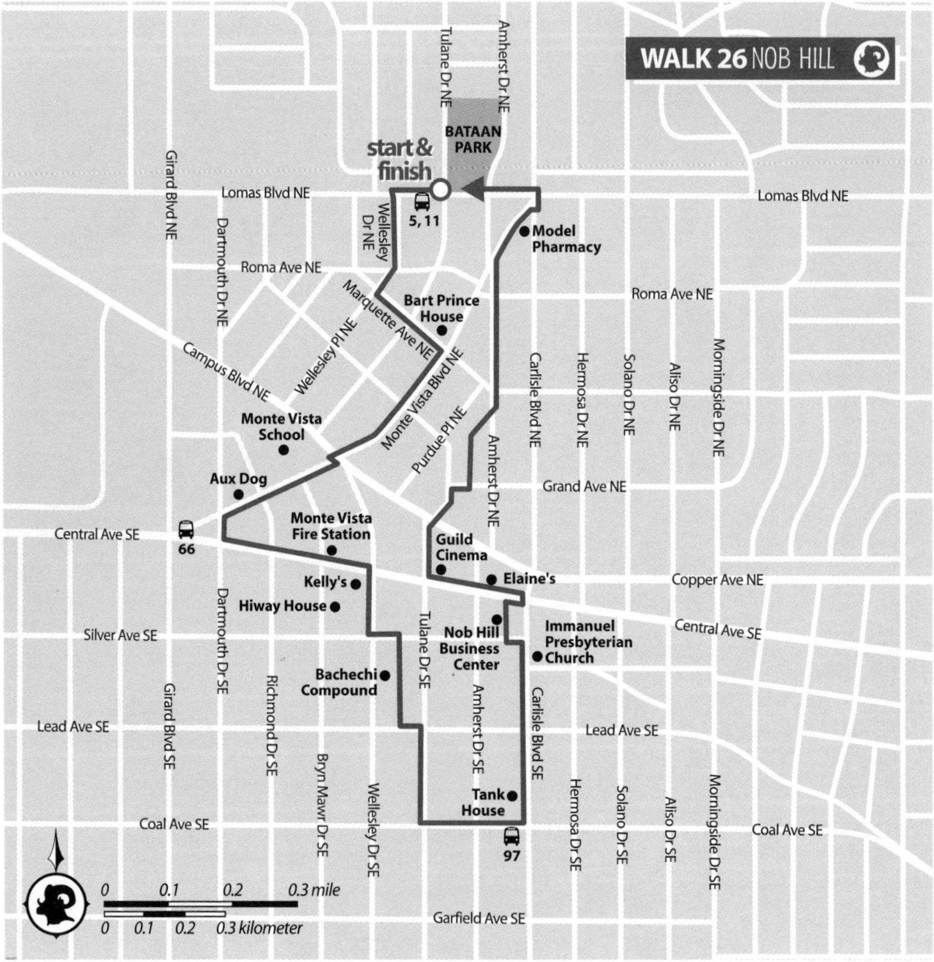
WALK 26 NOB HILL
start & finish
BATAAN PARK
Tulane Dr NE
Amherst Dr NE
Girard Blvd NE
Lomas Blvd NE
Lomas Blvd NE
5, 11
Wellesley Dr NE
Dartmouth Dr NE
Model Pharmacy
Roma Ave NE
Roma Ave NE
Marquette Ave NE
Bart Prince House
Wellesley Pl NE
Campus Blvd NE
Monte Vista Blvd NE
Purdue Pl NE
Carlisle Blvd NE
Hermosa Dr NE
Solano Dr NE
Aliso Dr NE
Morningside Dr NE
Monte Vista School
Amherst Dr NE
Aux Dog
Grand Ave NE
Monte Vista Fire Station
Central Ave SE
66
Guild Cinema
Elaine's
Copper Ave NE
Kelly's
Hiway House
Central Ave SE
Silver Ave SE
Nob Hill Business Center
Immanuel Presbyterian Church
Dartmouth Dr SE
Girard Blvd SE
Richmond Dr SE
Tulane Dr SE
Bachechi Compound
Amherst Dr SE
Carlisle Blvd SE
Lead Ave SE
Lead Ave SE
Bryn Mawr Dr SE
Wellesley Dr SE
Hermosa Dr SE
Solano Dr SE
Aliso Dr SE
Morningside Dr SE
Tank House
Coal Ave SE
Coal Ave SE
97
0 0.1 0.2 0.3 mile
0 0.1 0.2 0.3 kilometer
Garfield Ave SE

26 NOB HILL: HIPSTERS PARADISE

BOUNDARIES: **Lomas Blvd., Dartmouth Dr., Coal Ave., Carlisle Blvd.**
DISTANCE: **3.75 miles**
DIFFICULTY: **Moderate (hilly terrain)**
PARKING: **Free street parking at Bataan Park; metered parking along Central Ave.**
PUBLIC TRANSIT: **Buses 5 and 11 on Lomas Blvd. at Tulane Dr.; buses 66, 766, and 1618 along Central Ave.; bus 97 on Coal Ave. at Carlisle Blvd.**

Nob Hill is a collection of six neighborhood additions spanning from Lomas Blvd. to Zuni Rd., and from Girard Blvd. to Washington St. It's best known for its lively atmosphere of shopping and dining along Historic Route 66. Residential blocks north and south of the popular thoroughfare are showcases of eclectic, sometimes ostentatious architecture. It's self-billed as "Albuquerque's Most Fabulous Neighborhood," though also occasionally referred to as "Snob Hill," which seems less appropriate. Evidence of snootiness is scant. You're more likely to encounter charming denizens throughout this beauteous route. Be warned, however, that this progressive feast/pub crawl is not for amateurs. The number of options for cocktails and cuisine is staggering. Pace yourself accordingly.

- **Start at Bataan Memorial Park. In April 1942 about 12,000 Americans and 63,000 Filipinos captured by the Japanese were forced to walk to distant prison camps in what would become known as the Bataan Death March. In 1943, the city of Albuquerque vowed to build a memorial to the 1,800 New Mexico soldiers serving in defense of the Bataan Peninsula. The 4.5-acre memorial park received City Landmark status in 2012. Monuments are located on the south side of this verdant square.**

- **Walk west on Lomas Blvd. to the crosswalk. The area to the south is the Monte Vista Addition, platted in 1926 by William Leverett Sr. Because of the sloping terrain, Leverett hired a planner from Denver, Saco Rienk DeBoer, who interrupted the traditional grid pattern with subtle curves and diagonal streets. The innovative layout helped minimize seasonal flooding by channeling monsoon rains to Campus Blvd., which was then an arroyo. Monte Vista and its eastern neighbor College View were designated as a National Historic District in 2001.**

- Turn left to head south on Wellesley Dr., which soon bends southwest to intersect with Roma Ave. and Marquette Ave. The intersections create an unusual triangular lot. An isolated residence built on this private island is concealed behind fences and dense foliage.

- Turn left on Marquette Ave. Ahead on the corner of Monte Vista Blvd. is a ribbed capsule perched upon a tile tower. This otherworldly structure—complete with porthole windows; Arcosanti bells; clerestory windows; a masonry tower; and various antennae, posts, and masts—is the residence and studio of architect Bart Prince. Steel dinosaurs guard the driveway. Nearby residences seem to compete for attention in their own odd ways but don't come close to matching the oddity of the spaceship house, as it's locally known. Completed in 1984, it's one of a few new homes in the area. About 80% of the houses in Nob Hill were built before WWII. Popular styles include the regionally inspired Pueblo Revival and Territorial Revival. The Mediterranean Revival was popularized by the Panama-California Exhibition of 1915. Though each has its unique character, all houses in the neighborhood are set back from the street at a uniform distance.

- Turn right on Monte Vista Blvd. On the corner of Campus Blvd. is Monte Vista Elementary School, built in 1935. Leverett dedicated the land for the school to persuade families to move to the neighborhood. (Consider using the crosswalk here to ease your transition to Central Ave. later.) Ahead on the right is Aux Dog, one of the city's best venues to see live theater. This performance venue also houses X Gallery, a fine-arts exhibition space.

- Take a left on Dartmouth Dr., followed by another quick left on Central Ave. The area to the south is University Heights, developed by D. K. B. Sellers. Attracted by Albuquerque's Territorial Fair (Walk 27), Sellers arrived in 1903 following a stint of prospecting in the Klondike Gold Rush. In 1906 he began developing the western half of University Heights, directly south of the UNM campus, and named the streets for prominent universities. Sellers was a pioneering proponent of expanding Albuquerque onto the east mesa, where the air was supposedly healthier. His slogan—"Move out of the low zone and up to the ozone!"—appealed to the city's burgeoning population of tuberculosis patients or "lungers," who flocked to Albuquerque in search of a cure. In 1916 he platted the east half of University Heights, the first addition in what would become known as Nob Hill.

The Deco building on the corner of Dartmouth Dr. and Central Ave. has housed various eateries over the years. Rumor has it the next one will be Mendoza, an Argentinean-themed restaurant with ties to a couple of elite establishments that you'll see later on the walk. Next door is Buffalo Exchange, an upscale thrift store for hip/vintage/repurposed clothes. Another door down is Zinc Wine Bar & Bistro, with elegant dining on the main level and a cool little bar below. Next to that is the Lobo Theater, a former cinema hall that opened in 1938. A church took over the lease in 2000, but the classic marquee and neon still shine bright.

The 3100 block of Central Ave. is a colorful stretch of shops specializing in comics, hats, masks, body modifications, and other essential items. Skipping ahead to the 3200 block, Monte Vista Fire Station was built in 1936 under the auspices of the WPA and expanded in 1952 to accommodate longer trucks. Its resemblance to the Old Albuquerque Airport is no coincidence. Both were designed by architect Ernst Blumenthal, who incorporated a range of Spanish Pueblo–Revival details without compromising the functionality of the facilities. The fire station has since been repurposed into an elegant restaurant. The bar upstairs is favored for blues dancing.

Across the street, the Korean BBQ House might tempt you with the savory aroma of kalbi (grilled short ribs). If weather permits, take advantage of the patio seating. The restaurant occupies the front portion of Hiway House, a classic Route 66 motel built in the 1950s by former New York Yankees owner Del Webb. On the southwest corner at Wellesley Dr. is the former Jones Motor Company, built in 1939 in the Streamline Moderne style and repurposed as a brewpub in 2000. Kelly's has a large outdoor seating area that you'll likely find packed on any evening year-round.

- Turn right on Wellesley Dr. A colorful conglomeration called The Village is on the southwest corner at Silver Ave. There you'll find Limonata Italian Street Food Caffe, offering fresh baked goods and boutique grocery imports. The nearby P'Tit Louis is fashioned like a Paris bistro of the 1920s. Here you can pretend you're an expatriate author like Fitzgerald or Hemingway and drink wine until you run out of money. Or you can just enjoy a delicious duck confit sandwich with a side of rabbit paté.

- Turn left on Silver Ave. The concealed complex to the south is the Bachechi Compound. This Spanish Pueblo–Revival array of structures includes a main house, a pool and pool house, a barn, and three other residential units. The Bachechi family lived here from 1934–1959. German artist Carl Von Hassler, "Dean of the Albuquerque Art Colony," lived in the barn in the 1920s. The Bachechi Farm is a feature on Walk 14.

- Turn right into the first alley ahead. Built to access backyard garages, narrow corridors like this are common throughout Albuquerque neighborhoods developed during the early automotive era.

- Turn left on Lead Ave. and walk half a block east to Tulane Dr. The log cabin on the left was built in 1927 for Colonel Sellers. The 3,800-square-foot structure contains four bedrooms and three full baths on a one-third-acre lot. It sold in 2014 for about $517,000.

- Turn right on Tulane Dr. The most notable residence on the block, a "high style" Pueblo Revival home built in the 1930s, is seven doors down on the left. Look out for the lions guarding the driveway.

- Turn left on Coal Ave.

- Turn left on Carlisle Blvd. and note the cylindrical feature on the second house on the left. When Sellers platted the eastern half of University Heights, he constructed a ground-mounted water tank at the highest point to serve the new addition. Eventually, the city water utility replaced his private system, and in 1937 a house was constructed around the tank, which was repurposed as a living room.

  The Southwest Vernacular house at 300 Carlisle Blvd. was the residence of Mrs. K. B. Patterson, who platted the Granada Heights Addition in 1925. Immanuel Presbyterian Church, designed in the late 1940s by John Gaw Meem, marks the southwest corner of Granada Heights.

  Developer Robert Waggoman built New Mexico's first modern shopping center, Nob Hill Business Center, in 1947. Considering it too far from the downtown commercial area to attract business, critics dubbed it "Waggoman's Folly"—and were soon proven wrong.

- Turn left on Silver Ave. and follow the second crosswalk to a staircase that leads to the interior of the Nob Hill Business Center. Designed by architect Louis Hesselden, the U-shaped structure sports a predominantly Streamline Moderne style with rounded corners, decorative towers, and white stucco walls with horizontal bands of terra-cotta tile and brick. Today its anchor store is La Montañita Co-op Food Market. The nearby Mariposa Gallery is one of the oldest contemporary craft galleries in the country, though rumors indicate it's nearing the end of its long run. Many unusual boutiques occupy the business center, so explore it thoroughly. For excellent tapas in a casual atmosphere, try Gecko's. For a more upscale dining experience, there's the Scalo Northern Italian Grill, a 450-seat establishment with 100 employees. Steve Paternoster is the mastermind behind this legendary restaurant. He's also involved with the aforementioned Mendoza Restaurant, named for Scalo executive chef Garrick Mendoza, and the intimate yet ultrahip Elaine's, named for former Scalo general manager Elaine Blanco.

- Continue north to Central Ave. and turn right. The view east from the corner of Carlisle Blvd. may look vaguely familiar. It's the scene of Ernst Haas's famous 1969 photograph, "Albuquerque." The iconic shot was essentially duplicated in the climax of the 2007 neo-Western thriller *No Country for Old Men.* To re-create it yourself, go a few blocks west, attach a massive zoom lens to compress the background, and then wait for a late-afternoon monsoon.

- Cross Central Ave. and turn left. One outstanding establishment among the many ahead is Guild Cinema, currently the only independent movie theater in Albuquerque. Film curators of this 150-seat art house screen a brilliant selection of indies, foreign films, and thematic festivals.

- Turn right on Tulane Dr. At the end of the block, veer right onto Berkeley Pl. Time the walk right and you'll hear a bell-tower concerto emanating from Monte Vista Christian Church after 5 p.m.

- Turn right on Grand Ave., followed by a quick left into the first alley. This one bends east to bring you to Amherst Dr., where you'll take a left. The 400 block just might be the most endearing in the city. (No data to back that up, just a sentimental observation.)

- Turn right on Monte Vista Blvd. and follow it around the bend to Model Pharmacy. Its neon signage clues you in on what pharmacies once were and still should be. Inside you'll find a lunch counter with a soda fountain that serves up amazing sandwiches and milkshakes. Though the pharmacy might not be licensed to fill all prescriptions, it is stocked with an international selection of soaps, perfumes, and other hygienic sundries. And in case you didn't get enough to drink earlier, Jubilation across the street has an international selection of beer, wine, and spirits.

- Continue northeast to Carlisle Blvd. and follow the crosswalks counterclockwise to return to Bataan Park.

Concluding this walk, local sophisticate Steven J. Westman recollects: "Since 1982 I've made Nob Hill my home. Over the years I've watched it change and grow and even opened a business in the Nob Hill Shopping Center. I stay here because I like it. With its history and quirks, a walk down the streets is not just a stroll. You tend to discover something new with each step. Many of us still scratch our heads over what is going on inside the Bachechi Compound, and still miss the many legendary spots we used to frequent: Notes Cafe, the Silver Sunbeam, Pick Up Your Toys, Paul's Market, Tulane Street Deli, the Martini Grill. I could go on and on." Westman is the chief socialite for *Local iQ* magazine. Find out more about the latest happenings at local-iq.com.

POINTS OF INTEREST

Bataan Memorial Park cabq.gov, 3501 Lomas Blvd. NE, 505-768-5353

Aux Dog Theatre auxdog.com, 3011 Monte Vista Blvd. NE, 505-254-7716

Buffalo Exchange buffaloexchange.com, 3005 Central Ave. NE, 505-262-0098

Zinc Wine Bar & Bistro zincabq.com, 3009 Central Ave. NE, 505-254-9462

Monte Vista Fire Station Restaurant montevistafirestation.com, 3201 Central Ave. NE, 505-255-2424

Korean BBQ House and Sushi & Sake koreanbbqhousenm.com , 3200 Central Ave. SE, 505-338-2424

Hiway House Motel hiwayhousemotel.com, 3200 Central Ave. SE, 505-268-3971

Kelly's Brew Pub kellysbrewpub.com, 3222 Central Ave. SE, 505-262-2739

Limonata freshcitrus.us, 3222 Silver Ave. SE, 505-266-0607

P'tit Louis Bistro ptitlouisbistro.com, 3218 Silver Ave. SE, 505-314-1110

Immanuel Presbyterian Church rt66church.com, 114 Carlisle Blvd. SE, 505-265-7628

Nob Hill La Montañita Co-op Food Market lamontanita.coop, 3500 Central Ave. SE, 505-265-4631

Mariposa Gallery mariposa-gallery.com, 3500 Central Ave. SE, 505-268-6828

Gecko's Bar & Tapas geckosbar.com, 3500 Central Ave. SE, 505-262-1848

Scalo Northern Italian Grill scalonobhill.com, 3500 Central Ave. SE, 505-255-8781

Elaine's elainesnobhill.com, 3503 Central Ave. NE, 505-433-4782

Guild Cinema guildcinema.com, 3405 Central Ave NE, Albuquerque NM, 505-255-1848

Model Pharmacy modelpharmacy.com, 3636 Monte Vista Blvd. NE, 505-255-8686

Jubilation Wine & Spirits jubilationwines.com, 3512 Lomas Blvd. NE, 505-255-4404

route summary

1. Start at Bataan Memorial Park.
2. Walk west on Lomas Blvd. to the crosswalk.
3. Turn left on Wellesley Dr.
4. Turn left on Marquette Ave.
5. Turn right on Monte Vista Blvd.
6. Turn left on Dartmouth Dr.
7. Turn left on Central Ave.
8. Turn right on Wellesley Dr.
9. Turn left on Silver Ave.
10. Turn right into the first alley ahead.
11. Turn left on Lead Ave.
12. Turn right on Tulane Dr.
13. Turn left on Coal Ave.
14. Turn left on Carlisle Blvd.
15. Turn left on Silver Ave.
16. Turn right at the second crosswalk and go into Nob Hill Business Center.
17. Continue north to Central Ave. and turn right.
18. Cross Central Ave. and turn left.

19. Turn right on Tulane Dr.
20. Bear right onto Berkeley Pl.
21. Turn right on Grand Ave.
22. Turn left into the first alley. This one bends east to bring you to Amherst Dr.
23. Turn left on Amherst Dr.
24. Turn right on Monte Vista Blvd.
25. Continue northeast to Carlisle Blvd. and follow the crosswalks counterclockwise to return to Bataan Park.

Connecting the Walks

Walk 25 begins on the north side of Central near Cornell, six blocks west of Dartmouth.

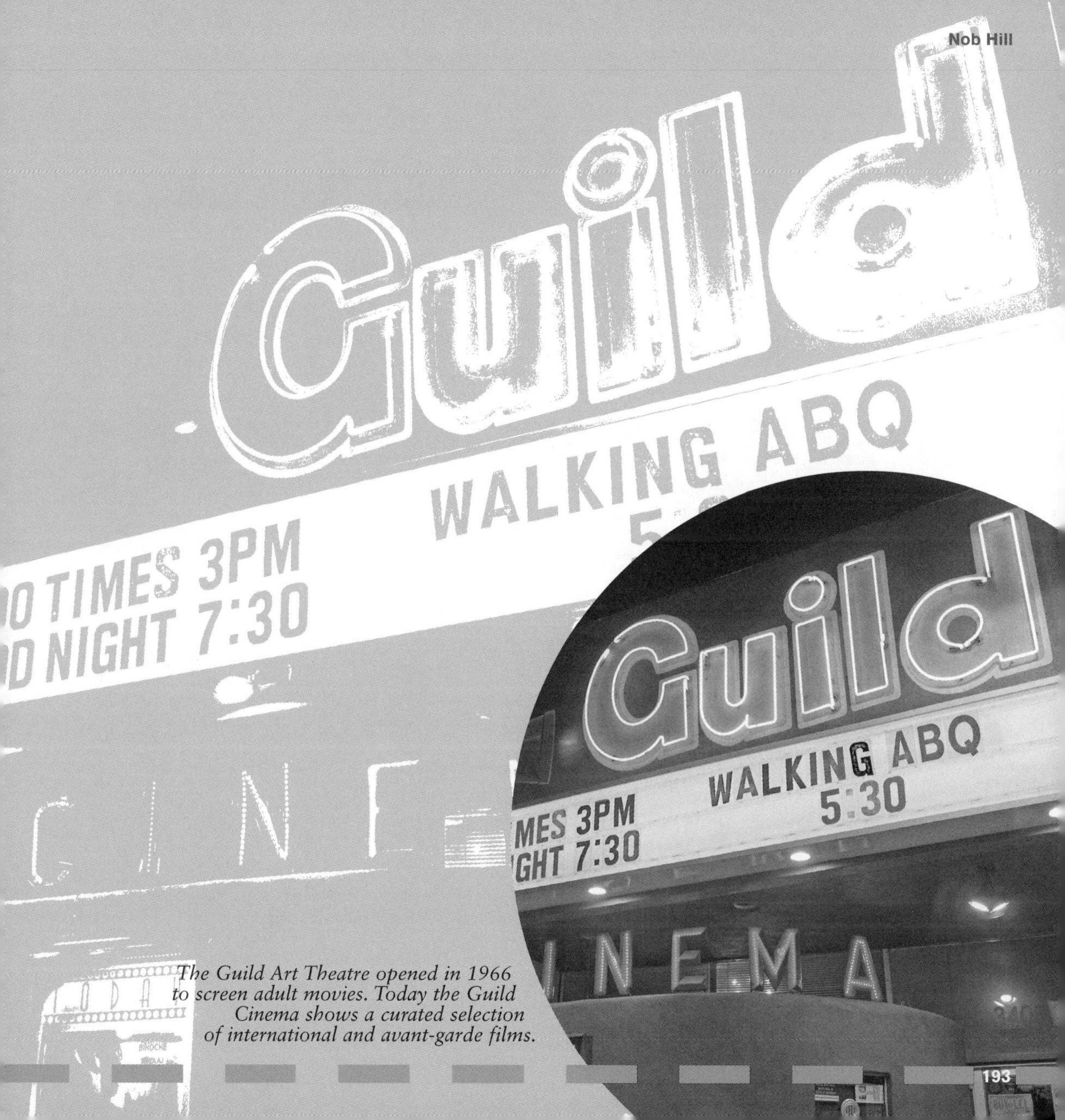

The Guild Art Theatre opened in 1966 to screen adult movies. Today the Guild Cinema shows a curated selection of international and avant-garde films.

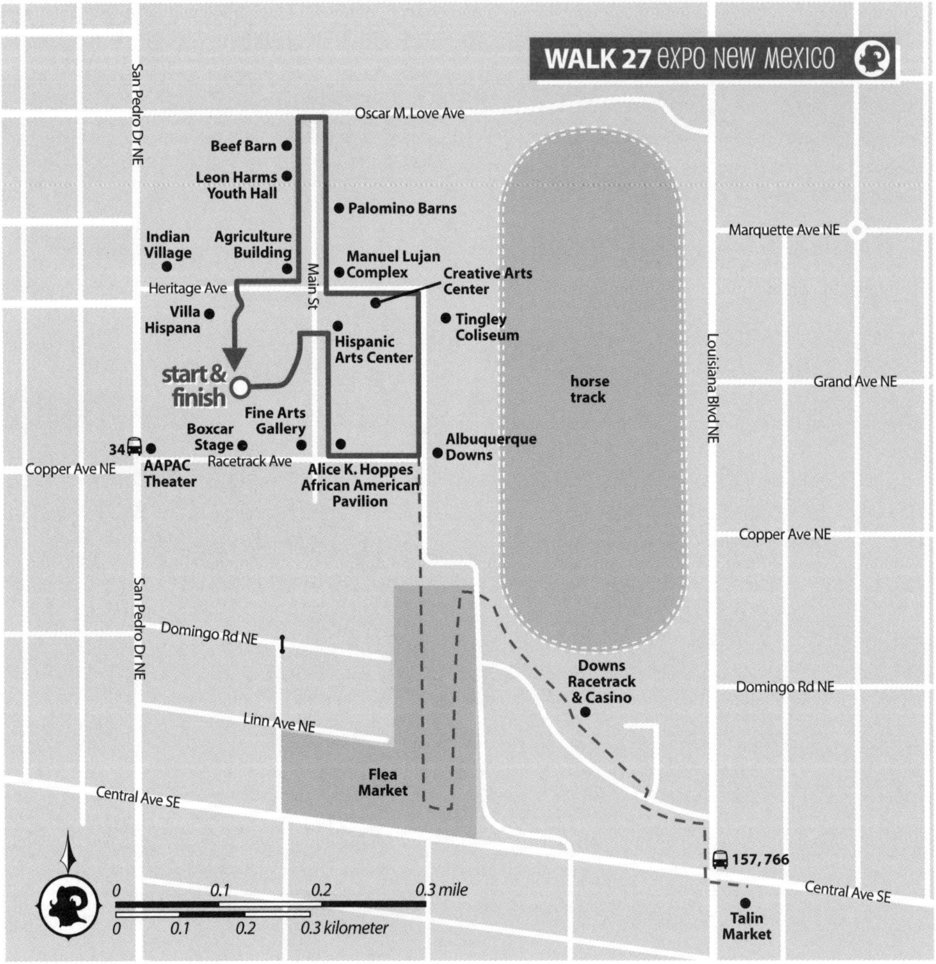
WALK 27 expo new mexico
Oscar M. Love Ave
San Pedro Dr NE
Beef Barn
Leon Harms Youth Hall
Palomino Barns
Indian Village
Agriculture Building
Main St
Manuel Lujan Complex
Creative Arts Center
Heritage Ave
Villa Hispana
Tingley Coliseum
Hispanic Arts Center
start & finish
Fine Arts Gallery
Boxcar Stage
34
AAPAC Theater
Copper Ave NE
Racetrack Ave
Alice K. Hoppes African American Pavilion
Albuquerque Downs
horse track
Marquette Ave NE
Grand Ave NE
Louisiana Blvd NE
Copper Ave NE
Domingo Rd NE
Downs Racetrack & Casino
Domingo Rd NE
Linn Ave NE
Flea Market
Central Ave SE
157, 766
Central Ave SE
Talin Market
0
0.1
0.2
0.3 mile
0
0.1
0.2
0.3 kilometer

27 Expo New Mexico: Beyond the Fair

BOUNDARIES: San Pedro Dr., Lomas Blvd., Louisiana Blvd., Central Ave.
DISTANCE: 1 mile; 2–3 miles with detour
DIFFICULTY: Easy
PARKING: Free–$10 on fairgrounds, depending on events; free parking on nearby streets
PUBLIC TRANSIT: Bus 34 on San Pedro Dr. at Copper Ave; buses 157 and 766 on Central Ave. at Louisiana Blvd.

In October 1881, the New Mexico Agricultural, Mineral and Industrial Exposition ran for five days in continuous rain. Despite the meager turnout, local business leaders recognized its potential and banded together to support the 1882 New Mexico Territorial Fair. In 1911, still several months before achieving statehood, the event was billed as the "30th Annual New Mexico Carnival and State Fair." With state funds increasingly scarce, the fair shut down from 1917 to 1937. Governor Clyde Tingley resurrected the fair at its current location in 1938. Today the grounds are known as Expo New Mexico and are run by the New Mexico State Fair Commission. On these 236 acres are more than two dozen venues that host 200 events throughout the year. Shows cater to a wide array of interests: antiques, jewelry, and fine arts; monster trucks and lowriders; health, home, and garden; cats, dogs, ponies, Arabian horses, and pygmy goats; and the ever-popular guns, swords, and knives. There's a beer fest, a pride fest, a chile fiesta, a folk festival, and more. These interim events draw about 400,000 visitors annually, slightly shy of the 12-day fair attendance in recent years. Check the expo website to coordinate your walk here with an event that catches your interest.

- **Start at the pedestrian entrance facing gate 4 for a welcome transition from craquelure parking lots to grassy lawns shaded by old-growth oak trees. On your right is the Boxcar Stage, so named for the French Gratitude Boxcars that serve as an onstage backdrop. After World War II, the French government sent a boxcar filled with gifts to each of the 48 continental United States. Historically disdainful of anything French, New Mexico promptly lost the gifts, stripped the car of its decorations and undercarriage, and used the box as a storage bin for grain. The French Boxcar Committee graciously procured a replica boxcar for New Mexico in 1986.**

- Follow the sidewalk, angling northeast past administration and the Indian arts building; then cross Main Street (also called the Avenue of the Governors). The Hispanic Arts Center is a traditional adobe with exposed vigas, wood-framed windows, double doors, and gloss-polished concrete flooring. Standing in the front lawn is the petroglyph-inspired wrought iron sculpture *Petro Circle* by Doug Weigel.

- Turn right and walk south. The neighboring oil well was installed in 1979 by the Mobil Oil Corporation as a reminder of royalties paid to the State Land Office in exchange for the massive amounts of oil and gas extracted from the state. Continue south toward Racetrack Ave. The building on the northwest corner was built in the early 1940s as State Fair Administration Offices and converted to the Fine Arts Gallery in the late 1950s. Today it hosts some of the most prestigious art shows in the region. It's also home to the state fair's extensive permanent collection, a showcase of New Mexico artists over the past eight decades. On the southeast corner is the Alice K. Hoppes African American Pavilion, named for a tenacious civil-rights leader and the first director of the Office of African American Affairs. At the dedication ceremony in 2004, Governor Bill Richardson remarked, "I can still hear Alice giving me hell."

- Turn left on Racetrack Ave. and walk east to the old Albuquerque Downs, a vintage simulcast gambling den with an updated grandstand that fronts the racetrack. Construction of the 1-mile racetrack began in 1936, with WPA workers shoveling 170,000 cubic yards of dirt to level a 20-foot dip in the terrain. Live races are held in August and September.

  Detour: This optional side trip works best on weekends, 7 a.m–6 p.m., when the flea market is running full tilt. At other times there's a bit too much empty space to cross to make it worth going the extra mile. With that in mind, go south from the old Downs to the state's oldest and largest open-air market. More than 1,300 vendors jam 25 acres to hawk clothing, jewelry, crafts, fresh produce, and auto parts. Wind through this enchanting bazaar of treasure and trash, and then make your way east to the new Downs Racetrack & Casino, open 365 days a year, 10 a.m.–1 a.m. Sunday–Thursday and 10 a.m.–4 a.m. Friday–Saturday. Inside this $25 million den of corruption, you'll find bars, lounges, a weekend nightclub, a trackside patio, simulcast betting, electronic casino games, and dining options ranging from casual to elegant.

- Continue southeast and exit through Gate 8 on Louisiana Blvd.

- Turn right and walk south to Central Ave. and into the heart of the International District. (The south side of the district is a feature on Walk 28.) On the southwest corner of Central and Louisiana, a giant lumberjack lords over a couple of Vietnamese restaurants. Some people refer to him as Paul Bunyan. To Cubans in the community, he is known as Fidel. He first appeared here in the 1960s, when the building beneath him housed the Duke City Lumber Company store. In 2014, he lost his ax when high winds ripped off his hands.

  On the southeast corner is Talin Market. This international grocer was established a block south of its current location in 1978 and now offers cooking classes, store tours, and a wider international selection organized by city. Looking for kimchi? Check the Seoul aisle. Need a steaming bowl of fresh ramen? Go next door to Gen Kai Japanese Restaurant, an expansion of the ramen bar formerly located inside the market.

  Also in the vicinity are some of the International District Pillars. The public art project consists of mosaic pillars and walls designed by Lori Roddick and produced by Margy O'Brien. Each represents a different culture of the world. Most are stationed along Louisiana between Central and Zuni, near the beautiful Thai/Laotian temple known as Wat Buddhamongkolnimit, or the Buddhist Temple of New Mexico. Finding them all adds an extra half mile to the detour. (Also keep an eye out for Roddick's granite dragon, which swims the sidewalk south of the Spanish pillar.) When you're done exploring the district, return to the old Downs.

- **Resuming the fairgrounds tour:** Continue north to Tingley Coliseum, a 380-foot-long, 240-foot-wide arena originally built for rodeos and 16,000 attendees. (Recent fire codes and handicap-access requirements have scaled seating capacity down to 10,000.) Roy Rogers and Dale Evans inaugurated the coliseum in 1957 for a $40,000 fee and 10 percent of the gate. Acts who have played here range from AC/DC to Jay-Z. Near the main entrance, 33 bronze relief flags representing the state's counties are part of a sculpture by Stephanie Huerta.

- Continue north to Heritage Ave. and turn left. The Creative Arts Center on the left and the Manuel Lujan Complex ahead on the right are the largest of the expo's exhibition facilities and host most of the art fairs and trade shows on the fairgrounds.

- Turn right on Main St. North of the Lujan Complex and its red-barn parking structure are the Palomino Barns. These adobe stables were the first structures built on the state fairgrounds. Construction began in 1936 and was completed in just over a year. In 2008, the barns were carefully dismantled brick by brick. Plumbing and structural components were brought to current code, and the adobe bricks were replaced in their original order.

- Cross Main St. to visit the Beef Barn. Completed shortly after the Palomino Barns and fully renovated in 2009, it's the second oldest structure on the fairgrounds. To its immediate south is the Leon Harms Youth Hall, named for the New Mexico State Fair's first general manager. Harms held his position for 30 years and long preached the value of youth involvement with the fair. The hall opened in 1948 to provide dormitories and a dining area for kids who traveled from distant farms to exhibit their animals. Next door, the Agriculture Building, also known as the Bolack Building, features a spacious horseshoe-shaped patio with a central flower garden.

- Turn right on Heritage Ave. and walk west past the School Arts Building and the Flower Arts Building to the entries to two amphitheaters. On the right, the Indian Village was completed in time for the 1964 fair and underwent renovations in 2009. The traditional hogan (dwelling) and [h]orno (oven), provided by the Indian Pueblo Cultural Center, enhance its rustic atmosphere. On the left, the Spanish Village opened in 1972 and was renamed Villa Hispana in 1978. It underwent a $2.3 million renovation in 2008 to enhance its upscale Spanish-style courtyard setting. Historical highlights on this site include campaign appearances by Ted Kennedy, Gerald Ford, Jimmy Carter, and Hillary Clinton.

- Go south from the Villa Hispana entrance to return to the Gate 4 parking area. One last point of interest before you go: The African American Performing Arts Center & Exhibition Hall was dedicated in 2008 to the intellectual and cultural history of African Americans in New Mexico and the Southwest. The AAPAC Theater hosts local stage productions, national touring companies, premier speaking engagements, and a variety of music concerts. The exhibition hall displays traveling exhibits such as Black Wings, a Smithsonian retrospective on African American aviators. The hall is open 10 a.m.–5 p.m. Tuesday–Friday and 10 a.m.–4 p.m. Saturday.

POINTS OF INTEREST

Expo New Mexico exponm.com, 300 San Pedro Blvd. NE, 505-222-9700

The Downs Racetrack & Casino abqdowns.com, 145 Louisiana Blvd. NE, 505-767-7171

Talin Market talinmarket.com, 88 Louisiana Blvd. SE, 505-268-0206

Gen Kai 110 B Louisiana Blvd NE, 505-255-0112

Wat Buddhamongkolnimit watnimit.blogspot.com, 320 Louisiana Blvd. SE, 505-268-4983

African American Performing Arts Center aapacnm.org, 310 San Pedro Dr. NE, 505-222-0785

ROUTE SUMMARY

1. Start at the pedestrian entrance facing gate 4.
2. Follow the sidewalk, angling northeast, and cross Main St.
3. Turn right and walk south to Racetrack Ave.
4. Turn left and walk east to the old Albuquerque Downs.
5. Turn left and walk north past Tingley Coliseum.
6. Turn left on Heritage Ave. and go west to Main St.
7. Turn right and walk north to Oscar M. Love Ave.
8. Cross Main St. and turn left.
9. Go south to Heritage Ave. and turn right.
10. Go south from the Villa Hispana entrance to return to the gate 4 parking area.

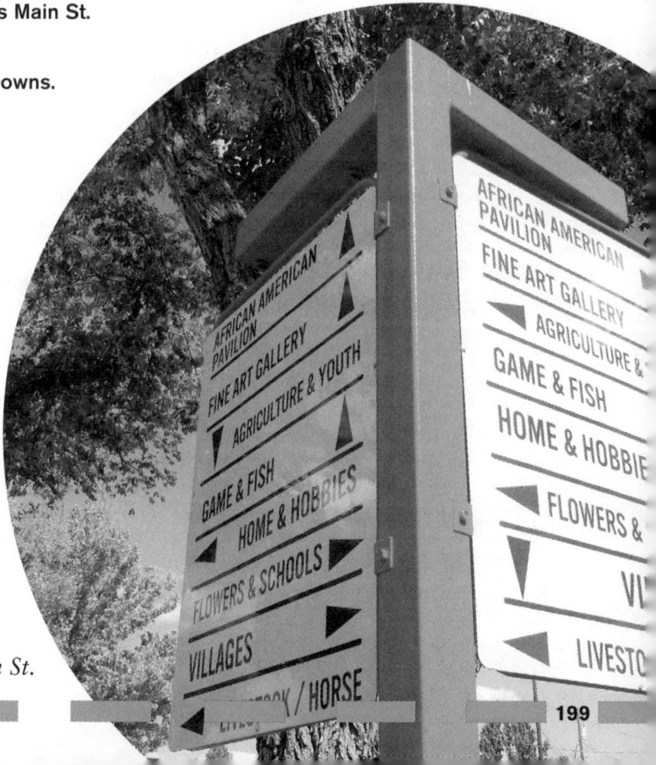

The corner of Heritage Ave. and Main St.

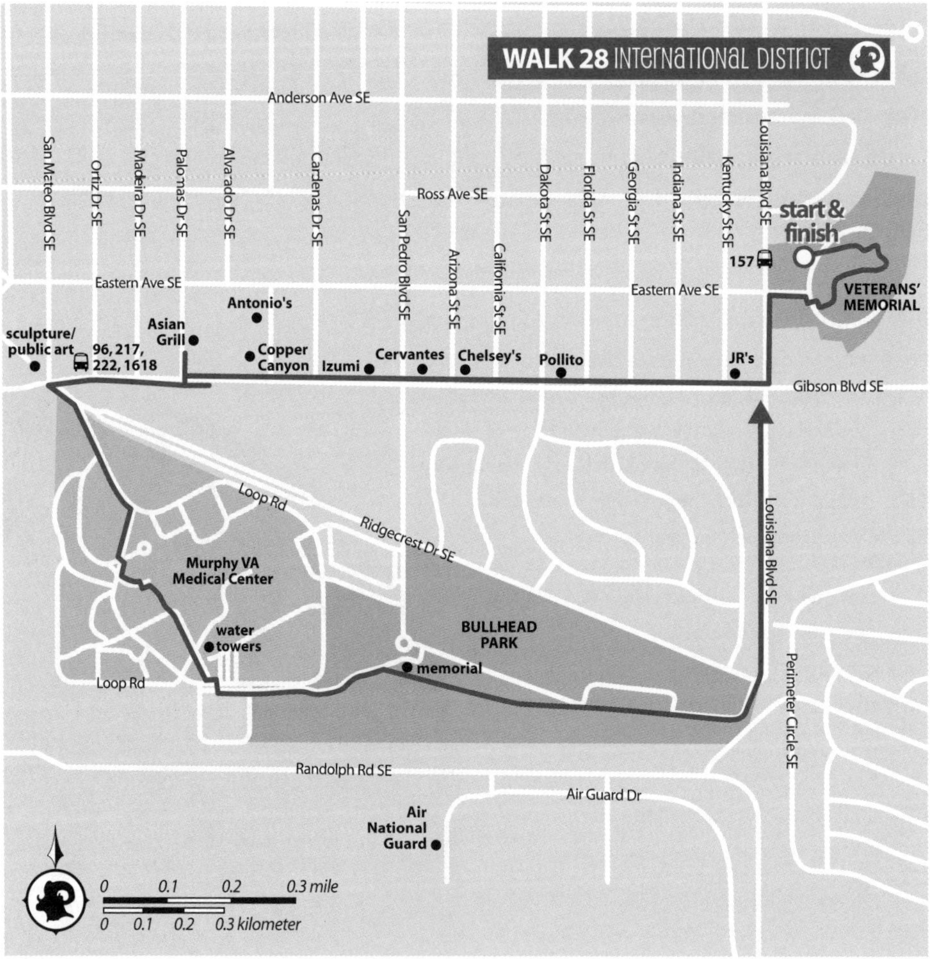
WALK 28 International District
Anderson Ave SE
San Mateo Blvd SE
Ortiz Dr SE
Madeira Dr SE
Palomas Dr SE
Alvarado Dr SE
Cardenas Dr SE
Ross Ave SE
San Pedro Blvd SE
Arizona St SE
California St SE
Dakota St SE
Florida St SE
Georgia St SE
Indiana St SE
Kentucky St SE
Louisiana Blvd SE
start & finish
157
VETERANS' MEMORIAL
Eastern Ave SE
Eastern Ave SE
Antonio's
Asian Grill
sculpture/ public art
96, 217, 222, 1618
Copper Canyon
Izumi
Cervantes
Chelsey's
Pollito
JR's
Gibson Blvd SE
Loop Rd
Ridgecrest Dr SE
Louisiana Blvd SE
Murphy VA Medical Center
water towers
BULLHEAD PARK
memorial
Loop Rd
Perimeter Circle SE
Randolph Rd SE
Air Guard Dr
Air National Guard
0 0.1 0.2 0.3 mile
0 0.1 0.2 0.3 kilometer

28 International District: Spoils of War

BOUNDARIES: **Louisiana Blvd., Randolph Rd., San Mateo Blvd., Gibson Blvd.**
DISTANCE: **3.5 miles**
DIFFICULTY: **Moderate (unpaved sections)**
PARKING: **Free parking at Veterans' Memorial and Bullhead Park**
PUBLIC TRANSIT: **Bus 157 on Louisiana Blvd. at Eastern Ave.; buses 96, 217, 222, and 1618 on Gibson Blvd. at San Mateo**

The International District, roughly bounded by Lomas, Wyoming, Gibson, and San Mateo Boulevards, is locally known as the War Zone due to areas of low income and high crime. To some degree it developed catering to tastes of personnel stationed at Kirtland, the sixth largest military installation in the U.S. Air Force, and its multinational population is largely a result of warfare overseas. From 1975 to 1978, for example, about 3,000 Vietnamese refugees were resettled in Albuquerque. In 1989, more arrived after the Vietnamese who had been interned in reeducation camps were released. The city's cultural diversity is further enriched by influxes of immigrants from Korea, El Salvador, Afghanistan, Somalia, and the Philippines. At Highland High School on the northeast side of the district, 27 languages are spoken. This walk skirts the south side of the district to explore memorial parks, historic buildings, a small sampling of international cuisine, and an unusual assortment of large objects mounted on pedestals.

- **Start at the New Mexico Veterans' Memorial. This 25-acre site is the southern extension of the 53-acre Phil Chacon Park. (To learn more about Officer Chacon, see Walk 5.) The Veterans' Memorial is open to the public, free of charge, 6 a.m.–10 p.m. year-round. At the visitor center, open Thursday–Monday, 9 a.m.–3 p.m., you'll find a modest museum and enthusiastic volunteers. The 50-page booklet ($2) is essential for a comprehensive tour of the grounds. The park takes a delicate approach to covering warfare from a New Mexico perspective. The monuments are subtle. The span of history is grand. It begins with a cycle of violence between indigenous and colonial powers that persisted for nearly 350 years. (See the Colonial War kiosk.) In the meantime, lesser wars were waged, such as the American Civil War. Near the visitor center, a small monument dedicated to buffalo soldiers mentions that "180,000 Blacks served in the Union Army and of these 33,000 died." Of course they all died,** eventually, but their adversaries at the time included such notable figures as Geronimo, Sitting Bull, Victorio, Lone Wolf, Billy the Kid, and Pancho Villa.

If pressed for time, check out just two monuments. The centrally located sculpture, *The Fallen Friend* (Jesús Moroles, 1997), consists of 84 white cement pylons set in four concentric circles. To its immediate east is *The Word from Home,* a collection of war letters etched in stone.

- Exit through the west gate and turn left on Louisiana Blvd.

- Turn right on Gibson Blvd. Many of the restaurants ahead serve as further reminders of past wars. The results of the Mexican War (1846–48) brought Texas into serious conflict with the federal government over the state's claim to a large portion of New Mexico. To this day, some Texans contend that their republic extends to the Rio Grande. In their view, half of Albuquerque belongs to the Lone Star State. JR's Bar-B-Que started in Houston and invaded Albuquerque in the late 1980s. Their slow-cooked ribs and brisket make a delicious peace offering.

Unlike Francisco Coronado, who started the first European conflict in New Mexico, Monica and Rene Coronado, owners of Pollito Con Papas, serve authentic Peruvian-style chicken that's spicy, savory, and immensely tasty. For those preferring American fare, the nearby Chelsey's Wings and Burgers is an excellent choice.

Prior to penning Don Quixote, Miguel de Cervantes served in the Spanish Navy. Cervantes Restaurant & Lounge borrows his name to evoke old-world Spanish traditions that influence the flavors in this well-established venue, a local favorite since 1973. Japan's contribution to the food scene, Izumi Sushi & Grill, is an enjoyable lunch option, though during dinner hours the teppan tables and sushi bar can get a bit boisterous.

Siesta Hills Shopping Center presents three more choices. Copper Canyon Café is dependable for a standard Mexican breakfast, lunch, or dinner, but their French dip is surprisingly good. Hidden directly behind Copper Canyon is Antonio's Café and Cantina, specializing in New Mexico fare. Nothing fancy on the menu, but the food is well above average. Asian Grill, no doubt supplied by neighboring 99 Bahn Oriental Market, serves outstanding cuisine from Vietnam. Their Singapore-style chow fun and Hong Kong chow mein are also well worth considering.

You can use the pedestrian overpass here to cross Gibson Blvd. Or stay on the north side of the street if you want a close look at Albuquerque's most iconic work of public art, *Cruising San Mateo I* (Barbara Grygutis, 1991). Nicknamed "Chevy on a Stick," the steel, stucco, and ceramic-tile monument depicts a full-scale 1965 Chevy atop an arched pedestal.

- Turn left on Ridgecrest Dr. A blacktop jogging path begins on the right side of the road just past the gatehouse. Follow it up to the Raymond G. Murphy VA Medical Center. Initially opened in 1932 as the Albuquerque Veterans Administration Medical Center, the old VA hospital was designed to resemble Taos Pueblo. The modified Pueblo-style structures feature tile-paved patios, deep porches, and massive exterior vigas. The buildings are grouped in an irregular circle, providing a partial enclosure, which you'll soon see.

- Walk around the right side of the main building, which currently serves as a behavioral health center. In 1983, 16 buildings in the complex were collectively listed on the National Register of Historic Places. In 2014 the hospital was added to the nationwide list of VA centers embroiled in the wait-list scandal.

- Exit the enclosure by following the sidewalk between buildings 53 (Veterans Services Office) and 4 (Human Resources), and continue straight past the water towers on Sandia Rd.

- Go through the gate ahead and turn left into the parking lot. The roofs in the covered parking area on your left are solar panels, and the high-pitched whine you hear is coming from the attached generators. Continue east through USS Bullhead Memorial Park, passing baseball fields along the way. Directly ahead, three torpedoes mounted on concrete pedestals memorialize the USS *Bullhead* SS-332. Named after the large-headed catfish, the submarine was lost on August 6, 1945, the same day the first atomic bomb was dropped on Hiroshima. It was the last U.S. Navy ship sunk by enemy action during World War II.

  Less than a quarter mile south of the torpedoes, two aircraft are mounted on steel pedestals behind a perimeter fence. The one on the right is a North American F-100 Super Sabre, a supersonic jet fighter that served with the Air Force from 1954 to 1971 and with the Air National Guard until 1979. The F-100 was the Air Force's primary close air-support jet in Vietnam until replaced by the Ling-Temco-Vought A-7 Corsair II, which is the jet on the right. The A-7 is a carrier-capable subsonic aircraft that initially entered service with the U.S. Navy in 1967. Built for a combined cost of roughly $10 million in today's dollars, the jets now serve to decorate the grounds of the Air National Guard, a relatively small facility on an 80-square-mile military installation.

Construction of Kirtland Army Air Field began in 1941. On Christmas Eve that year, the base was designated as an advanced flying school to train pilots for the new B-17 "Flying Fortress." One of the flight instructors was First Lieutenant Jimmy Stewart. Other notable actors of the day, including Pat O'Brien, Randoph Scott, and Eddie Albert, arrived for the filming of *Bombardier.* The 1943 movie foreshadowed massive firebombing campaigns on civilian populations in 1944–45. In 1945, Kirtland Field introduced flight training for the B-29, the "Superfortress" deployed to drop atomic bombs on Japan later that year.

In 1947, when the U.S. Army Air Forces became the U.S. Air Force, Kirtland received its Air Force Base designation. A fuel facility installed in 1953 began leaking almost immediately and to date has spilled an estimated 24 million gallons of jet fuel into the surrounding soil. The plume, first detected in 1999, continues to spread toward municipal wells that supply the city's drinking water. Depending on wind conditions, the smell of petroleum and aircraft exhaust can be noticeable on the park's soccer fields and playgrounds.

- Continue east to the far end of the park and turn left to exit through the gate. Walk north on Louisiana Blvd. and cross Gibson to return to the Veterans' Memorial.

For fascinating exhibits on New Mexico's role in the atomic age, visit the National Museum of Nuclear Science & History. The family-friendly museum, a Smithsonian Affiliate member, is located at 601 Eubank Blvd. NE—just 2 aerial miles from the Veterans' Memorial Park, though walking between the two is not recommended. For more info: 505-245-2137, nuclearmuseum.org.

POINTS OF INTEREST

New Mexico Veterans' Memorial nmvetsmemorial.org, 1100 Louisiana Blvd. SE, 505-256-2042

JR's Bar-B-Que jrs-barbeque.com, 6501 Gibson Blvd. SE, 505-268-1676

Pollito Con Papas pollitoconpapas.com, 6105 Gibson Blvd. SE, 505-765-5486

Chelsey's Wings and Burgers 5901 Gibson Blvd. SE, 505-266-6223

Cervantes Restaurant & Lounge cervantesabq.com, 5801 Gibson Blvd. SE, 505-262-2253

Izumi Sushi & Grill izumisushiandgrillabq.com, 5701 Gibson Blvd. SE, 505-260-0011

Copper Canyon Café coppercanyoncafe.com, 5455 Gibson Blvd. SE, 505-266-6318

Antonio's Café and Cantina thebirddelivers.com, 5409 Gibson Blvd. SE, 505-255-3151

Asian Grill asiangrillabq.com, 5303 Gibson Blvd. SE, 505-265-4702

Raymond G. Murphy VA Medical Center albuquerque.va.gov, 1501 San Pedro Dr. SE, 505-265-1711

USS Bullhead Memorial Park cabq.gov, 1606 San Pedro Blvd. SE, 505-291-6239

route summary

1. **Start at New Mexico Veterans' Memorial.**
2. **Exit through the west gate and turn left on Louisiana Blvd.**
3. **Turn right on Gibson Blvd.**
4. **Turn left on Ridgecrest Dr.**
5. **Walk around the right side of the old VA hospital and go straight past the water towers.**
6. **Go through the gate ahead and turn left into the parking lot.**
7. **Walk east through USS Bullhead Memorial Park.**
8. **Turn left at the far end of the parking lot and exit through the gate.**
9. **Continue north on Louisiana Blvd. and cross Gibson Blvd. to return to New Mexico Veterans' Memorial.**

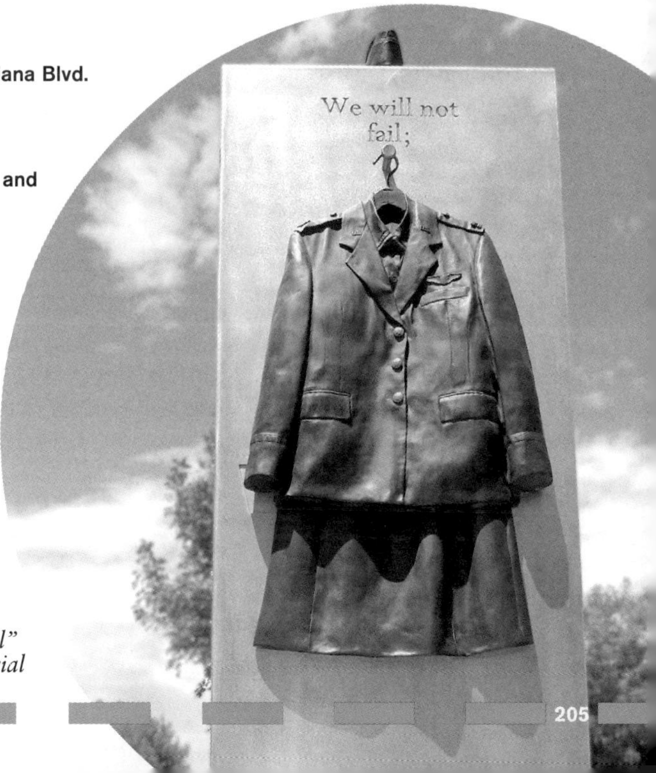

Bronze sculpture in "The Call" venue at the Veterans' Memorial

WALK 29 Menaul Trailhead
Morris St NE
Juan Tabo Blvd NE
Tramway Blvd NE
Camino de la Sierra NE
Candelaria Rd NE
Candelaria Rd NE
7
Chelwood Park Blvd NE
LYNNEWOOD PARK
Deli-Berry
ROSS ENCHANTED PARK
Piedra Lisa Trailhead
Blue Eagle
Ayurvedic Institute
Menaul Blvd NE
8
Nagomi
PIEDRA LISA PARK
SANDIA FOOTHILLS
Menaul Blvd NE
Collet Park Elementary School
Dagmars
DON JUAN de OÑATE PARK
Brentwood Hills Blvd NE
Taste of Italy
Bikram Yoga
start & finish
CRESTVIEW HEIGHTS PARK
Morrow Ave NE
Indian School Rd NE
1
6
Monte Largo Dr NE
Morris St NE
Juan Tabo Blvd NE
Chelwood Park Blvd NE
Tramway Blvd NE
Indian School Rd NE
Constitution Ave NE
0 0.2 0.4 0.6 mile
0 0.2 0.4 0.6 kilometer

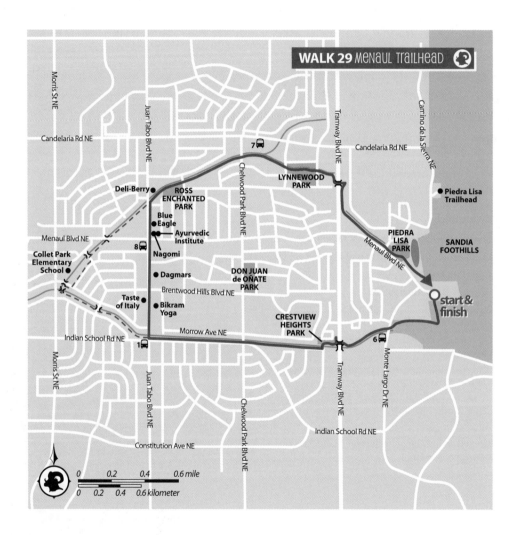

29 Menaul Trailhead: Hard Channel Navigation

BOUNDARIES: Menaul Blvd., Indian School Rd., Juan Tabo Blvd., (Morris St. on 5-mile option), Candelaria Rd.
DISTANCE: 4.5- and 5-mile options
DIFFICULTY: Difficult (unpaved surfaces, steep terrain)
PARKING: Trailhead parking lot closes at 9 p.m. April–October, 7 p.m. November–March
PUBLIC TRANSIT: Bus 6 on Monte Largo Dr. at Rover Ave.; bus 1 on Indian School Rd. at Juan Tabo Blvd.

This route explores bicycle/pedestrian routes in the Northeast Heights, starting from the Menaul Trailhead (as it appears on maps) at the east end of Menaul Blvd. A sign at the gate identifies the area as Embudo Canyon Trailhead, which is actually another half mile southeast at the end of Indian School Rd. Most people come here to bike along the north–south Open Space trails or hike into the adjoining wilderness area. For additional walking options, a map of the Sandia Ranger District is helpful for navigating the network of trails east of the trailhead, and a city bike map is useful for exploring urban routes to the west. See **www.fs.usda.gov/cibola** for Sandia maps. The bike maps are available at most bike stores, or use the interactive map on **cabq.gov.**

- **Start on the east side of the Menaul Trailhead parking lot. According to local legend, an old hermit lived in a cave somewhere in these hills. He had a habit of bringing prostitutes to his lair and, in lieu of payment for their services, murdering them. The story may have roots in the era when mining camps dotted the Sandias. To this day hikers report phantom footsteps in the night and ghostly apparitions carrying a lantern. If you happen to witness any paranormal phenomena, it probably means you're out when Open Space Foothills are closed, the gate is locked, and your car is stuck inside for the night. Daylight hours are a better time to enjoy the foothills. Numerous drainages support a wide variety of shrubs, including chamisa, Apache plume, three-leaf sumac, and oak. Common wildlife includes mule deer, rabbits, rock squirrels, and lots of lizards. Canyon towhee, house finch, Western scrub jay, greater roadrunner, Cooper's hawk, and Say's phoebe are a few of the birds that can be seen any time of year. But watch your step: rattlesnakes, harvester ants, and a variety of cacti are among the hazards.**

- Go through the gate on the east side of the parking lot and turn right on Trail 401. This dirt path, designated for hiking long before the advent of the Internet, still shows up as Menaul Blvd. on certain Web-based maps.

- Make another quick right on Trail 288 and follow it west, then south to a Y junction.

- Bear right and walk west along the north side of the drainage, Embudo Arroyo. Spanish for "funnel," Embudo Canyon indeed funnels runoff through a narrow pass before downsizing to an arroyo. This and other drainages carried vast amounts of sediments to create the alluvial outwash plain upon which the Northeast Heights are built. They also serve as wildlife corridors. When food gets scarce in the mountains, bobcats, coyotes, mountain lions, and black bears wander down the arroyos to hunt and forage in nearby neighborhoods. Sightings west of Tramway are rare.

  Embudo Arroyo becomes a concrete trapezoidal channel before reaching the first cross street. By this point you're surrounded by residential developments. The rapid onset of suburbia was a result of the city's population boom in the 1950s and Federal Housing Authority programs that encouraged platted subdivisions with identical tract houses. Some developers attempted to vary residential types and styles, but the FHA wasn't too keen on designs that deviated from their conservative guidelines. The result was homogenous housing with superficial variations. "Dressing up a box" is a common description for housing designs in the Heights.

- Cross Monte Largo Dr. and follow the hard channel down to Tramway Trail, a paved multiuse path that's closed to motor traffic. Popular with cyclists and joggers, it runs along the east side of Tramway Blvd. for 8.5 miles from Central Ave. north to Tramway Rd.

  The Heights are laid out on a grid of arterial roads spaced 1 mile apart. The placement of these major roads is based on the Public Land Survey System. This mathematical mapping method came to New Mexico in 1855 to define the land in terms of parcels, townships, and ranges. A basic unit in the PLSS is a section, which measures 1 square mile. With rare exceptions, the arterial roads in the Heights simply follow section boundaries. Tramway Blvd. is the easternmost arterial road, hence the first you'll encounter on the walk. To cross it, use the arched wooden bridge officially known as the Tramway-Rover Crossing Structure. Crestview Heights Park, a 2-acre green space with a playground and shade structure, awaits on the far side.

In 1955, the city commission passed the City Park Dedication Ordinance, which required developers to donate a percentage of their land to the city for parks. They often chose to allocate land that was unsuitable for housing, namely parcels on arroyos. Crestview Heights Park isn't a city park, but it follows the same principle, as do the other three parks on this route. This park also marks the beginning of the Embudo Channel Trail, a paved multiuse path that's closed to motor traffic.

Albuquerque writer Mike Smith has spent many trips exploring the length of Embudo Arroyo and its tributaries, often with his young children on cloudless days, and says that the arroyo is full of interesting surprises. "One of my favorite things about it is the colorful street art and buoyant tags you can find beneath many of Embudo Arroyo's bridges," he says. "But my favorite surprise the arroyo holds is its secret caches of what I call arroyo glass—windshield glass from various car accidents, washed into crevices and potholes of the arroyo and then weathered smooth, like beach glass, by years of seasonal flooding."

- Follow the Embudo Channel Trail to Juan Tabo Blvd. Here you have a choice to stay on the trail for a 5-mile loop or take a shortcut through a commercial district that's typical of arterial roads in the Northeast Heights.

- For the shortcut: Turn right on Juan Tabo Blvd. It is not a particularly scenic street, and its namesake is a mystery. Speculation on Juan Tabo varies. He could've been a shepherd, miner, or priest who lived in nearby Tijeras Canyon, which shows up on a 1748 document as "La Cañada de Juan Tabo." But then it's unclear why a city planner in the 1950s would reference an obscure document from the 18th century. In any case, a few unique establishments punctuate the three-quarter-mile stretch of boulevard between the Embudo and Piedra Lisa arroyos. Bikram Yoga is the first studio in Albuquerque to maintain a 105°F temperature and 40% humidity for the exquisite torture known as hot yoga. The Ayurvedic Institute was established in Santa Fe in 1984 and relocated here in 1986 to teach and offer traditional medicine and therapies of India. Core programs are taught by the renowned author and ayurvedic physician Vasant Lad. For additional enlightenment, visit the nearby Blue Eagle Metaphysical Emporium, your one-stop shop for energy crystals, magickal herbs, Wiccan spells, Celtic amulets, tarot cards, and incense burners. Dining options along the way also cater to international tastes. For gyros, subs, and pasta by the bucket, try A Taste of Italy. For German cuisine and

European pastries, go to Dagmar's Restaurant & Strudel Haus, For sushi, Nagomi. And for fresh deli sandwiches and frozen yogurt, Deli-Berry is on the north bank of Piedra Lisa Arroyo. Turn right on the Paseo de las Montañas Trail on the south bank.

- For the 5-mile option: Continue straight on Embudo Channel Trail to a footbridge and cross it to start on Paseo de las Montañas Trail. This paved motor-free path is briefly interrupted with a detour around a playground via Snow Heights Blvd., Gretta St., and Martha St. The playground belongs to Collet Park Elementary School, built in 1962. Snow Heights is named for Edward H. Snow, one of the developers responsible for the early phases of suburbanizing the Northeast Heights. Other major players include Dale Bellamah and Sam Hoffman. New techniques in mass-produced housing in the 1950s made Hoffman's enterprise the world's fourth largest home construction company, while Bellamah's ranked sixth worldwide.

  The extended route rejoins the shortcut after a school crossing on Juan Tabo Blvd. Close ahead, Ross Enchanted Park is a 5.5-acre site with a playground, picnic tables, and a soccer field. The arroyo and trail bend south before entering Lynnewood Park. This 9.5-acre site, with tennis courts, a basketball court, a soccer field, a playground, and picnic tables, is by far the most pleasant of the four. What makes it unique are the well-established trees shading the contoured landscape along the shallow concrete channel. The canyon from which it flows also happens to be one of the best hiking spots in the foothills. You'll see its (usually dry) waterfall when you cross the wooden bridge over Tramway Blvd. ahead. (For a closer look at the dry falls, go to Piedra Lisa Canyon Trailhead, just half a mile directly east of the bridge.)

- Turn right on Tramway Trail and walk south to the Piedra Lisa Storm Drain. (If you reach Menaul Blvd., you missed it.)

- Turn left on the dirt path on the south side of the storm drain and follow it to Piedra Lisa Park. This 3.3-acre facility features a playground, a basketball court, and memorial trees. The park entrance is a sculptural series of concrete panels that echo the shape of the mountains. Gaze through the geometric windows in the panels for different perspectives of the park. Titled *Mountain Waves,* the work was completed in 1986 by David Witherspoon. On the far side of the park, Nancy Young's 1996 mural, *Morning Allegory,* is painted on the retaining wall of the Piedra Lisa Dam.

- **Continue straight on the trail past the south side of the dam to return to the Menaul Trailhead parking lot.**

POINTS OF INTEREST

Bikram Yoga bikramabq.com, 1930 Juan Tabo Blvd. NE, 505-296-9642

A Taste of Italy atasteofitalynm.com, 1945 Juan Tabo Blvd. NE, 505-275-8334

Dagmar's dagmarsrestaurant.com, 2120 Juan Tabo Blvd. NE, 505-293-1982

The Ayurvedic Institute ayurveda.com, 11311 Menaul Blvd. NE, 505-291-9698

Nagomi 400 Juan Tabo Blvd. NE, 505-298-3081

Blue Eagle Metaphysical Emporium blueeaglemetaphysical.com, 2422 Juan Tabo Blvd. NE, 505-298-3682

Deli-Berry deli-berry.com, 2520 Juan Tabo Blvd. NE, 505-508-0487

Ross Enchanted Park cabq.gov, 2519 Algodones St. NE, 505-452-5200

Lynnewood Park cabq.gov, 2799 Marie Park Dr. NE, 505-452-5200

Piedra Lisa Park cabq.gov, 12901 Menaul Blvd. NE, 505-452-5200

ROUTE SUMMARY

1. **Start at the Menaul Trailhead parking lot and go east through the gate.**
2. **Take two quick rights onto Trail 288 and follow it west, then south to a Y junction.**
3. **Go right at Y and walk west to Monte Largo Dr.**
4. **Continue west on the paths alongside the concrete channel.**
5. **Turn right on Juan Tabo Blvd. (For the 5-mile option, continue straight to Piedra Lisa Arroyo.)**
6. **Turn right on the path alongside Piedra Lisa Arroyo and follow it back to Tramway Blvd.**
7. **Go south on the bike trail to the next channel.**
8. **Turn left and follow the channel to Piedra Lisa Park.**
9. **Continue straight back to the parking area.**

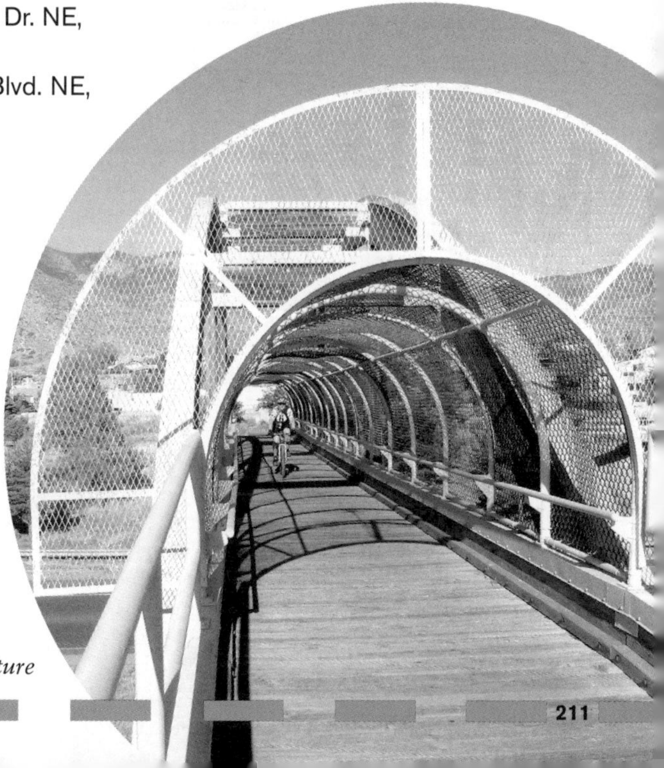

Tramway-Rover Crossing Structure

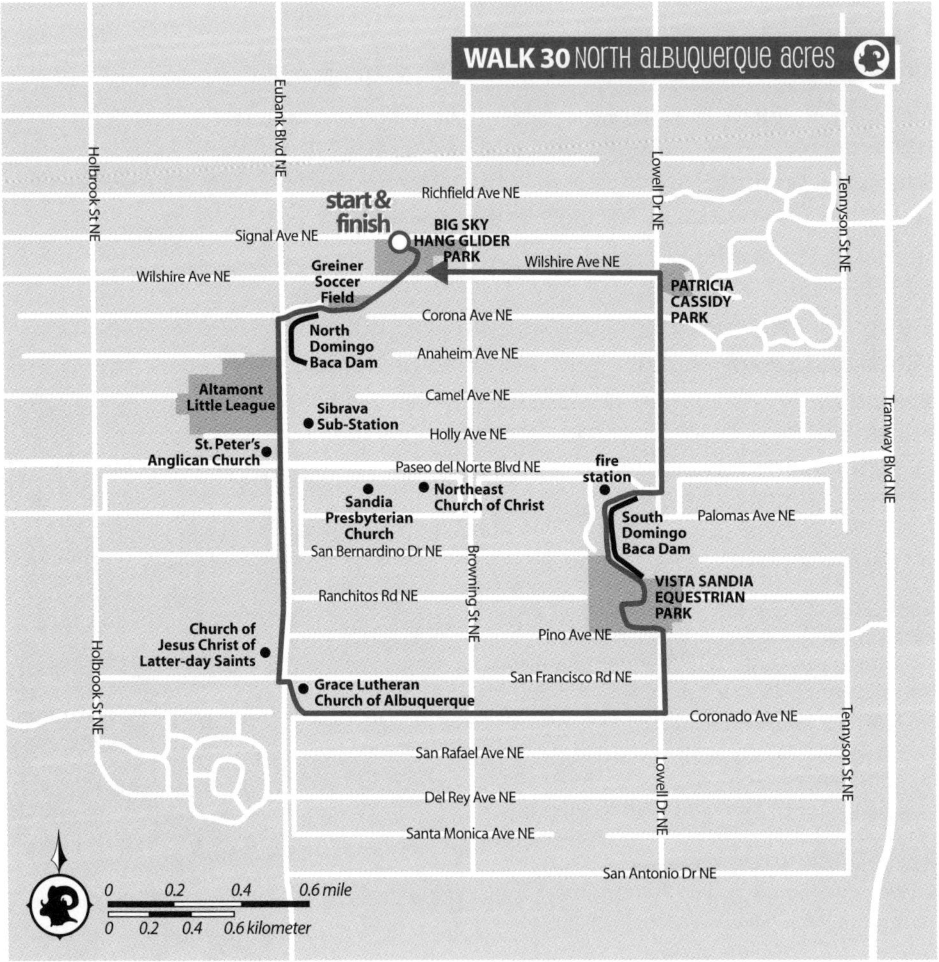

WALK 30 NORTH ALBUQUERQUE ACRES
start & finish
BIG SKY HANG GLIDER PARK
Richfield Ave NE
Signal Ave NE
Wilshire Ave NE
Greiner Soccer Field
Corona Ave NE
North Domingo Baca Dam
Anaheim Ave NE
Altamont Little League
Camel Ave NE
Sibrava Sub-Station
Holly Ave NE
St. Peter's Anglican Church
Paseo del Norte Blvd NE
fire station
Northeast Church of Christ
Sandia Presbyterian Church
South Domingo Baca Dam
Palomas Ave NE
San Bernardino Dr NE
Ranchitos Rd NE
VISTA SANDIA EQUESTRIAN PARK
Pino Ave NE
Church of Jesus Christ of Latter-day Saints
San Francisco Rd NE
Grace Lutheran Church of Albuquerque
Coronado Ave NE
San Rafael Ave NE
Del Rey Ave NE
Santa Monica Ave NE
San Antonio Dr NE
PATRICIA CASSIDY PARK
Holbrook St NE
Eubank Blvd NE
Browning St NE
Lowell Dr NE
Tennyson St NE
Tramway Blvd NE
0 0.2 0.4 0.6 mile
0 0.2 0.4 0.6 kilometer

30 North Albuquerque Acres: Places to Play and Pray

BOUNDARIES: **Signal Ave., Eubank Blvd., Coronado Ave., Lowell Dr.**
DISTANCE: **4.5 miles**
DIFFICULTY: **Moderate (unpaved sections, narrow road shoulders, elevation 5,700–5,950 ft.)**
PARKING: **Free at all parks. Summer, 6 a.m.–10 p.m.; winter, sunrise–sunset**
PUBLIC TRANSIT: **None**

Chances are you've never heard of North Albuquerque Acres, even if you live there. It's one of those development names that only real estate agents and neighborhood associations find useful. The boundary resembles Delaware turned on its side and without the coastal curves. Platted in grid fashion, North Albuquerque Acres fills in the northeast section of the Northeast Heights west of Tramway Blvd. With uniform blocks, each running 0.5 mile east–west and 0.10 mile north–south, its street map resembles a spreadsheet. The curves in the walking route here come courtesy of the Domingo Baca Watershed, usually dry arroyos trenched by stormwater that occasionally streams off the mountains. Collectively they drain the 11.3 square miles into the North Diversion Channel between Paseo del Norte and Alameda Blvd. (To learn where it flows from there, check out Walk 13.) The arroyos and channels downstream are concrete lined, but here they remain in a relatively natural state, with some exceptions. The Albuquerque Metropolitan Arroyo Flood Control Authority (AMAFCA) maintains three dams in this watershed, allowing for development downstream where a floodplain would otherwise exist. What remains of the floodplain is obviously unsuitable for commercial or residential development. To make the most of their empty acreage in the usually dry dam basins, AMAFCA teamed up with Bernalillo County's Park and Recreation Department to develop joint-use facilities. With numerous parks and colossal churches, North Albuquerque Acres is largely for play and great sects.

- **Start at the parking lot of the U.S. Senator Harrison H. Schmitt Big Sky Hang Glider Park. This 11-acre facility serves as a landing zone for hang gliders that soar down from Sandia Peak. It's named for a former geologist, pilot, astronaut, and of course**

Back Story: The Mormon Battalion March and the Long Walk of the Navajo

Two legendary walking routes overlap in Albuquerque, both heroic and tragic in their own ways.

At the onset of the Mexican–American War, Mormon leader Brigham Young offered a unit of 500 men to serve a year in exchange for U.S. Government assistance with helping Mormons settle in the west. The Mormon Battalion—the only religiously based military unit in U.S. history—set off from Council Bluffs, Iowa, in July, 1846. They picked up the Santa Fe Trail in Kansas and arrived at its terminus in early October. Once in Santa Fe the infirm were sent to Fort Pueblo, Colorado, while 397 men continued the march to Albuquerque, essentially following the modern-day route of I-25. They lingered in the area for a few weeks, perhaps hesitant to continue, knowing the worst was yet to come. By November 9, they'd followed the Rio Grande about 150 miles south to what is now Truth or Consequences, where a final sick detachment was sent back to Fort Pueblo, leaving 337 men to continue the journey to San Diego. To their good fortune, they soon encountered Kit Carson. With the legendary frontiersman as their guide, they reached their destination in January 1847, thus completing their 1,850-mile journey—the longest infantry march in U.S. history. Today, an obscure monument to the Mormon Battalion stands in an otherwise empty field off I-25 about 15 miles northeast of Albuquerque, near the village of Budaghers.

In July 1863, Colonel Carson launched a campaign against the Navajo, burning their villages, destroying crops and livestock, and contaminating their water, all in an effort to facilitate General James Carleton's plan to round them up and bring an end to the Indian Wars. Between September 1863 and January 1864, an estimated 9,000 Navajos and 500 Mescalero Apaches were driven through Albuquerque on the 400-mile march to concentration camps at Bosque Redondo. In 1868, few more than 7,300 passed through town again on the long walk home. Today, an elementary school and a city park along the Albuquerque section of the route are named in honor of Kit Carson.

senator. Schmitt walked on the moon and took the famous "Blue Marble" photo of Earth during the Apollo 7 mission in 1972.

- Turn left on the asphalt loop and follow it clockwise. It soon bends southwest and runs alongside La Cueva Arroyo Diversion Channel, a concrete trapezoidal channel that flows into the North Domingo Baca Dam. Continue straight at the Y ahead and follow the path to Ben Greiner Memorial Soccer Field, named for a pilot who crashed 3 miles northwest of here in 1996. The 5-acre park includes a picnic shelter and playground. A multipurpose field is perched on the rim of the 40-foot-deep basin. A ball kicked out of bounds here might be difficult to retrieve. At the base of the dam is a ported outlet structure. Stormwater-quality debris facilities like this annually prevent an average of 60,000 cubic yards of sediment and 50,000 cubic yards of trash from reaching the Rio Grande.

- Continue west through the parking lot to exit the park.

- Turn left on Eubank Blvd. Directly south of the house with the private tennis court are the public North Domingo Baca Tennis Courts. Directly south of that is Altamont Little League, a 17-acre park with a picnic area and nine ball fields of varying sizes for kids of varying ages. Rules and regulations also vary slightly for each field. Sports-field complexes like this are a relief for parents who would otherwise have to shuttle their kids to ballparks spaced throughout the Heights.

  Across the road, on the northeast corner of Eubank Blvd. and Holly Ave., is the Lt. William Sibrava Memorial Sub-Station. In 1994, after 19 years with the Bernalillo County Sheriff's Department and one year shy of retirement, Lieutenant Sibrava was shot and killed by the son of former state senator Joe Mercer.

  Near the northwest corner, St. Peter's Anglican Church occupies a modest doublewide. Two larger church complexes—Sandia Presbyterian and Northeast Church of Christ—are approximately a quarter mile east on the south side of Paseo del Norte. The intersection here may seem like a crossroads of faiths. Actually, in the course of this walk, you'll pass within a half mile of nine different churches. You've got your Episcopalians, your Roman Catholics, and seven other denominations (including your non-denominationalists)—all within a 1-mile radius. Rules and regulations for each church vary somewhat, as do their sizes. The biggest one (in terms of parking spaces and square footage) is straight ahead.

- Continue walking south and use caution crossing Paseo del Norte. As of 2014, the Church of Jesus Christ of Latter-day Saints boasts 74 temples worldwide in exotic locations like Tonga, the Congo, and Hong Kong. The Albuquerque Temple was announced in 1997 and dedicated in 2000. The classic modern, single-spire design features an exterior finish of desert-rose precast concrete trimmed with Texas pearl granite, and a total floor area of 34,245 square feet. Rooms inside include a baptistry, a celestial room, two ordinance rooms, three sealing rooms, and a cafeteria. The complex occupies an 8.5-acre site on the west side of Eubank Blvd. The west-facing entrance makes a grander statement than the façade seen from the sidewalk.

  Grace Lutheran Church of Albuquerque is part of the Missouri Synod, a traditional denomination founded in Chicago in 1847. Notable on the edifice is the bronze jumbo Jesus flattened against its west tower. Other ecclesiastical artworks on display include a unique Trinity reredos by local artist Byron Wickstrom and 16 stained glass windows illustrating scenes from such popular Biblical hits as *The Three Men in the Fiery Furnace* and *Naaman's Leprosy Healed.*

- Turn left on Coronado Ave. It doesn't intersect with Eubank Blvd., so it's easiest to reach by exiting through the south side of the Lutheran parking lot. Note the sharp bend in the road behind you and the lack of sidewalks ahead, and use caution accordingly. For all the spaciousness this neighborhood offers, the absence of paved walkways seems less an oversight than a deliberate attempt to discourage pedestrian traffic. Property fence lines are often pushed close to the road, especially where scrub grows thick on the shoulder. At times you'll have no choice but to walk on the street. Fortunately, traffic tends to be light and numerous speed bumps keep it running slow.

  As you may have noticed by now, particularly if it's summer, there's precious little shade on this route. Trees don't fare well up here. Sheep overgrazed the land long before the houses arrived. And now with dams and channels, water has little chance to disperse except through lawn sprinklers. Even with extensive irrigation installed, an orchard of 100 apple trees struggled on the northeast corner of Coronado Ave. and Lowell Dr. for more than 20 years before owners chopped it down and sold it as firewood in 2014.

- Turn left on Lowell Dr. Again, no sidewalks, but retreated fence lines afford more walking room, and safety is enhanced at intersections that use both stop signs and roundabouts to direct traffic. The scents of hay and horses emanate from the stables and corrals ahead. Continue straight through the second roundabout to enter Vista Sandia Equestrian Park. The playground near the parking lot overlooks the South Domingo Baca Dam. The black gravel path on top is part of the South Domingo Baca Dam Trail. You'll need to take that to reach the next section of Lowell Dr.

- Walk west and follow the dirt trail down to the big corral.

- Turn right and follow the gravel trail on top of the dam. The best views of both the mountains and the city are along this stretch of the walk. Continue past the fire station and exit through the pedestrian access on the left side of the gate ahead.

- Turn left on Lowell Dr. Five blocks north of Paseo del Norte, you'll see Patricia Cassidy Park on your right. It's a small park with a remarkably minuscule library. The first of the Free Little Libraries appeared in Hudson, Wisconsin, in 2009, with the simple idea of "take a book, leave a book." Since then, more than 10,000 of the handcrafted exchange boxes have popped up around the world, each one measuring 36 by 36 by 36 inches or less. The one in the park here stocks mostly children's books, along with a title by Arnold Palmer, which probably won't be checked out anytime soon. On the south side of the park, a path runs alongside North Domingo Baca Arroyo, creating a secluded natural corridor that extends about half a mile to Tramway Blvd. Explore it if you like, or return to Lowell Dr.

- Walk west on Wilshire Ave. Cross the arroyo at the end of road, or turn right and find an easier place to cross, if necessary, and return to the parking lot.

POINTS OF INTEREST

U.S. Senator Harrison H. Schmitt Big Sky Hang Glider Park bernco.gov/parks, 10900 Signal Ave. NE, 505-314-0400

Ben Greiner Soccer Field bernco.gov/parks, 8500 Eubank Blvd. NE, 505-314-0400

North Domingo Baca Tennis Courts bernco.gov/parks, 8401 Eubank Blvd. NE, 505-314-0400

Altamont Little League altamontlittleleague.org, 8301 Eubank Blvd. NE, 505-828-9712

St Peter's Anglican Church stpeters-hccar.com, 8100 Eubank Blvd. NE, 505-822-1192

Northeast Church of Christ giftofeternallife.org, 1000 Paseo del Norte NE, 505-797-3025

Sandia Presbyterian Church sandiapres.org, 10704 Paseo del Norte Blvd. NE, 505-856-5040

The Church of Jesus Christ of Latter-day Saints lds.org, 10301 San Francisco Dr. NE, 505-822-5110

Grace Lutheran Church of Albuquerque gracelutheran-nm.org, 7550 Eubank Blvd. NE, 505-823-9100

Vista Sandia Equestrian Park bernco.gov/parks, 11809 Pino Ave. NE, 505-314-0400

Patricia Cassidy Park bernco.gov/parks, 11900 Summer Wind Pl. NE, 505-314-0400

route summary

1. **Turn left on the asphalt loop and follow it clockwise.**
2. **Continue straight at the Y and follow the path to Eubank Blvd.**
3. **Turn left on Eubank Blvd.**
4. **Turn left on Coronado Ave., the first road south of Grace Lutheran Church.**
5. **Turn left on Lowell Dr.**
6. **Turn left at the Vista Sandia parking lot and follow the dirt path down to the big corral.**
7. **Turn right and follow the trail on top of the dam around to Lowell Dr.**
8. **Turn left on Lowell Dr.**
9. **Turn left on Wilshire Ave.**
10. **Cross the arroyo at the end of Wilshire Ave. and turn right to return to the parking lot.**

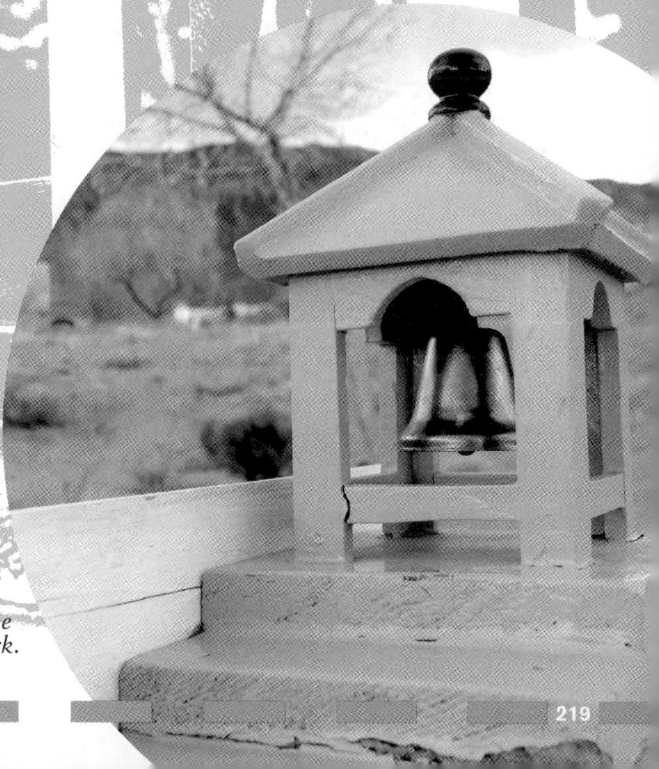

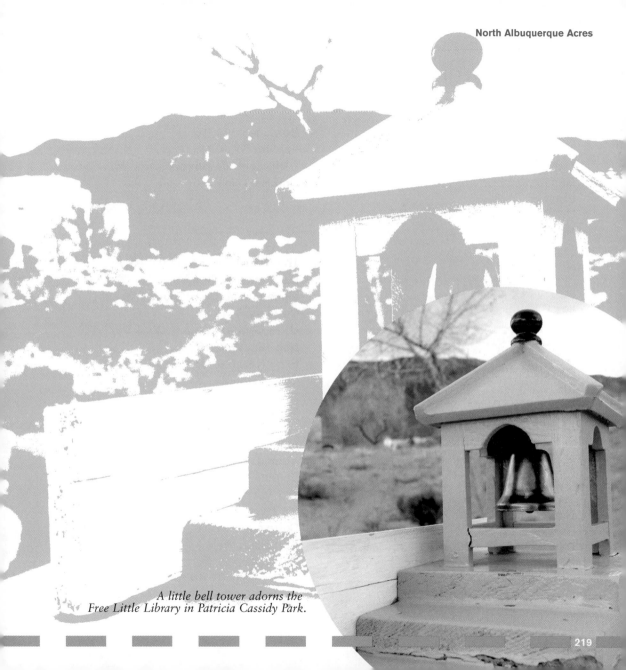

A little bell tower adorns the Free Little Library in Patricia Cassidy Park.

Appendix 1: Walks by Theme

Absolute Favorites (Sensational Six)

The Downtown Scene (Walk 1)
Old Town (Walk 6)
Museum and Courthouse (Walk 7)
Corrales (Walk 16)
UNM Central Campus (Walk 25)
Nob Hill (Walk 26)

Agriculture (Urban Pastures)

Los Duranes (Walk 9)
Los Poblanos (Walk 11)
El Rancho Plaza (Walk 12)
Alameda Bridge (Walk 14)
Corrales (Walk 16)
Rio Bravo (Walk 18)
Valle de Oro (Walk 20)
Pajarito (Walk 21)

Architecture (Built for Style)

The Downtown Scene (Walk 1)
Huning Highland (Walk 2)
Barelas (Walk 3)
Downtown to the Country Club (Walk 4)
Downtown to Old Town (Walk 5)
Old Town (Walk 6)
Museum and Courthouse (Walk 7)
Los Poblanos (Walk 11)
Corrales (Walk 16)
Pajarito (Walk 21)
UNM Central Campus (Walk 25)
Nob Hill (Walk 26)

Art (On/Off the Wall)

The Downtown Scene (Walk 1)
Barelas (Walk 3)
Museum and Courthouse (Walk 7)
Corrales (Walk 16)
UNM Central Campus (Walk 25)
Nob Hill (Walk 26)
Expo New Mexico (Walk 27)

Food (Progressive Feasts)

The Downtown Scene (Walk 1)
Huning Highland (Walk 2)
Barelas (Walk 3)
Old Town (Walk 6)
Pat Hurley Park–BioPark (Walk 8)
Corrales (Walk 16)
Bernalillo (Walk 17)
Nob Hill (Walk 26)
International District (Walk 28)
Menaul Trailhead (Walk 29)

Industrial (Major Infrastructure)

Barelas (Walk 3)
Pat Hurley Park–BioPark (Walk 8)
Martineztown–Santa Barbara (Walk 10)
Balloon Fiesta (Walk 13)
Alameda Bridge (Walk 14)
Rio Bravo (Walk 18)
Mountain View (Walk 19)
Mesa del Sol (Walk 22)
UNM South Campus (Walk 24)
Expo New Mexico (Walk 27)
Menaul Trailhead (Walk 29)

Nature (Wild in the City)

Pat Hurley Park–BioPark (Walk 8)
Los Poblanos (Walk 11)
Alameda Bridge (Walk 14)
Volcano Trails (Walk 15)
Corrales (Walk 16)
Rio Bravo (Walk 18)
Mountain View (Walk 19)
Valle de Oro (Walk 20)
Pajarito (Walk 21)
Mesa del Sol (Walk 22)
Menaul Trailhead (Walk 29)

Shopping (Hey, Big Spender)

The Downtown Scene (Walk 1)
Barelas (Walk 3)
Old Town (Walk 6)
Corrales (Walk 16)
Nob Hill (Walk 26)
Expo New Mexico (Walk 27)

Spirituality (Pondering the Afterlife)

Barelas (Walk 3)
Old Town (Walk 6)
Martineztown–Santa Barbara (Walk 10)
El Rancho Plaza (Walk 12)
Volcano Trails (Walk 15)
Corrales (Walk 16)
Fairview Memorial Park (Walk 23)
International District (Walk 28)
North Albuquerque Acres (Walk 30)

Appendix 2: Points of Interest

Bars and Nightclubs

Albuquerque Press Club qpressclub.com, 201 Highland Park Cir. SE, 505-243-8476 (Walk 2)

Anodyne theanodyne.com, 409 Central Ave. NW, 505-244-1820 (Walk 1)

Burt's Tiki Lounge 313 Gold Ave. SW, 505-247-2878 (Walk 1)

Chama River Microbar chamariverbrewery.com, 106 2nd St. SW, 505-842-8329 (Walk 1)

***Launchpad** launchpadrocks.com, 618 Central Ave. SW, 505-764-8887 (Walk 1)

Sandia Bar 4445 Corrales Rd., 505-897-7577 (Walk 16)

Silva's Saloon 955 S. Camino del Pueblo, 505-867-9976 (Walk 17)

Sister Bar sisterthebar.com, 407 Central Ave. NW, 505-242-4900 (Walk 1)

Cinema, Theater, and Concert Halls

African American Performing Arts Center aapacnm.org, 310 San Pedro Dr. NE, 505-222-0785 (Walk 27)

Aux Dog Theatre auxdog.com, 3011 Monte Vista Blvd. NE, 505-254-7716 (Walk 26)

Carlisle Performance Space Elizabeth Waters Center for Dance theatre.unm.edu, 505-277-4332 (Walk 25)

The Cell fusionabq.org, 700 1st St. NW, 505-766-9412 (Walk 1)

Century Theatres cinemark.com/theatre-447, 100 Central Ave. SW, 505-243-9555 (Walk 1)

Expo New Mexico exponm.com, 300 San Pedro Blvd. NE, 505-222-9700 (Walk 27)

Guild Cinema guildcinema.com, 3405 Central Ave. NE, 505-255-1848 (Walk 26)

***Isleta Amphitheater** isletaamphitheater.net, 5601 University Blvd. SE, 505-452-5100 (Walk 22)

(*major attraction)

Keller Hall music.unm.edu, 203 Cornell Dr. NE, 505-277-4569 (Walk 25)

***KiMo Theater** kimotickets.com, 421 Central Ave. NW, 505-768-3522 (Walk 1)

***Popejoy Hall** popejoypresents.com, 203 Cornell Dr. NE, 505-277-8010 (Walk 25)

El Rey Theater elreytheater.com, 622 Central Ave. SW, 505-242-2353 (Walk 1)

Rodey Theatre theatre.unm.edu, 203 Cornell Dr. NE, 505-277-4332 (Walk 25)

***Sunshine Theater** sunshinetheaterlive.com, 120 Central Ave. SW, 505-764-0249 (Walk 1)

Theatre X theatre.unm.edu, 203 Cornell Dr. NE, 505-277-4332 (Walk 25)

Warehouse 508 warehouse508.org, 508 1st St. NW, 505-296-2738 (Walk 1)

DINING

Abuelita's New Mexican Kitchen abuelitasnmkitchen.com, 621 S. Camino del Pueblo, 505-867-9988 (Walk 17)

Abuelita's New Mexican Kitchen 6083 Isleta Blvd. SW, 505-877-5700 (Walk 21)

Antonio's Café and Cantina thebirddelivers.com, 5409 Gibson Blvd. SE, 505-255-3151 (Walk 28)

Artichoke Cafe artichokecafe.com, 424 Central Ave. SE, 505-243-0200 (Walk 2)

Asian Grill asiangrillabq.com, 5303 Gibson Blvd. SE, 505-265-4702 (Walk 28)

Barelas Coffee House 1502 4th St. SW, 505-843-7577 (Walk 3)

Blake's Lotaburger lotaburger.com, 6600 Edith Blvd. NE, 505-344-7105 (Walk 12)

Boiler Monkey Bistro boilermonkeybistro.com, 724 Mountain Rd. NW, 505-315-0567 (Walk 7)

Casa Rondeña Winery casarondena.com, 733 Chavez Rd. NW, 505-344-5911 (Walk 11)

Cervantes Restaurant & Lounge cervantesabq.com, 5801 Gibson Blvd. SE, 505-262-2253 (Walk 28)

(*major attraction)

DINING (CONTINUED)

El Charritos Mexican Restaurant 4703 Central Ave. NW, 505-836-2464 (Walk 8) Chelsey's Wings and Burgers 5901 Gibson Blvd. SE, 505-266-6223 (Walk 28)

Cocina Azul cafeazul.com, 1134 Mountain Rd. NW, 505-831-2500 (Walk 7)

Copper Canyon Café coppercanyoncafe.com, 5455 Gibson Blvd. SE, 505-266-6318 (Walk 28)

La Crêpe Michel lacrepemichel.com, 400 San Felipe St. NW #C2, 505-242-1251 (Walk 6)

Dagmar's dagmarsrestaurant.com, 2120 Juan Tabo Blvd. NE, 505-293-1982 (Walk 29)

Deli-Berry deli-berry.com, 2520 Juan Tabo Blvd. NE, 505-508-0487 (Walk 29)

Dog House Drive In 1216 Central Ave. NW, 505-243-1019 (Walk 4)

Elaine's elainesnobhill.com, 3503 Central Ave. NE, 505-433-4782 (Walk 26)

Flying Star Cafe flyingstarcafe.com, 200 S. Camino del Pueblo, 505-404-2100 (Walk 17)

Flying Star Cafe lyingstarcafe.com, 723 Silver Ave. SW, 505-244-8099 (Walk 4)

Firenze Pizzeria firenzepizzeria.com, 900 Park Ave., 505-242-2939 (Walk 4)

La Fonda del Bosque lafondadelbosque.com, 1701 4th St. SW, 505-247-9480 (Walk 3)

Gecko's Bar & Tapas geckosbar.com, 3500 Central Ave. SE, 505-262-1848 (Walk 26)

Gen Kai 110 B Louisiana Blvd NE, 505-255-0112 (Walk 27)

Golden Crown goldencrown.biz, 1103 Mountain Rd. NW, 505-243-2424 (Walk 7)

Grove Cafe & Market thegrovecafemarket.com, 600 Central Ave. SE, 505-248-9800 (Walk 2)

La Hacienda Restaurant haciendadelriocantina.com, 302 San Felipe St. NW, 505-243-3131 (Walk 6)

High Noon Restaurant & Saloon highnoonrestaurant.com, 425 San Felipe St. NW, 505-765-1455 (Walk 6)

Indigo Crow Cafe indigocrowcafe.com, 4515 Corrales Rd., 505-898-7000 (Walk 16)

Izumi Sushi & Grill izumisushiandgrillabq.com, 5701 Gibson Blvd. SE, 505-260-0011 (Walk 28)

Java Joe's downtownjavajoes.com, 906 Park Ave. SW, 505-765-1514 (Walk 4)

JR's Bar-B-Que jrs-barbeque.com, 6501 Gibson Blvd. SE, 505-268-1676 (Walk 28)

(*major attraction)

Juanita's Comida Mexicana 910 4th St. SW, 505-843-9669 (Walk 3)

***Kelly's Brew Pub** kellysbrewpub.com, 3222 Central Ave. SE, 505-262-2739 (Walk 26)

Korean BBQ House and Sushi & Sake koreanbbqhousenm.com, 3200 Central Ave. SE, 505-338-2424 (Walk 26)

Limonata freshcitrus.us, 3222 Silver Ave. SE, 505-266-0607 (Walk 26)

Little Red Hamburger Hut littleredsburgers.tripod.com, 1501 Mountain Rd. NW, 505-304-1819 (Walk 7)

MÁS hotelandaluz.com, 125 2nd St. NW, 505-923-9080 (Walk 1)

El Modelo 1715 2nd St. SW, 505-242-1843 (Walk 3)

Model Pharmacy modelpharmacy.com, 3636 Monte Vista Blvd. NE, 505-255-8686 (Walk 26)

Monte Carlo Liquors & Steak House 3916 Central Ave. SW, 505-831-2444 (Walk 8)

Monte Vista Fire Station Restaurant montevistafirestation.com, 3201 Central Ave. NE, 505-255-2424 (Walk 26)

Nagomi 2400 Juan Tabo Blvd. NE, 505-298-3081 (Walk 29)

Perea's Restaurant 4590 Corrales Rd., 505-898-2442 (Walk 16)

Pollito Con Papas pollitoconpapas.com, 6105 Gibson Blvd. SE, 505-765-5486 (Walk 28)

Pro's Ranch Market prosranch.com, 4201 Central Ave. NW, 505-833-1765 (Walk 8)

P'tit Louis Bistro ptitlouisbistro.com, 3218 Silver Ave. SE, 505-314-1110 (Walk 26)

Quarters BBQ thequartersbbq.com, 801 Yale Blvd. SE, 505-843-6949 (Walk 23)

The Range Cafe rangecafe.com, 925 Camino del Pueblo, 505-867-1700 (Walk 17)

Rose's Table Cafe rosestablecafe.com; 5700 University Blvd. SE, Suite 130; 505-433-5772 (Walk 22)

Red Ball Café redballcafe.com, 1301 4th St. SW, 505-247-9438 (Walk 3)

Roma Bakery and Deli romabakeryanddeli.com, 501 Roma Ave. NW, 505-843-9418 (Walk 5)

***Scalo Northern Italian Grill** scalonobhill.com, 3500 Central Ave. SE, 505-255-8781 (Walk 26)

Slate Street Café slatestreetcafe.com, 515 Slate Ave. NW, 505-243-2210 (Walk 7)

Standard Diner standarddiner.com, 320 Central Ave. SE, 505-243-1440 (Walk 2)

(*major attraction)

DINING (CONTINUED)

St. James Tearoom stjamestearoom.com; 320 Osuna Rd. NE, Suite D; 505-242-3752 (Walk 12)

Sushi Hana sushihananm.com, 521 Central Ave. NW, 505-842-8700 (Walk 1)

Sushi King sushikingnm.com, 118 Central Ave. SW, 505-842-5099 (Walk 1)

Tango Café tangocafeabq.com, 800 Bradbury Dr. SE, 505-224-2980 (Walk 24)

A Taste of Italy atasteofitalynm.com, 1945 Juan Tabo Blvd. NE, 505-275-8334 (Walk 29)

Tucanos Brazilian Grill tucanos.com, 110 Central Ave. SW, 505-246-9900 (Walk 1)

Villa di Capo villadicapo.com, 722 Central Ave SW, 505-242-2006 (Walk 4)

Zinc Wine Bar & Bistro zincabq.com, 3009 Central Ave. NE, 505-254-9462 (Walk 26)

EDUCATION AND INSTRUCTION

The Ayurvedic Institute ayurveda.com, 11311 Menaul Blvd. NE, 505-291-9698 (Walk 29)

Central New Mexico Community College cnm.edu, 525 Buena Vista Dr. SE, 505-224-3000 (Walk 24)

Interdisciplinary Film and Digital Media Program ifdm.unm.edu, 5700 University Blvd. SE, 505-277-2286 (Walk 22)

Manufacturing Training and Technology Center stc.unm.edu, 800 Bradbury Dr. SE, 505-272-7310 (Walk 24)

Menaul School menaulschool.com, 301 Menaul Blvd. NE, 505-345-7727 (Walk 10)

Los Ranchos Agri-Nature Center losranchosnm.gov, 4920 Rio Grande Blvd. NW, 505-344-9426 (Walk 11)

Special Collections Library abclibrary.org/specialcollections, 423 Central Ave. NE, 505-848-1376 (Walk 2)

GALLERIES AND MUSEUMS

516 Arts 516arts.org, 516 Central Ave. SW, 505-242-1445 (Walk 1)

(*major attraction)

***Albuquerque Museum of Art and History** cabq.gov/culturalservices/albuquerque-museum, 2000 Mountain Rd. NW, 505-242-4600 (Walk 7)

American International Rattlesnake Museum rattlesnakes.com, 202 San Felipe St. NW, 505-242-6569 (Walk 5)

***Anderson-Abruzzo Albuquerque International Balloon Museum** balloonmuseum.com, 9201 Balloon Museum Dr. NE, 505-768-6020 (Walk 13)

Downtown Contemporary Gallery downtowncontemporary.com, 105 4th St. SW, 505-363-3870 (Walk 1)

***Explora!** explora.us, 1701 Mountain Rd. NW, 505-224-8300 (Walk 7)

Gutiérrez-Hubbell House gutierrezhubbellhouse.org, 6029 Isleta Blvd. SW, 505-244-0507 (Walk 21)

Harwood Art Center harwoodartcenter.org, 1114 7th St. NW, 505-242-6367 (Walk 7)

Herzstein Latin American Gallery, Zimmerman Library library.unm.edu, 505-925-9554, (Walk 25)

Holocaust & Intolerance Museum of New Mexico nmholocaustmuseum.org, 616 Central Ave. SW, 505-247-0606 (Walk 1)

***Indian Pueblo Cultural Center** indianpueblo.org, 2401 12th St. NW, 505-843-7270 (Walk 9)

John Sommers Gallery finearts.unm.edu; UNM Main Campus, Art Building; 505-277-5861 (Walk 25)

Mariposa Gallery mariposa-gallery.com, 3500 Central Ave. SE, 505-268-6828 (Walk 26)

Masley Art Gallery, Masley Hall unm.edu/~arted, 505-277-4112 (Walk 25)

***Maxwell Museum** maxwellmuseum.unm.edu; UNM Main Campus, Anthropology Building; 505-277-4405 (Walk 25)

Museum of Southwestern Biology msb.unm.edu; UNM Main Campus, CERIA Building; 505-277-1360 (Walk 25)

***National Hispanic Cultural Center** nhccnm.org, 1701 4th St. SW, 505-242-5289 (Walk 3)

(*major attraction)

Galleries and Museums (continued)

***National Museum of Nuclear Science & History** nuclearmuseum.org, 601 Eubank Blvd. NE, 505-245-2137 (Walk 28)

***New Mexico Museum of Natural History and Science** nmnaturalhistory.org, 1801 Mountain Rd. NW, 505-841-2800 (Walk 7)

Silver Family Geology Museum, Northrop Hall epswww.unm.edu, 505-277-4204 (Walk 25)

Small Engine Gallery smallenginegallery.com, 1413 4th St. SW (Walk 3)

Tamarind Institute tamarind.unm.edu, 2500 Central Ave. SE, 505-277-3901 (Walk 25)

The TANNEX facebook.com/thetannex, 1417 4th St. SW (Walk 3)

Telephone Museum of New Mexico telecomhistory.org, 110 4th St. NW, 505-842-2937 (Walk 1)

UNM Arts Lab artslab.unm.edu, 1601 Central Ave. NE, 505-277-2253 (Walk 25)

***UNM Art Museum** unmartmuseum.org, 203 Cornell Dr. NE, 505-277-4001 (Walk 25)

Unser Racing Museum unserracingmuseum.com, 1776 Montaño Rd. NW, 505-341-1776 (Walk 11)

Wheels Museum wheelsmuseum.org, 1100 2nd St. SW, 505-243-6269 (Walk 3)

Graveyards

Bernalillo Cemetery Off Calle Gabrielle (Walk 17)

Fairview Memorial Park facebook.com/HistoricFairviewCemetery, 700 Yale Blvd. SE, 505-262-1454 (Walk 23)

Mount Calvary Cemetery archdiocesesantafe.org, 1900 Edith Blvd. NE, 505-243-0218 (Walk 10)

Mount Carmel Cemetery Edith Blvd. NE (Walk 12)

Our Lady of Sorrows Cemetery Off S. Hill Rd. (Walk 17)

San Carlos Cemetery Alameda Blvd. (Walk 13)

Sunset Memorial Park sunset-memorial.com, 924 Menaul Blvd. NE, 505-345-3536 (Walk 10)

(*major attraction)

LODGING

Bottger Mansion bottger.com, 110 San Felipe St. NW, 505-243-3639 (Walk 5)

Downtown Historic B&B downtownhistoric.com, 207 High St., 505-842-0223 (Walk 2)

Hiway House Motel hiwayhousemotel.com, 3200 Central Ave. SE, 505-268-3971 (Walk 26)

Hotel Andaluz hotelandaluz.com, 125 2nd St. NW, 505-242-9090 (Walk 1)

Hotel Blue thehotelblue.com, 717 Central Ave. NW, 505-924-2400 (Walk 4)

Hotel Parq Central hotelparqcentral.com, 806 Central Ave. SE, 505-242-0040 (Walk 2)

Los Poblanos Inn lospoblanos.com, 4803 Rio Grande Blvd. NW, 505-344-9297 (Walk 11)

Mauger Estate B&B Inn maugerbb.com, 701 Roma Ave. NW, 800-719-9189 (Walk 5)

Route 66 Hostel rt66hostel.com, 1012 Central Ave. SW, 505-247-1813 (Walk 4)

Sandia Peak Inn sandiapeakinnmotel.com, 4614 Central Ave. SW, 505-831-5036 (Walk 8)

Sarabande Bed and Breakfast sarabandebnb.com, 5637 Rio Grande Blvd. NW, 888-506-4923 (Walk 11)

Parks & Open Space

***ABQ BioPark** cabq.gov/culturalservices/biopark, 505-764-6200

- **Aquarium and Botanic Garden** 2601 Central Ave. NW (Walk 8)
- **Tingley Beach** 1800 Tingley Dr. (Walk 4)
- **Zoo** 903 10th St. SW (Walk 4)

Alameda/Rio Grande Open Space cabq.gov, 1401 Alameda Blvd. NW, 505-452-5200(Walk 14)

Ambassador Edward L. Romero Park bernco.gov/parks, 310 Rossmoor Rd. SE, 505-314-0400 (Walk 18)

Bachechi Open Space bernco.gov/bachechi-3978, 9521 Rio Grande Blvd. NW, 505-314-0398 (Walk 14)

Bataan Memorial Park cabq.gov, 3501 Lomas Blvd. NE, 505-768-5353 (Walk 26)

Durand Open Space bernco.gov, 4750 Isleta Blvd. SW, 505-314-0400 (Walk 21)

(*major attraction)

Parks & Open Space (continued)

Hailey Ratliff Trails Park cabq.gov/parksandrecreation, Treeline Ave. and Rainbow Blvd., 505-857-8650 (Walk 15)

Hartnett Park losranchosnm.gov/services, 6718 Rio Grande Blvd., 505-344-6582 (Walk 11)

Lynnewood Park cabq.gov, 2799 Marie Park Dr. NE, 505-452-5200 (Walk 29)

Martineztown–Santa Barbara Park cabq.gov/parksandrecreation, 1825 Edith Blvd. NE (Walk 10)

New Mexico Veterans' Memorial nmvetsmemorial.org, 1100 Louisiana Blvd. SE, 505-256-2042 (Walk 28)

Pajarito Open Space bernco.gov, 6000 Beck Rd. SW, 505-314-0400 (Walk 21)

Pat Hurley Park cabq.gov, 350 Yucca Dr. NW, 505-768-2000 (Walk 8)

Patricia Cassidy Park bernco.gov/parks, 11900 Summer Wind Pl. NE, 505-314-0400 (Walk 30)

Piedra Lisa Park cabq.gov, 12901 Menaul Blvd. NE, 505-452-5200 (Walk 29)

Los Poblanos Open Space cabq.gov/parksandrecreation, 1701 Montaño Rd. NW, 505-768-5353 (Walk 11)

Ross Enchanted Park cabq.gov, 2519 Algodones St. NE, 505-452-5200 (Walk 29)

Rio Bravo Riverside Picnic Area cabq.gov, Poco Loco Frontage Rd. SE, 505-452-5200 (Walks 18, 19)

Rio Grande Community Farm riograndefarm.org, 1701 Montaño Rd. NW, 505-510-1837 (Walk 11)

***Rio Grande Valley State Park** cabq.gov/parksandrecreation, 505-897-8831 (Walks 8, 14, 18–20)

Valle del Oro National Wildlife Refuge fws.gov/refuge/valle_de_oro or facebook.com/valledeoronationalwildliferefuge, 7851 2nd St. SW, 505-933-2708 (Walk 20)

Roosevelt Park cabq.gov/parksandrecreation, 525 Sycamore St. SE, 505-857-8650 (Walk 24)

USS Bullhead Memorial Park cabq.gov, 1606 San Pedro Blvd. SE, 505-291-6239 (Walk 28)

(*major attraction)

recreation and sports

Albuquerque Country Club albuquerquecountryclub.org, 601 Laguna Blvd. SW, 505-247-4111 (Walk 4)

Altamont Little League altamontlittleleague.org, 8301 Eubank Blvd. NE, 505-828-9712 (Walk 30)

Ben Greiner Soccer Field bernco.gov/parks, 8500 Eubank Blvd. NE, 505-314-0400 (Walk 30)

Bernalillo County Regional Recreation Complex bernco.gov, 5601 University Blvd. SE, 505-314-0400 (Walk 22)

Bernalillo Recreation Center townofbernalillo.org/depts/recreation, 370 Rotary Park Rd., 505-771-2078 (Walk 17)

Bikram Yoga bikramabq.com, 1930 Juan Tabo Blvd. NE, 505-296-9642 (Walk 29)

Carley Adventure Studios 4765 Corrales Rd., 505-897-4874 (Walk 16)

City of Albuquerque Golf Training Center cabq.gov/parksandrecreation, 9401 Balloon Museum Dr. NE, 505-857-8437 (Walk 13)

The Downs Racetrack & Casino abqdowns.com, 145 Louisiana Blvd. NE, 505-767-7171 (Walk 27)

Duke City BMX dukecitybmx.org, 1011 Buena Vista Dr. SE, 505-890-1269 (Walk 24)

Los Duranes Park & Community Center cabq.gov, 2920 Leopoldo Rd. NW, 505-848-1338 (Walk 9)

Harrison H. Schmitt Big Sky Hang Glider Park bernco.gov/parks, 10900 Signal Ave. NE, 505-314-0400 (Walk 30)

Horses Unlimited (Rancho de los Sueños) horsesunlimited.us, 850 Salida Sandia SW, 505-873-9043 (Walk 20)

***Isotopes Park** abqisotopes.com, 1601 Avenida César Chávez SE, 505-924-2255 (Walk 24)

Mountain View Community Center bernco.gov, 201 Prosperity Ave. SE, 505-314-0297 (Walk 19)

North Domingo Baca Tennis Courts bernco.gov/parks, 8401 Eubank Blvd. NE, 505-314-0400 (Walk 30)

(*major attraction)

recreation and sports (continued)

***The Pit** golobos.com, 1414 Bradbury Dr. SE, 505-925-5608 (Walk 24)

Rio Grande Pool cabq.gov/parksandrecreation, 1410 Iron Ave. SW, 505-848-1397 (Walk 4)

Routes Bicycle Rentals & Tours routesrental.com, 404 San Felipe St. NW, 505-933-5667 (Walk 6)

***University Stadium** unmtickets.com, 1111 Avenida César Chávez SE, 505-664-8661 (Walk 24)

Vista Sandia Equestrian Park bernco.gov/parks, 11809 Pino Ave. NE, 505-314-0400 (Walk 30)

SHOPPING

Albuquerque Water Gardens 2704 Duranes Rd. NW, 505-246-8278 (Walk 9)

B. Ruppe Drugs facebook.com/bruppedrugsinc, 807 4th St. SW, 505-243-6719 (Walk 3)

Blue Eagle Metaphysical Emporium blueeaglemetaphysical.com, 2422 Juan Tabo Blvd. NE, 505-298-3682 (Walk 29)

Buffalo Exchange buffaloexchange.com, 3005 Central Ave. NE, 505-262-0098 (Walk 26)

Camino Real Antiques 1100 S. Camino del Pueblo, 505-867-7448 (Walk 17)

Gertrude Zachary's Castle Antiques gertrudezachary.com, 416 2nd St. SW, 505-244-1320 (Walk 3)

Gertrude Zachary Jewelry Etc. gertrudezachary.com, 1501 Lomas Blvd. NW, 505-247-4442 (Walk 5)

Joy Junction Thrift Store joyjunction.org, 107 Bowers Rd. SW, 505-873-8372 (Walk 19)

Jubilation Wine & Spirits jubilationwines.com, 3512 Lomas Blvd. NE, 505-255-4404 (Walk 26)

Judy's Trading Post & Auction judystradingpost.com, 6016 Isleta Blvd. SW, 505-877-6000 (Walk 21)

Little Shops on Rio Grande littleshopsonriogrande.com, 1507 Rio Grande Blvd. NW, 505-765-5489 (Walk 9)

(*major attraction)

Nob Hill La Montañita Co-op Food Market lamontanita.coop, 3500 Central Ave. SE, 505-265-4631 (Walk 26)

New Mexico Earth Adobes newmexicoearth.com, 310 El Pueblo Rd. NE, 505-898-1271 (Walk 12)

La Paloma Greenhouse arcaorganics.org, 181 E. La Entrada Ln., 505-897-2184 (Walk 16)

Plant World plantworldinc.com, 250 El Pueblo Rd. NE, 505-898-9627 (Walk 12)

Prized Possessions prizedpossessionsjewelryantiques.com, 4534 Corrales Rd., 505-899-4800 (Walk 16)

***Rail Yards Market** railyardsmarket.org, 777 1st St. SW, 505-203-6200 (Walk 3)

Steadfast Soldiers steadfastsoldiers.com, 328 San Felipe St. NW, 505-247-2310 (Walk 6)

Sunwest Silver sunwestsilver.com, 324 Lomas Blvd. NW, 505-243-3781 (Walk 7)

Talin Market talinmarket.com, 88 Louisiana Blvd. SE, 505-268-0206 (Walk 27)

Valencia Farms valenciafarms.com, 119 Yucca Tr., 505-899-5336 (Walk 16)

Wagner Farms Market wagnerfarmscorrales.com, 5000 Corrales Rd., 505-898-3903 (Walk 16)

SPIRITUALITY

Antioch Baptist Church antiochbc-abq.cwwsites.com, 305 47th St. NW, 505-831-2088 (Walk 8)

Canossian Spirituality Center canossianspiritualitycenter.org, 5625 Isleta Blvd. SW, 505-452-9402 (Walk 21)

The Church of Jesus Christ of Latter-day Saints lds.org, 10301 San Francisco Dr. NE, 505-822-5110 (Walk 30)

First United Methodist Church fumconline.org, 314 Lead Ave. SW, 505-243-5646 (Walk 3)

Grace Lutheran Church of Albuquerque gracelutheran-nm.org, 7550 Eubank Blvd. NE, 505-823-9100 (Walk 30)

Immanuel Presbyterian Church rt66church.com, 114 Carlisle Blvd. SE, 505-265-7628 (Walk 26)

(*major attraction)

Spirituality (continued)

Islamic Center of New Mexico icnm-abq.org, 1100 Yale Blvd. SE, 505-256-1450 (Walk 23)

Mission San Jose de los Duranes 2110 Los Luceros Rd. NW, 505-243-4628 (Walk 9)

Northeast Church of Christ giftofeternallife.org, 1000 Paseo del Norte NE, 505-797-3025 (Walk 30)

Our Lady of Kazan Monastery kazanmonastery.org, 324 Hazeldine Ave. SW, 505-242-6186 (Walk 3)

Our Lady of Mt. Carmel Church 7813 Edith Blvd. NE (Walk 12)

Our Lady of Sorrows olosbernalillonm.org, 301 S. Camino del Pueblo, 505-867-5252 (Walk 17)

***San Felipe de Neri Parish** sanfelipedeneri.org, 2005 N. Plaza St. NW, 505-243-4628, (Walk 6)

San Ignacio Catholic Church 1300 Walter St. NE, 505-243-4287 (Walk 10)

Sandia Presbyterian Church sandiapres.org, 10704 Paseo del Norte Blvd. NE, 505-856-5040 (Walk 30)

St. George Greek Orthodox Church stgeorgenm.org, 308 High St. SE, 505-247-9411 (Walk 2)

St. Peter's Anglican Church stpeters-hccar.com, 8100 Eubank Blvd. NE, 505-822-1192 (Walk 30)

Wat Buddhamongkolnimit watnimit.blogspot.com, 320 Louisiana Blvd. SE, 505-268-4983 (Walk 27)

Visitor and Information Centers

***Las Imágenes Visitor Center** nps.gov/petr, 6510 Western Trail NW, 505-899-0205 (Walk 15)

Old Town Visitors Center albuquerqueoldtown.com, 303 Romero St. NW, 505-243-3215 (Walk 6)

Sandoval County Visitor Center sandovalcounty.org, 264 S. Camino del Pueblo, 505-867-TOUR or 800-252-0191 (Walk 17)

Student Support & Services Center unm.edu, 1155 University Blvd. SE, 505-277-8503 (Walk 24)

Student Union Building sub.unm.edu, 505-277-2331 (Walk 25)

(*major attraction)

INDEX

S

T

U

V

W

Y

Z

about the author

STEPHEN AUSHERMAN is the author of *60 Hikes within 60 Miles: Albuquerque*. He moved to Albuquerque in 1996 and has written extensively about it for both local and national publications. He received a New Visions Award for experimental film from the New Mexico Film Office and has exhibited his video compositions in galleries, museums, and theaters throughout Albuquerque, Santa Fe, and elsewhere in the world.